Bayard Webster

XLX85 00

ANNALS OF
THE NEW YORK ACADEMY
OF SCIENCES

Volume 353

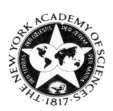

EDITORIAL STAFF
Executive Editor
BILL BOLAND
Managing Editor
JOYCE HITCHCOCK
Associate Editor
WERNER SIMON

The New York Academy of Sciences
2 East 63rd Street
New York, New York 10021

AIRBORNE CONTAGION

ANNALS OF THE NEW YORK ACADEMY OF SCIENCES
Volume 353

AIRBORNE CONTAGION

Edited by Ruth B. Kundsin

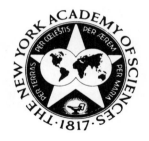

The New York Academy of Sciences
New York, New York
1980

Library of Congress Cataloging In Publication Data

Main entry under title:

Airborne contagion.

(Annals of New York Academy of Sciences; v. 353)
Papers presented at a conference held Nov. 7-9, 1979, by New York Academy of Sciences.
1. Airborne infection—Congresses.   2. Epidem-
iology—Congresses.   I. Kundsin, Ruth B., 1916
II. Series: New York Academy of Sciences.   Annals;
v. 353.
Q11.N5   vol. 353   [RA642.A5]   500s   80-27061
ISBN 0-98766-095-1   [614.4'3]
ISBN 0-89766-096-X (pbk.)

SP
Printed in the United States of America
ISBN-0-89766-095-1 (cloth)
ISBN-0-89766-096-X (paper)

ANNALS OF THE NEW YORK ACADEMY OF SCIENCES
VOLUME 353
December 5, 1980

AIRBORNE CONTAGION*

Editor and Conference Chair
RUTH B. KUNDSIN

Organizing Committee
LLOYD G. HERMAN, RICHARD L. RILEY, and CARL W. WALTER

CONTENTS

*This series of papers is the result of a conference entitled Airborne Contagion held 7–9 November, 1979 by The New York Academy of Sciences.

Financial assistance was received from:

- BOEHRINGER INGELHEIM LTD.
- JOHNSON & JOHNSON PRODUCTS, INC.
- MERCK SHARP & DOHME RESEARCH LABORATORIES
- A. H. ROBBINS COMPANY
- NATIONAL INSTITUTE OF ALLERGY AND INFECTIOUS DISEASES—
    FOGARTY INTERNATIONAL CENTER
- OFFICE OF NAVAL RESEARCH

OPENING REMARKS

Ruth B. Kundsin

Brigham and Women's Hospital and Harvard Medical School
Boston, Massachusetts 02115

In the context of this conference, airborne contagion has been very broadly defined. Wells originally described airborne contagion as the chain reaction indoors resulting from person-to-person transfer of droplet nuclei implicated in respiratory tract infection. The magnitude of this is cited by the National Center for Health Statistics, Office of Health Research, Statistics, and Technology, Public Health Service, U.S. Department of Health, Education, and Welfare, in statistics for 1977–1978.[1] The incidence of acute respiratory conditions was 117 per 100 persons with 4.5 days of restricted activity and 2.4 days in bed per person.

For the purpose of this conference, the concept of airborne contagion has been expanded to include aerosols from inanimate sources such as air conditioners, dental drills, fungal spores from soil and insulating material, as well as long range outdoor transfer of microorganisms. Air as a vehicle for dissemination of microorganisms is the theme, whether dynamic contagion is involved with a geometric increase in cases or static infection arising from a single source and whether humans, animals or plants are implicated as hosts.

There are three important reasons for holding a conference on airborne contagion at this time.

First, Threshold Limit Values for chemical substances and physical agents in a workroom environment as well as for outdoor air were established when the Threshold Limit Values were published in the Federal Register in 1971. Three categories of Threshold Limit Values were described:

1. Threshold Limit Value—a Time Weighted Average that is the time-weighted average concentration for a normal eight hour workday or a 40 hour work week to which nearly all workers may be repeatedly exposed, day after day, without adverse effect.

2. Threshold Limit Value—A Short-Term Exposure Limit that is the maximal concentration to which workers can be exposed for a period up to 15 minutes continuously without suffering from irritation, chronic or irreversible tissue change.

3. Threshold Limit Value Ceiling—That level of concentration that should not be exceeded even instantaneously.

Viable particles have no threshold level either indoors or outdoors for any period of exposure. Industry and laboratories can liberally spew out bacterial, viral or fungal particles into the air and into the sewer system. There has been recent concern with DNA recombinant research and degrees of isolation were described. However, no threshold levels of viable particles that may be emitted or to which humans can be exposed are in existence. The area of human exposure to viable particles in the environment has been totally disregarded.

The second reason why this conference has urgency is that our present emphasis on energy conservation will necessitate greater proportions of recirculated air indoors, whether heated or air-conditioned, and less make up outdoor air in order to conserve the energy required to cool or heat intake air. There is, however, no standard for viable particles that would determine how much

1

0077-8923/80/0353-001 $01.75/0 © 1980, NYAS

outdoor air intake, how much recirculation is essential for the safety of aggregations of people in the indoor environment.

This conference will, therefore, be an attempt to collate from experience as well as from experimental human and animal studies what information we have on viable particles hazardous to life. With this information we can begin to make intelligent decisions about actions we have to take to initiate changes. Temperature and humidity control which have heretofore been the only conditions to be controlled are not life threatening. Viable particles can be. Standards need to be defined for microorganisms in the air. Whether these standards will depend on an indicator microorganism from the respiratory tract, such as *Streptococcus viridans*, just as *Escherichia coli* is the indicator organism for enterics in water, or on total count of all microorganisms, should be determined. Standards, once established, should be enforced.

Third, this conference is a tribute to William Firth Wells sixteen years after his death in the Veteran's Hospital in Baltimore, Maryland. He first called attention to airborne contagion in the nineteen thirties. While the concept was not generally accepted by the scientific community, it nevertheless stimulated a burst of interest in airborne infection.

Airborne transmission is the most important mode of transmission of respiratory infections from person to person indoors. It may well be the most important mode of transmission for other human infections not considered as primarily respiratory. There is published evidence of droplet nuclei transmission of hepatitis B virus, smallpox, rabies, chicken pox, mumps, measles as well as tuberculosis.

I am deeply grateful to Dr. Lloyd G. Herman, Dr. Richard L. Riley, and Dr. Carl W. Walter for their interest, support, and total dedication to the theme of this conference: airborne contagion.

REFERENCE

1.   NATIONAL CENTER FOR HEALTH STATISTICS: Acute Conditions: Incidence and Associated Disability, United States, July 1977–June 1978: 7–12. U.S. Department of Health, Education, and Welfare. Public Health Service. Office of Health Research, Statistics, and Technology. National Center for Health Statistics. Washington, D.C.

HISTORICAL BACKGROUND

Richard L. Riley*

Petersham, Massachusetts 01366

The Smith papyrus, dating back to 1600 B.C., states that the first of the incantations to the gods of sickness was devoted to cleansing "winds" of the "pest of the year."[1] Twelve hundred years later, in 400 B.C., Hippocrates taught that "airs, waters and places" influenced the health of populations,[1] and in the second century A.D. Galen gave forth the ominous pronouncement, "When many sicken and die at once, we must look to a single common cause, the air we breathe."[2] In the 14th century epidemic plague, the Black Death, marked according to Winslow,[2] "the nearest approach to a definite break in the continuity of history that has ever occured." It produced almost universal conversion to a belief in the communicability of disease. In the 16th century Fracastorius anticipated the microbiological era with his talk of contagious "seminaria"; a century later Sydenham extended this thought by saying that it was not the air itself, but "pestilential particles" carried by the air that convey disease; and another two centuries later, in 1840, Jacob Henle claimed that the pestilential particles were not inert but "animate, indeed endowed with individual life."[2] Then, in the second half of the nineteenth century, after more than 3,000 years of recorded thoughts about airborne contagion, came a sudden rush of scientific and public health activity which added both insight and confusion.

In 1862 Pasteur published his "Memoir on the organized corpuscles that exist in the atmosphere" in which he demonstrated that organisms appearing the next day in a sterile culture medium standing open on a laboratory bench arise not from spontaneous generation but because the medium is inoculated by dust-borne organisms settling into it.[3] This scientific experiment, repeated many many times with ingenious modifications, sanctified the age-old belief that disease was airborne and led the most brilliant minds into the most imaginative overstatements. Here is John Tyndall in 1876:

> I have spoken of the floating dust of the air, of the means of rendering it visible (the Tyndall beam), and of the perfect immunity from putrefaction which accompanies the contact of germless infusions and moteless air. Consider the woes which these wafted particles, during historic and prehistoric ages, have inflicted on mankind; consider the loss of life in hospitals from putrefying wounds; consider the loss in places where there are plenty of wounds, but no hospitals, and in the ages before hospitals were anywhere founded; consider the slaughter which has hitherto followed that of the battlefield, when those bacterial destroyers are let loose, often producing a mortality far greater than that of the battle itself; add to this the other conception that in times of epidemic disease the self-same floating matter has mingled with it the special germs which produce the epidemic, being thus enabled to sow pestilence and death over nations and continents—consider all this, and you will come with me to the conclusion that all the havoc of war, ten times multiplied, would be evanescent if compared with the ravages due to atmospheric dust.[3]

Whenever I am tempted to overstate the case for airborne contagion, I am

*Professor Emeritus, Department of Environmental Health Sciences, The Johns Hopkins School of Hygiene and Public Health, Baltimore, Maryland.

0077-8923/80/0353-003 $01.75/0 © 1980, NYAS

consoled by this quote from the great John Tyndall! But while Tyndall was imagining the public health implications of airborne organisms, hard epidemiological evidence of a contrary nature was accumulating. In 1854 an outbreak of cholera in London was studied by Snow and traced to the notorious Broad Street well.[4] With increasing awareness of the importance of water, food and milk in the transmission of enteric diseases and the demonstration of control by sanitary measures, this important group of diseases was removed from the airborne category.

Then in 1893 Smith and Kilborne showed the part played by ticks in the transmission of Texas cattle fever; in 1895 Ross watched the development of the malarial parasite in mosquitoes, and during the 1880s and 90s Finlay carried on his experimental work on mosquitoes and yellow fever.[5] After the occupation of Cuba by the United States in 1898, the War Department applied all that was known about sanitation and isolation in an unsuccessful effort to reduce yellow fever in Havana. Only after the Yellow Fever Commission, consisting of Reed, Carroll, Agramonte and Lazear, accomplished mosquito control were malaria and yellow fever wiped out, first in Havana and later in the Panama Canal Zone. This achievement was a classic in the annals of public health and provided convincing proof that malaria and yellow fever were not airborne in the usual sense of the word. And, of course, everyone knew that venereal diseases were not airborne.

Thus, with enteric diseases, insect-borne diseases, and venereal diseases removed from the airborne category, the pendulum moved to the other extreme: the denial that airborne infection was of any importance at all.

The man who completed the antiairborne swing of the pendulum was a scholarly health officer from Providence, Rhode Island, Charles V. Chapin. In *Sources and Modes of Infection*, published in 1910,[6] he states: "Bacteriology teaches that former ideas in regard to the manner in which diseases may be airborne are entirely erroneous; that most diseases are not likely to be dust-borne, and they are spray-borne only for 2 or 3 feet, a phenomenon which after all resembles contact infection more than it does aerial infection as ordinarily understood." And again "Without denying the possibility of such (airborne) infection, it may be fairly affirmed that there is no evidence that it is an appreciable factor in the maintenance of most of our common contagious diseases. We are warranted then, in discarding it as a working hypothesis and devoting our chief attention to the prevention of contact infection." Then he adds a fascinating proviso that shows the pragmatic state of mind of the health officer. "It will be a great relief to most persons to be freed from the spector of infected air, a spector which has pursued the race from the time of Hippocrates, and we may rest assured that if people can as a consequence be better taught to practice strict personal cleanliness, they will be let to do that which will more than anything else prevent aerial infection also, if that should in the end be proved to be of more importance than now appears."

With respect to tuberculosis Chapin was cautious. He was aware that Klein had infected guinea pigs by exposure in the ventilating shaft of Brompton Hospital. He considered tuberculosis more likely to be airborne than any other disease. Concerning influenza, a disease that was then considered "chiefly airborne, and airborne to great distances, even across the Atlantic," he found that "in no instance did the disease develop except as the result of contact with the sick or (in the case of deep sea fishermen) within two or three days after leaving shore." Even the great influenza pandemic of 1918 came and went with little change in the ideas enunciated by Chapin. Contagion meant direct contact, as its Latin root indicated.

William F. Wells was the man who brought new insights to bear on the transmission of contagious disease. Without a doctoral degree, he started out as a commissioned officer in the Public Health Service, served in the Sanitary Corps in World War I, had extensive experience with community water works, and investigated sources of shellfish contamination. He resigned from the commissioned service to become Instructor in Sanitary Science at the Harvard School of Public Health and redirected his research toward bacterial contamination of air. In 1931 he developed an instrument for the bacterial examination of air (the Wells centrifuge) which was his basic tool. This apparatus was described in the first of three publications on airborne infection that appeared in 1933 and 34.[7] In the second, entitled *Droplets and Droplet Nuclei*, Wells sketched briefly the salient aerodynamic characteristics of droplet nuclei,[8] "It appears, therefore, that transmission of infection through air may take one of two forms depending upon the size of the infected droplet. The form first recognized and most obvious is droplet infection proper. It applies to droplets larger than a tenth millimeter in diameter, which are rapidly removed from the air by gravity, before they can dry, and within a short distance of the source. The second form may be called air-borne infection, and deals with dried infected droplet nuclei, derived directly from droplets less than a tenth millimeter diameter, depending primarily upon air for the buoyancy which keeps them suspended for long times and carries them long distances."

Wells had the greatest respect for the logic and scholarly approach of Chapin. He considered droplet nucleus transmission an extension of contact infection in that both required close proximity between host and victim. Chapin had accepted the two to three foot range of respiratory droplets as an extended form of contact, and Wells extended the concept of contact to include sharing the same indoor atmosphere. Chapin quite rightly rejected the concept of transmission by air over long distance outdoors. Wells paid his respects to the requirements of close proximity by insisting on the term "airborne contagion," by which he meant close enough contact for exchange or organisms by air between the sick and the well.

Droplet nuclei, being invisible and widely dispersed, were exceedingly difficult to demonstrate. Wells made the analogy to polluted water:[8] "Failure to discover air-borne infection bacteriologically no more proves its absence, therefore, than failure to isolate B. *typhosus* from a sewage-polluted water proves that typhoid fever cannot be conveyed by drinking water." Wells' first demonstration that droplet nuclei were responsible for epidemic spread of disease under normal conditions of community life was indirect. Having discovered that ultraviolet (UV) radiation was effective in ridding the air of infectious droplet nuclei,[9] he installed UV fixtures in certain grade schools in suburban Philadelphia. Shortly thereafter a major epidemic of measles struck the control school which did not have UV air disinfection. The UV irradiated schools were almost completely spared.[10] In this experiment opportunities for direct contact were the same in test and control schools, so the reduced spread of infection in the UV irradiated schools could be attributed to the single factor that was different, namely, the concentration of airborne virus. To accept this conclusion, one had to accept UV air disinfection before being convinced of the airborne transmission of measles. This was more than the scientific community was ready to accept, but the study renewed interest in airborne contagion and stimulated attempts at confirmation.

One such study was carried out by Perkins, Bahlke and Silverman in schools in upstate New York.[11] It was a failure in that the number of cases of measles in the UV irradiated school was not reduced. However, in the irradiated school there was a long drawn out endemic pattern of disease in contrast to the peaked epidemic pattern that occurred in the unirradiated school. It is difficult to see how this could have been caused by anything other than the UV lights. Most of the children were bussed to the UV irradiated school, and it seems likely that measles may have been propagated at a slow rate in the unirradiated buses, even though checked in the classrooms. Nevertheless, the study, as performed, did not provide a practical answer to the control of measles. The extenuating circumstances were forgotten and the negative side remembered.

Other epidemiologic studies of UV air disinfection were also flawed by the confounding effects of exposures in unirradiated atmospheres. In an important study under the auspices of the British Medical Research Council,[12] UV lights were installed in schools in the Southall district of London. There were almost unlimited opportunities for contacts in the crowded surrounding community, and again the attempt to control airborne contagion failed. During and after World War II there were studies of UV lights and of dust supressive measures at Camp Sampson and Great Lakes Naval Training Stations.[26] These studies achieved a moderate degree of control of respiratory contagion even though the experimental conditions were not ideal. Dust suppressive measures in Army barracks were of marginal benefit.[27]

Wells, ever ready to put his theories to the test, attempted to control airborne contagion in the entire community of Pleasantville, New York. He and Holla[13] installed UV fixtures in schools, churches, clubs, the theater, certain stores, and other places of assembly of children, but not including private houses. The town of Mt. Kisco served as a control. In Pleasantville infection shifted from irradiated atmospheres to unirradiated atmospheres, with little effect upon the total incidence of airborne infection. For Wells, the study was a valuable survey of channels of airborne contagion throughout the community, using UV light as a tool for blocking selected channels. For others, it was simply another failure.

Thus, following a burst of enthusiasm in the 1930s and 40s, belief in airborne contagion was at a low ebb in the early 50s. Failure to control the spread of infection with UV was interpreted by many as disproof of the droplet nucleus theory. In the case of enteric diseases, control by pure community water had demonstrated that the infections were waterborne. Pure community air, not coming from a central source, could not be provided, and isolated UV installations proved to be inadequate. With the exception of Wells' early study in schools in suburban Philadelphia, efforts to control airborne contagion among people free to move about in the community had failed. Airborne contagion had to be demonstrated directly, by the presence of airborne disease, rather than indirectly, by the absence of disease with air disinfection.

By the late 1950s such demonstrations began to appear. At the Veterans Administration Hospital in Baltimore a large colony of guinea pigs breathed air from a tuberculosis ward.[14,15] On the average, three animals a month caught tuberculosis. This direct demonstration of airbone infection was widely accepted, but only for tuberculosis.

A decade later in 1968, Schulman demonstrated natural airborne transmission of influenza in mice.[16] In 1970, following an outbreak of smallpox in a West German hospital in which a single patient infected 19 others whom he had never seen, no less prestigious a scientific journal than *Newsweek* reported:[17] "With the aid of a smoke bomb—and the use of deductive skills worthy of a homicide squad—they (W.H.O.) demonstrated for the first time that smallpox, like flu, can be wafted by air currents." Thus, if *Newsweek* reflects the popular mind, airborne contagion was staging a comeback. Parenthetically, smallpox has now been wiped out, not by air disinfection but by isolation and vaccination (surveillance-containment).[18]

My brother, Edward Riley will shortly discuss a measles outbreak in a school where, as in the smallpox episode, the index case never even occupied the same room as most of the secondaries but infected them nevertheless by way of the ventilating system.[19]

In these direct demonstrations, infection was airborne indoors from the respiratory tract of an infectious individual to the respiratory tract of a susceptible recipient. This was aerial contact, or airborne contagion, in the Wellsian sense, and thoroughly consistent with transmission by droplet nuclei.

While some were attempting to control airborne contagion in the community, others were applying these concepts to the more circumscribed hospital environment. The surgeons were first, following in the steps of Lister and his carbolic spray. According to Wells,[1] "Hardly had the potency of ultraviolet light against airborne organisms been disclosed in the laboratory than Deryl Hart, without awaiting more detailed study, equipped his operating room." This was at Duke University Hospital in 1936.[20] I am pleased to see that Dr. Leonard Goldner of Duke University is on the program of this conference. Dr. Overholt at the New England Deaconess Hospital was next.[21] Then followed UV installations in nurseries, children's wards, burns units, convalescent homes, emergency wards, tuberculosis wards, and others. Chemical disinfection, usually with glycol vapors was also tried during the 1940s but proved difficult to manage.[22] Most of the early studies reported favorable results, indicating that genuine protection against airborne contagion was provided for patients remaining in protected atmospheres continuously. We will be brought up to date on airborne infection in hospitals later in this conference.

The development of the technique of air disinfection is a story in itself. The net result, however, has been relatively little progress since the UV barriers and fixtures for upper air irradiation first developed by Wells. The interaction between ventilation and upper air irradiation is a little better understood,[23] and more quantitative information has been obtained on the relative sensitivity to UV of different species of organisms.[24] Failure of cooperation between architects, engineers, microbiologists, and people developing the technique of air disinfection has held back progress. The medical profession remains confused and, by and large, has not given its blessing to air disinfection in hospitals.

At this conference other forms of airborne infection will be discussed where an infectious human host may not be the source and where transmission may not be limited to indoor atmospheres. I will make no attempt to sketch the historical background of these aspects but am delighted that they are included in the conference. It will broaden the horizons of those of us with a parochial medical background.

So, for the moment, the theory of airborne contagion appears to have outstripped practice. In contrast to the practice of water purification and insect control, which proved the theory of waterborne and insectborne diseases, air disinfection has not been widely practiced even though the theory of airborne contagion is accepted.

We are now at a point in the history of airborne contagion where the accumulated evidence forces us to shun the excessive enthusiasm of Tyndall and the excessive negativism of Chapin. But the very increase in our understanding increases our awareness of things that remain obscure. This characteristic of scientific progress was stated succinctly by Joseph Priestley in 1781:[25] "The greater is the circle of light, the greater is the boundary of darkness by which it is confined."

REFERENCES

1. WELLS, W. F. 1955. Airborne Contagion and Air Hygiene. Harvard University Press. Cambridge, Mass.
2. WINSLOW, C. E. A. 1943. Conquest of Epidemic Diseases. Princeton University Press. Princeton, N.J.
3. CONANT, J. B. 1957. Pasteur's and Tyndall's study of spontaneous generation. Case 7 in Harvard Case Histories in Experimental Science 2. Harvard University Press. Cambridge, Mass.
4. CHAPIN, C. V. 1910. Infection by food and drink. In Sources and Modes of Infection: Chap. 7. John Wiley and Sons. New York, N.Y.
5. CHAPIN, C. V. 1910. Infection by insects. In Sources and Modes of Infection: Chap. 8. John Wiley and Sons. New York, N.Y.
6. CHAPIN, C. V. 1910. Infection by air. In Sources and Modes of Infection: Chap. 6. John Wiley and Sons, New York, N.Y.
7. WELLS, W. F. 1933. Apparatus for study of the bacterial behavior of air. Am. J. Public Health 23: (1).
8. WELLS, W. F. 1934. On air-borne infection. Study II. Droplets and droplet nuclei. Am. J. Hygiene 20 (3): 611–618.
9. WELLS, W. F. & G. M. FAIR. 1935. Viability of B. coli exposed to ultraviolet radiation in air. Science 82: 280–281.
10. WELLS, W. F., M. W. WELLS & T. S. WILDER. 1942. The environmental control of epidemic contagion. I. An epidemiologic study of radiant disinfection of air in day schools. Am. J. Hygiene 35 (1): 97–121.
11. PERKINS, J. E., A. M. BAHLKE & H. F. SILVERMAN. 1947. Effect of ultraviolet irradiation of classrooms on the spread of measles in large rural central schools. Am. J. Public Health 37: 529–537.
12. MEDICAL RESEARCH COUNCIL. 1954. Air disinfection with ultraviolet irradiation; its effect on illness among school children. Special Report Series No. 283. London, England.
13. WELLS, W. F. & W. A. HOLLA. 1950. Ventilation in flow of measles and chickenpox through community. Progress report, Jan. 1, 1946 to June 15, 1949, airborne infection study. Westchester County Department of Health. J. Am. Med. Assoc. 142: 1337–1344.
14. RILEY, R. L., W. F. WELLS, C. C. MILLS, W. NYKA & R. L. MCLEAN. 1957. Air hygiene in tuberculosis: quantitative studies of infectivity and control in pilot ward. Am. Rev. Tuber. & Pulm. Dis. 75: 420–431.
15. RILEY, R. L., C. C. MILLS, F. O'GRADY, L. U. SULTAN, F. WITTESTADT, & D. N. SHIVPURI. 1962. Infectiousness of air from a tuberculosis ward: ultraviolet irradiation of infected air: comparative infectiousness of different patients. Am. Rev. Resp. Dis. 84: 511–525.
16. SCHULMAN, J. L. 1968. The use of an animal model to study transmission of influenza virus infection. Am. J. Public Health 58: 2092–2096.
17. NEWSWEEK. 1970. Nov. 16 issue.
18. HENDERSON, D. A. 1976. The eradication of smallpox. Sci. Am. 235: 25–33.
19. RILEY, E. C., G. MURPHY & R. L. RILEY. 1978. Airborne spread of measles in a suburban elementary school. Am. J. Epidem. 107: 421–432.
20. HART, D. 1936. Sterilization of the air in the operating room by special bactericidal radiant energy. J. Thoracic Surg. 6: 45–81.
21. OVERHOLT, R. H. & R. H. BETTS. 1940. A comparative report on infection of thoraco-plasty wounds. J. Thoracic Surg. 9: 520–529.

22. ROBERTSON, O. H., E. BIGG, B. F. MILLER & Z. BAKER. 1941. Sterilization of air by certain glycols employed as aerosols. Science **93:** 213-214.
23. RILEY, R. L. & S. PERMUTT. 1971. Room air disinfection by ultraviolet irradiation of upper air. Arch. Environ. Health **22:** 208-219.
24. RILEY, R. L., M. KNIGHT & G. MIDDLEBROOK. 1976. Ultraviolet susceptibility of BCG and virulent tubercle bacilli. Am. Rev. Resp. Dis. **113:** 413-418.
25. CONANT, F. B. 1957. Plants and the atmosphere. Case 5 in Harvard Case Histories in Experimental Science **2.** Harvard University Press. Cambridge, Mass.
26. WILLMON, T. L., A. HOLLAENDER & A. D. LANGMUIR. 1948. Studies of the control of acute respiratory diseases among naval recruits: A review of a four-year experience with ultraviolet irradiation and dust supressive measures, 1943-1947. Am. J. Hyg. **48:** 227-232.
27. LOOSLI, C. G. & O. H. ROBERTSON. 1945. Recent studies on the control of dust-borne bacteria by treatment of floors and bedclothes with oil. Am. J. M. Sc. **209:** 166-172.

SPREAD OF TUBERCULOSIS VIA RECIRCULATED AIR IN A NAVAL VESSEL: THE *BYRD* STUDY

Vernon N. Houk

Environmental Health Services Division
Bureau of State Services
Center for Disease Control
Atlanta, Georgia 30333

The Greek physician Hippocrates was the first to offer a clear description of tuberculosis, and in the fifth century B.C., Isocrates suggested that tuberculosis was transmitted from person to person. However, there was no tangible evidence of a means of transmission, and so interest in this theory declined.

Then, in 1882, Robert Koch's discovery of the tubercle bacillus reawakened speculation about the communicability of tuberculosis. The mechanism of infection with *Mycobacterium tuberculosis* became a subject of serious and, at times, intensive investigation.

By 1966, these investigations had led to the generally held theory that tuberculosis infection was acquired from the inhalation of the tubercle bacillus in a droplet-nucleus form. It was at this time that we were suddenly presented with an excellent opportunity to test this theory and shed more light on the epidemiology of tuberculosis infection.

REPORT OF A CASE

Over a year earlier, in May, 1965, aboard the U.S.S. *Richard E. Byrd*, a Navy ship with over 350 enlisted members and officers, a seaman had converted his five tuberculin unit (TU) tuberculin skin test from negative to positive. At that time, the seaman's chest roentgenogram was normal and his medical officer elected not to place him on isoniazid chemoprophylaxis.

Ten months later, in March, 1966, the seaman began to exhibit significant symptoms. Though he attended sick call on three occasions, the illness was diagnosed as a virus infection. A chest roentgenogram was not done until late August, 1966, about six months after the appearance of the significant symptoms. At that point, a diagnosis of tuberculosis was made, and the seaman was transferred from the ship to the U.S. Naval Hospital at St. Albans, New York.

The chest roentgenogram of the seaman disclosed a five centimeter cavity that could be classified as far advanced. His pulmonary secretions contained many acid-fast bacilli on direct smear. He had a significant cough. It was estimated that his disease had been active for at least six months. Therefore, it was concluded that the remainder of the personnel aboard the U.S.S. *Byrd* had been at high risk of contracting tuberculosis over the past six months.

Because of the unique circumstances surrounding the initial case, it was recognized that here was an excellent opportunity for an in-depth and detailed study aimed at elucidating the epidemiology of tuberculosis infection in a closed

10

0077-8923/80/0353-0010 $01.75/0 © 1980, NYAS

environment. The facilities of the East Coast Tuberculosis Treatment Center for the Navy were quickly made available for this study.

STUDY OF THE SHIP

All officers and enlisted personnel of the U.S.S. *Byrd* were admitted to the U.S. Naval Hospital at St. Albans where a complete physical examination was given and a complete medical history obtained.

Virtually every one of the individuals on board the U.S.S. *Byrd* had had a tuberculin skin test just six months earlier as part of the U.S. Navy's annual tuberculin skin testing program. Individuals reporting on board the ship after that time had also been tested. Therefore, it was possible to conclude that a change in any individual's tuberculin skin test from negative to positive was due to events and conditions aboard the U.S.S. *Byrd* over the past six months.

Before the officers and enlisted personnel were reunited with the ship and it was returned to active duty, the ship was completely decontaminated so that no mycobacteria could survive. Periodic followup was carried out over the next 12 months on all those who had been on the U.S.S. *Byrd* during the epidemic and on any individual who reported for duty on the ship subsequently.

Along with this medical data, detailed information concerning the sleeping location and its duration for each individual at risk was obtained. An individual at risk was defined as a previously known tuberculin negative individual. For each individual, the degree and closeness of contact with the initial case and with others on board who had active disease were ascertained. This included contact during work hours, nonwork hours, and closeness of social contacts both on and off the ship. Information concerning the use of the same equipment at work such as telephones and other communication sets was also obtained.

It was also necessary to make a detailed study of the ship's ventilation system. The U.S.S. *Byrd* has an overall ventilation system that allows for complete, closed recirculation of air. Within this overall system, there is cross-ventilation between various compartments in the ship. But the ventilation systems of some areas of the ship are not connected with the systems of other areas, and thus no cross-ventilation occurs between these areas. The connections between the ventilation systems of various compartments or the absence of such connections were examined in detail. The number and location of inlets and exhausts in the various compartments were also noted.

BACKGROUND

It was hoped that this mass of medical and environmental data would enable us to determine whether tuberculosis infection on board the U.S.S. *Byrd* was acquired from the inhalation of the tubercle bacillus in droplet-nucleus form and to trace the paths along which this infection spread in the closed environment of the ship. This theory of the transmission of tuberculosis infection had already received substantial support from the work of several past researchers.

W. F. Wells and his colleagues[1] had demonstrated in 1948 that the size of the inhaled particle is important. In their experiments, it was shown that rabbits inhaling two or three bovine tubercle bacilli dispersed as single units contracted more pulmonary tuberculosis than when inhaling 10,000 bacilli dispersed in larger aggregates. The larger clumps did not reach the alveolar lining membranes on lung tissue sections. But smaller particles of single bacilli were deposited on the alveolar surface of similar lung tissue sections. Here conditions are most favorable for the organism to proliferate.

In the early 1950s, the studies of Ratcliffe and Palladino[2,3] had shown that almost all tubercle bacilli inhaled as single organisms reached the alveolus and produced a tubercle. They noted that it was most unusual for more than a single organism to be deposited at any given site. They postulated that airborne tuberculosis in animals develops by inhalation of a single bacillus contained in the droplet nucleus that is the residual of the droplet after evaporation and contains any organism originally present in the droplet.[4]

In their classic experiments, Riley and his colleagues[5,6] in the late 1950s demonstrated that tubercle bacilli in droplet-nuclei form infected guinea pigs and other animals. These droplet nuclei were shown to occur in the room air of certain patients with tuberculosis. It was also found that the number of tubercle bacilli discharged into the atmosphere by a tuberculosis patient depends not only on the number of bacilli in his sputum but also upon such conditions as the fluidity of his sputum, the nature and forcefulness of his cough, and whether he covers his mouth during a cough or sneeze. Other factors are probably also important.

In 1965 Bates et al.[7] presented convincing evidence that inhalation of the tubercle bacillus in droplet-nucleus form was an important method of human infection. Droplet nuclei are less than five microns in diameter and are rapidly and randomly dispersed throughout closed atmospheres. Bates also postulated that singing may produce a fine particle aerosol in the infected individuals by the action of vibrating vocal chords.

An article in Medical World News[8] in 1965 suggested that a rock and roll group in the Netherlands probably infected hundreds, if not thousands, of their fans with Mycobacterium tuberculosis. Two of the singing group had "acute tuberculosis." From them, at least 40 fans developed active disease, and many others who did not have roentgenographic disease demonstrated a positive tuberculin test. Similarly, Protheroe[9] described an epidemic in an Army band, postulating that since band members exhale more forcefully and keep droplets airborne for a longer period of time, a greater concentration of airborne tubercle bacilli are produced. Many other examples were cited by Edith Lincoln[10] in her review of 109 separate epidemics.

It was against this background of previous observation and theory that we proceeded to analyze our own data.

RESULTS AND COMMENT

Sleeping locations of the enlisted personnel on the ship at the time of the initial study are presented in FIGURES 1–7. These diagrams are not drawn to scale, and because of security reasons, the proximity of berthing spaces and compartments is not detailed. These omissions, however, detract in no way from the impact of the data. It can be said that, in general, individuals from particular divisions who worked together also berthed in the same compartment.

Each large rectangle in the diagram represents a berthing space of three bunks placed atop one another. FIGURE 8 explains the symbols used in these diagrams.

The location of ventilation system inlets is also detailed in each diagram. Again, for security reasons, the overall system cannot be drawn in detail, but when appropriate, connections within the ventilation system between various compartments will be cited.

The figures depict the sleeping locations for 308 enlisted crew members at risk; of these, 140 individuals or 45.5 percent converted their five TU tuberculin reactions from a previously known negative to a positive at the time of the initial study. In addition, there were seven individuals who had clinically active disease with abnormal chest roentgenograms.

All of those with active disease, with one exception, worked and berthed in

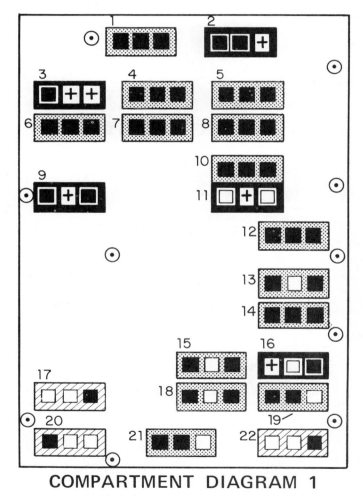

COMPARTMENT DIAGRAM 1

FIGURE 1. Compartment that berthed six of the seven individuals with active disease.

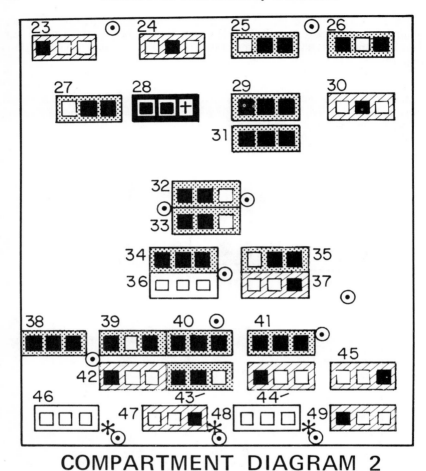

COMPARTMENT DIAGRAM 2

FIGURE 2. Another highly infected compartment. Ventilation comes from the same system as for Compartment One.

immediate proximity to each other. These individuals also spent considerable time together during their nonworking hours. They were frequently together when on liberty. One individual with active disease who did not berth with the others and did not work closely with them was a close personal friend and spent a great deal of time with them.

A more significant pattern, however, appears when we look at those who became infected with the tubercle bacillus. From the data gathered, it is apparent that nearly 50 percent of the ship's company was infected as a result of the failure to detect early the one individual who had disease. Of the enlisted personnel at risk who were berthed in the various compartments, the percentage of infected individuals was as follows: In Compartment One, 52 of 66 individuals or 78.8

percent (FIGURE 1); in Compartment Two, 46 of 81 individuals or 56.8 percent (FIGURE 2); in Compartment Three, 17 of 42 individuals or 40.5 percent (FIGURE 3); in Compartment Four, 12 of 39 individuals or 30.8 percent (FIGURE 4); in Compartment Five, 11 of 37 individuals or 28.2 percent (FIGURE 5); and in Compartments Six and Seven, 9 of 42 individuals or 21.4 percent (FIGURES 6 and 7).

At that time the overall incidence of positive tuberculin tests in the U.S. Navy approached 8 percent, a figure derived from the 1966 skin test surveys of ships,

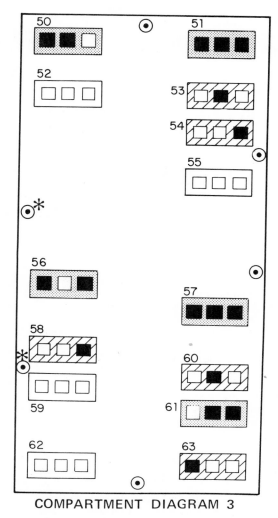

COMPARTMENT DIAGRAM 3

FIGURE 3. Individuals berthed in this compartment worked with individuals berthed in Compartment One, but in a different division.

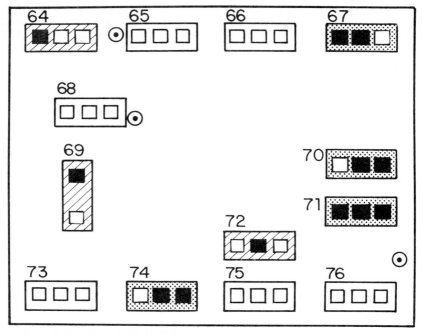

COMPARTMENT DIAGRAM 4

FIGURE 4. Lower rated personnel of the ship were berthed in this compartment.

including nearly 250,000 individuals. In 1965, the incidence of positive skin tests (defined as more than 9 millimeters induration produced by five test units of purified protein derivative (PPD-standard) for recruits entering the Navy was 3.4 percent. In the period 1961 through 1966 when any ship had been surveyed and the tuberculin positive rate found to be in excess of 20 percent, an individual with active tuberculosis had been found on board that ship. In light of these typical percentages, the percentages found on board the U.S.S. *Byrd* were extremely significant.

It is not surprising that individuals who had close contact with the initial case demonstrated tuberculous infection. As noted in FIGURE 1, each group of three-tiered bunks in the compartment in which the initial case slept had at least one tuberculous infection, and the majority had more than one. Forty-six of 66 individuals at risk in this compartment converted their tuberculin skin test and six had active disease. The initial case had slept for seven months in the middle bunk of space 3 in this compartment. Patients with active disease were grouped together; they lived together, shared close working spaces, and had off-duty social contacts.

Also of interest are the individuals in this compartment who were tuberculin negative at the time of the initial survey and who occupied a berthing space with one individual who had active disease. This was in space 11 in the diagram (FIGURE 1). Both of these individuals subsequently developed positive tuberculins, yet at the time of the initial study they had been on board the U.S.S. *Byrd* less than 4 weeks. Since they converted their tuberculin tests within 6 weeks of the initial study, they must have been infected soon after coming on board. This droplet nuclei containing tubercle bacilli must have abounded in this compartment.

The seven individuals in this same compartment who had been on board a substantial time and who remained uninfected must have had a real, natural immunity to the infection. None of these individuals had skin test sensitivity to mycobacteria other than *Mycobacterium tuberculosis*. This was evidenced by

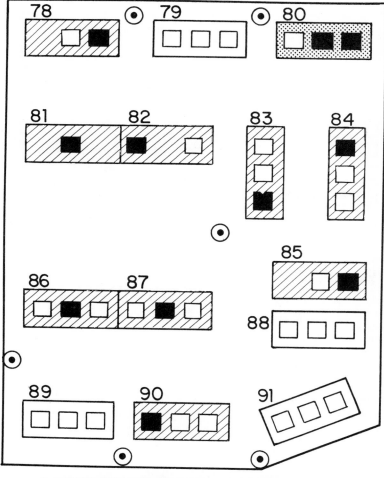

COMPARTMENT DIAGRAM 5

FIGURE 5. Crew's quarters for enlisted personnel in the supply division, including cooks.

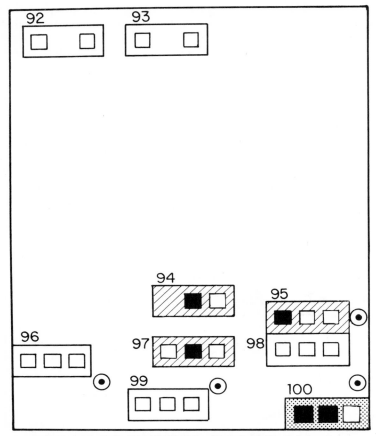

COMPARTMENT DIAGRAM 6

FIGURE 6. Quarters for more senior enlisted ratings.

lack of reactivity to either PPD-Battey or PPD-Gause upon entry into the Naval Service and a lack of reactivity to PPD-Gause during the initial period of this study. None had previously been vaccinated with BCG vaccine. Therefore, a naturally occurring immunity seems a more likely explanation than protection from a previous so-called atypical infection which had been cited by Palmer et al.[11]

The flow of air in the compartment was generally from the inlets noted in the diagram to exhaust openings near the center of the compartment. This probably explains why there was less infection in those berths located at the bottom of the diagram, the area upstream in the air flow pattern.

Of extreme significance in this study are the individuals berthed in the second compartment (FIGURE 2). Of the 81 individuals at risk, 45 converted their tuberculin skin test, and there was one case of active disease. These individuals had little in common in any respect and had little, if any, contact with individuals berthed in Compartment One. Their work duties and work locations were entirely different, and there was almost no off-duty close contact with the individuals in Compartment One. Nor did they employ the same equipment in the performance of their duties.

The only common source of contact between the individuals in Compartment One and Compartment Two was the ventilation system. Infected individuals in Compartment Two are for the most part located in the area where the systems for

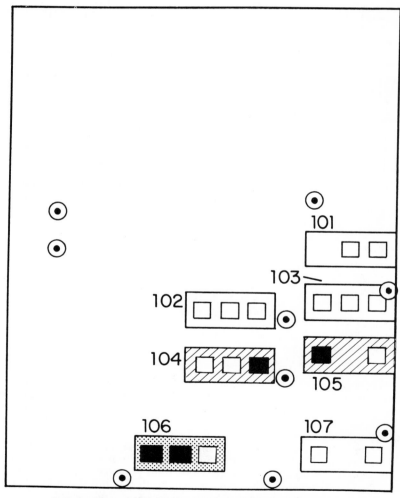

COMPARTMENT DIAGRAM 7

FIGURE 7. Quarters for more senior enlisted ratings.

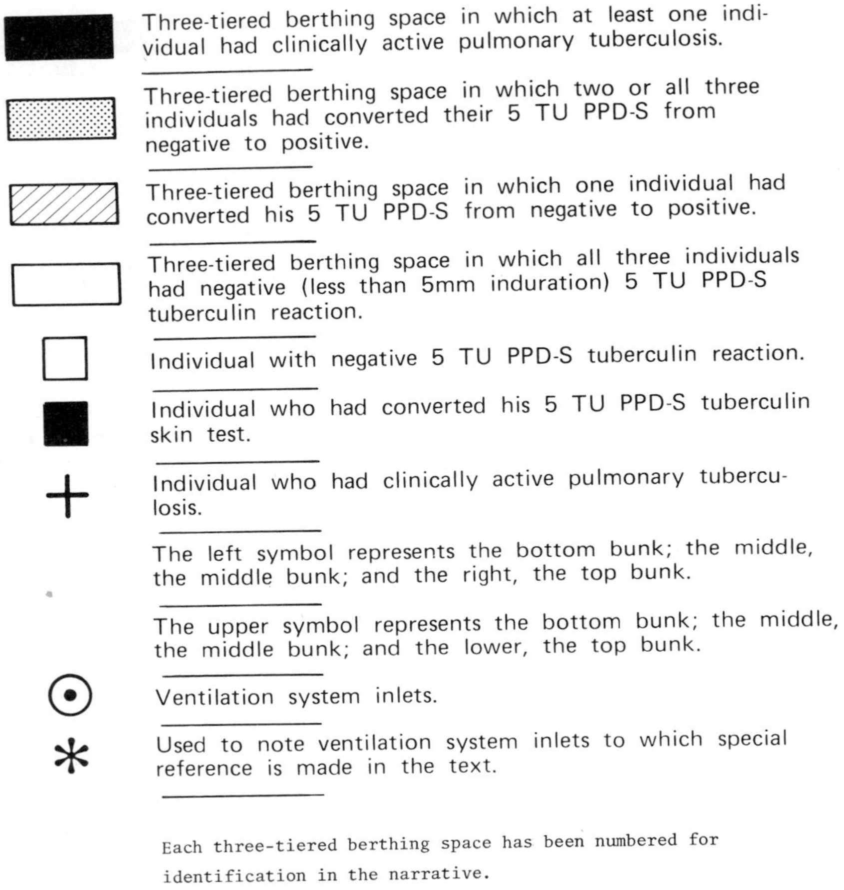

■ Three-tiered berthing space in which at least one individual had clinically active pulmonary tuberculosis.

▦ Three-tiered berthing space in which two or all three individuals had converted their 5 TU PPD-S from negative to positive.

▧ Three-tiered berthing space in which one individual had converted his 5 TU PPD-S from negative to positive.

▭ Three-tiered berthing space in which all three individuals had negative (less than 5mm induration) 5 TU PPD-S tuberculin reaction.

□ Individual with negative 5 TU PPD-S tuberculin reaction.

■ Individual who had converted his 5 TU PPD-S tuberculin skin test.

+ Individual who had clinically active pulmonary tuberculosis.

The left symbol represents the bottom bunk; the middle, the middle bunk; and the right, the top bunk.

The upper symbol represents the bottom bunk; the middle, the middle bunk; and the lower, the top bunk.

⊙ Ventilation system inlets.

✳ Used to note ventilation system inlets to which special reference is made in the text.

Each three-tiered berthing space has been numbered for identification in the narrative.

FIGURE 8. Explanation of symbols used in Figures 1 through 7 to depict berthing areas, converters, and ventilation systems.

the two compartments are interconnected. In the area where ventilation is supplied from another, nonrelated system (the inlets marked by an asterisk in the figure), only two of 12 individuals were tuberculin converters. There appears to be a dilution factor in this compartment when the airflow and air mixing are taken into consideration.

The one individual in this compartment with active disease had a minimal infiltrate. *Mycobacterium tuberculosis* was recovered in small numbers from his sputum. One of three gastrics grew five colonies of *Mycobacterium tuberculosis*; three induced sputa were sterile. He had been berthed in this area for only three weeks and was entirely asymptomatic with no cough.

Therefore, it seems unlikely that this individual with active disease infected the 45 other infected individuals in this compartment. It is more likely that their infection came via a droplet nuclei carried in the ventilation system from Compartment One.

The fact that Compartment Two was heavily contaminated prior to the basic decontamination of the ship is evidenced by the subsequent tuberculin conversion of two of the three individuals berthed in space 36, who had been on board less than six weeks at the time of the initial survey.

It was the data gathered in this particular compartment which gives strongest support to the theory that the ventilation system of the ship was the primary pathway of infection and that the means of transmission of infection was by droplet nuclei.

The next greatest incidence of infection occurred in those individuals berthed in Compartment Three (FIGURE 3). Seventeen of 42 individuals at risk in this compartment (or 40.5%) converted their skin tests from a previously known negative to positive. These individuals worked closely with the individuals from Compartment One and had many off-duty and social contacts with them.

The individual with active disease discussed earlier, who had moved to Compartment Two just three weeks prior to the initial study, had berthed the five previous months in Space 54 in this compartment. However, since this individual had only minimal disease, it seems unlikely that he was the source of infection for the 17 other infected individuals in this compartment.

The ventilation into this compartment came in part from the system that supplied Compartment One. The inlet openings are again denoted in the diagram (FIGURE 3). The inlets marked by an asterisk at the left of the diagram are not from the same system. It is interesting that the majority of infections were in individuals berthed along the right wall where the exhaust opening was located.

The one berthing space, number 55, along the right side that had no infection was occupied by three individuals who were berthed there in excess of six months. Two of these individuals had skin test sensitivity to PPD-Battey upon entering the Naval Service. This may explain the lack of infection with *Mycobacterium tuberculosis*.[12]

In all areas of heavy infection (that is, Compartments One, Two, and Three), the areas where the greatest number of infected individuals occurred were nearest the exhaust system. In Compartment One the area between spaces 9 and 11 was the exhaust area (FIGURE 1). More infection occurred in areas depicted at the top of the diagram of Compartment One than at the bottom. In Compartment Two, the exhaust was located near space 37 (FIGURE 2). Increasing infection is seen as we move toward this site, and decreasing infection occurs as we move toward more peripheral locations. The dilution effect from a noncontributory ventilation system is most evident in this diagram. These data further support the concept of droplet-nucleus infection postulated and demonstrated by Riley *et al.* in 1957 and 1959.[5,6]

In Compartment Four, 12 of 39 individuals at risk (or 30.8%) were infected (FIGURE 4). No connections existed between the ventilation system of this compartment and that of Compartments One and Two, but it did use the same exhaust system as Compartment Three. There was also moderate contact between infected individuals in this compartment and those from Compartments One and Two. A high percentage of the tuberculin converters in tests subsequent to the initial study came from individuals berthed in this compartment.

It is interesting to speculate on the source of these late infections. The U.S.S. *Byrd*, including its ventilation system, had been thoroughly decontaminated by an aerosol method following the discovery of active disease on board the ship. It is doubtful that dried nuclei from the ventilation system would account for these late infections. But it is possible that these late infections resulted from the shedding of a few tubercle bacilli from those tuberculin converters who did not manifest roentgenographic evidence of the disease. Another possible explanation for the late infections found in this compartment is that the initial case, who had cause to enter the compartment with great frequency to reach certain operational machinery in its center, could have infected the individuals who converted their tuberculins six weeks later; however, it is difficult to envision that he was directly responsible for conversions that occurred after the fourth month.

Compartment Five, which had an infection rate of 28.2 percent (that is, 11 of 37 individuals at risk) was not connected by means of its ventilation system with Compartments One, Two, or Three, and there was little contact between individuals berthed there and other individuals who had been infected (FIGURE 5).

There was, however, one exception to this which may be significant. One individual who did have extensive contact with the initial case did not have and did not subsequently develop roentgenographic disease, but his pulmonary secretions contained tubercle bacilli in significant numbers. On two of the three days on which his pulmonary secretion was cultured, confluent growth was evidenced on the culture media. It is interesting that this individual, who was berthed in space 80, was an amateur singer and sang for the benefit of those in his compartment. Besides the pleasure of his singing, they may also have acquired tuberculous infection during these musical interludes.

This individual initially denied cough, but when he returned for reevaluation after the postive cultures were obtained he stated that he had had a "cold" and cough for six weeks and had lost six pounds in weight. His chest roentgenogram (including tomography) remained normal. In fairness, however, we must note that these symptoms were elicited after intensive questioning and may have been iatrogenic rather than real.

However, one is led to speculate that such individuals, although they do not evidence roentgenographic disease, may be capable of transmitting the infection to susceptible individuals. Most of these individuals shed but few bacilli. However, a few have been demonstrated to shed organisms in significant numbers. The noise of the ship would make shouting and loud talking occasionally common. In fact, these individuals may be found to shout more than others in a more sedentary situation. Thus, one can demonstrate not only the organisms but also the possible method of dissemination. If a single bacillus is capable of producing a tubercle in human beings as it appears to do in lower animals,[2,3] then this concept of the transmission of infection by those without active disease has merit.

The higher rated personnel, who berthed in Compartments Six and Seven, had only supervisory contact with individuals in the other compartments (FIGURES 6 and 7). In general, skin test converters among this group (9 of 42 at risk or 21.4%) had closer contacts with each other than with nonconverters. There were no ventilation cross-connections with the other compartments. One individual, berthed in space 100, had, as his only contact, the use of the same headset used by the initial case. These communication headsets have mouthpiece microphones which are less than a centimeter away from the individual's mouth. An attractive, though speculative hypothesis, is that infection was transmitted by means of this headset. An individual shedding tubercle bacilli might cough and deposit a droplet on the microphone; that droplet may dry leaving a residual nucleus that contains the tubercle bacillus. The bacillus may then be inhaled by a susceptible individual and thus infection is transmitted.

CONCLUSIONS

In a study published in 1960, Walter and Kundsin[13] had demonstrated that a hospital floor may act as a source of droplet nuclei even after thorough cleansing. In 1962, Ochs[14] theorized that in a closed environment dried nuclei not exposed to sunlight may be infectious for a long period of time. He felt that contaminated particles deposited in certain areas may be resuspended in the air under certain circumstances. Then in 1966, Kent's[15] review of several epidemics in the U.S. Navy supported this theory of the resuspension of particles. It was pointed out that in most of the outbreaks of tuberculosis observed in the U.S. Navy, new infections continued to occur long after the active disease had been removed from the ship. The majority of the new tuberculin converters had been previously nonreactive to five test units of PPD-Standard, PPD-Battey, and PPD-Gause. It is unlikely therefore that all of these new tuberculin converters resulted from the booster effect of repeated tuberculins,[12] though their reaction to 100 Test Units was not known.

On the other hand, *Mycobacterium tuberculosis* had been grown from some of the individuals who became infected despite the fact that active disease had been removed.[16] It is possible that dried nuclei resuspended in the air are responsible for the new infections as Ochs postulated. However, available evidence[17] suggests that tubercle bacilli lodged on fomites do not constitute a significant infection hazard since most of them die quickly through the action of drying, heat, and sunlight. Dried secretions are very difficult to fragment and suspend in air, and furthermore, the airborne particles which do arise from surfaces are ordinarily innocuous. They are too large to penetrate the lung. In addition, in this study, the ship was thoroughly decontaminated. It is difficult to envision contaminated particles remaining after a complete decontamination. And yet new infections did occur several months after decontamination.

A more attractive concept, though not proven by these epidemiologic data, is that "converters" who have no roentgenographic disease, but who shed organisms in their pulmonary secretions, may be responsible for the continued tuberculosis infections, as was theorized by Kent et al.[16] in 1967. It is possible in virtually every individual who converts his skin test within a specified period to culture *Mycobacterium tuberculosis* from his pulmonary secretions if these secretions are cultured frequently enough.[16] We feel that this concept may be important in certain conditions of a closed environment when air is being recirculated within that environment. However, with more normal ventilation such as in a room or in the general community, it is doubted that those individuals who have normal chest roentgenograms constitute significant risk for the remaining uninfected population.

In summary, we were able to conclude that the vast majority of infection found aboard the U.S.S. *Richard E. Byrd* during this epidemic came by way of droplet nuclei. These droplet nuclei measure from two microns to 10 microns and are rapidly and evenly dispersed throughout a closed environment with a recirculation ventilation system. These droplets may infect others who have little or no contact with the infected individual who is shedding *Mycobacterium tuberculosis* in his pulmonary secretions. It is also possible that some individuals, that is, tuberculin skin test converters who have normal roentgenograms but whose pulmonary secretions contain *Mycobacterium tuberculosis*, may be capable of transmitting the infection to susceptible individuals.

REFERENCES

1. WELLS, W. F., H. L. RATCLIFFE & C. CRUMB. 1948. On mechanics of droplet-nuclei infection; quantitative experimental airborne tuberculosis in rabbits. Am. J. Hyg. **47:** 11–28.
2. RATCLIFFE, H. L. 1952. Tuberculosis induced by droplet-nuclei infection; pulmonary tuberculosis of predetermined initial intensity in mammals. Am. J. Hyg. **55:** 36–48.
3. RATCLIFFE, H. L. & V. S. PALLADINO. 1953. Tuberculosis induced by droplet-nuclei infection; initial homogeneous response of small mammals (rats, mice, guinea pigs, and hamsters) to human and to bovine bacilli and rate and pattern of tubercle development. J. Exp. Med. **97:** 61–68.
4. RILEY, R. L. & F. O'GRADY. 1961. Airborne Infection, Transmission and Control. Macmillan and Company. New York City, N.Y.
5. RILEY, R. L. *et al.* 1957. Air hygiene in tuberculosis: quantitative studies of infectivity and control in a pilot ward. Am. Rev. Tuberc. **75:** 420–431.
6. RILEY, R. L. *et al.* 1959. Aerial dissemination of pulmonary tuberculosis, a two-year study of contagion in a tuberculosis ward. Am. J. Hyg. **70:** 185–196.
7. BATES, J. H., W. E. POTTS & M. Lewis. 1965. Epidemiology of primary tuberculosis in an industrial school. N. Engl. J. Med. **272:** 714–717.
8. Med. World News. December 10, 1965. New twist on TB spread. **6:** 34.
9. PROTHEROE, C. 1957. Epidemic of pulmonary tuberculosis in a closed community. Br. Med. J. **1:** 80–82.
10. LINCOLN, E. M. 1965. Epidemics of tuberculosis, fascicle 21: advanced tuberculosis research. Bibl. Tuberc. **14:** 157–201.
11. PALMER, C. E. & M. LONG. 1966. Effects of infection with atypical mycobacteria on BCG vaccination and tuberculosis. Am. Rev. Respir. Dis. **94** (October): 553–568.
12. SMITH, D. T. 1967. New aspects of mycobacterial skin tests. Arch. Environ. Health **14:** 569–579.
13. WALTER, C. W. & R. B. KUNDSIN. 1960. Floor as a reservoir of hospital infections. Surg. Gynecol. Obstet. **111** (October): 412–422.
14. OCHS, C. W. 1962. The epidemiology of tuberculosis. J. Am. Med. Assoc. **179:** 247–252.
15. KENT, D. C. 1967. Tuberculosis as a military epidemic disease and its control by the Navy tuberculosis control program. Dis. Chest. **52:** 588–594.
16. KENT, D. C. *et al.* 1967. Tuberculin conversion: the iceberg of tuberculosis pathogenesis. Arch. Environ. Health **14:** 580–584.
17. 1967. Statement of National Tuberculosis Association Committee on Treatment of Tuberculous Patients in General Hospitals. Am. Rev. Respir. Dis. **96** (October): 836–837.

THE ROLE OF VENTILATION IN THE SPREAD OF MEASLES IN AN ELEMENTARY SCHOOL

Edward C. Riley

Box 340, Route 1
Bokeelia, Florida 33922

I am delighted to participate in this conference on airborne contagion and compare notes on dissemination mechanisms. In the early 1930s, before I studied medicine, I worked with Professor William F. Wells at Harvard. First we studied airborne organisms around the Cambridge sewage treatment plant and later the effect of contaminated humidifying water on airborne organisms in textile mills in Massachusetts. After we left Boston, our paths separated; I went to medical school in New York City and Professor Wells moved his laboratory to Philadelphia, Pennsylvania, and later to Baltimore, Maryland. Not until I retired in 1970 did I return to the study of airborne contagion; but in Baltimore, my brother, Doctor Richard Riley, and Professor Wells collaborated for many years prior to Wells' death in 1963 in the Baltimore Veterans Administration Hospital.

For several years while in Philadelphia, Professor Wells and his wife, Mildred Wells, M.D., studied epidemics of contagious diseases in primary and secondary schools. These studies were designed to demonstrate the potential of ultraviolet irradiation of the upper portion of classrooms for the control of airborne disease. The irradiation changed the rate and pattern of spread, but the results were inconsistent and there was no satisfactory explanation for the failure of some installations to prevent airborne spread of disease. Although not directly involved in these studies, I shared Wells' conviction that many contagious diseases were airborne and that sterilization of the ambient air should prevent airborne infections.

For many years, either the Soper equation or the Reed-Frost modification has provided the conceptual model for the spread of contagious disease.

$$C = rIS \qquad \text{Soper}$$
$$C = S(1 - e^{-Ir}) \qquad \text{Reed-Frost} \tag{1}$$

Analogy to the basic law of mass action, so successfully applied to chemical reactions, seemed appropriate and there was no convincing explanation for the failure of observed epidemic patterns to conform to the simple equation $C = rIS$. A careful analysis of the mechanism of airborne spread of infection from person to person identified the factors which must be included in a realistic mathematical model. These are: 1. The number of infectious organisms dispersed into a closed system which remain airborne long enough to be breathed by a susceptible subject, 2. The volume of air into which these organisms are dispersed and 3. The number of infectious organisms breathed by susceptible subjects during 4. The time that infectors and susceptibles share a closed system during one generation of epidemic spread. In order to include these factors in the mathematical model, they must be introduced through r, the effective contact rate. Equation 2 defines r in terms of four variables.

0077-8923/80/0353-0025 $01.75/0 © 1980, NYAS

$$r = pqt/Q \tag{2}$$

where $p =$ pulmonary ventilation rate (susceptible)

        $q =$ dissemination rate (infector)

                The rate at which an infector disseminates infectious particles which remain airborne long enough to be inhaled by a susceptible subject.

        $t =$ exposure time

                Time that infector(s) and susceptibles share a confined space or ventilating system during one generation.

        $Q =$ dilution rate (germ-free air)

                Applicable only to ventilating systems with good mixing under steady state conditions. Any consistent system of units may be used.

This definition involving four parameters which vary during a single generation of exposure indicates why r is not a constant and why a single value is an unrealistic oversimplification and has not produced consistent simulations of observed epidemic patterns.

Before quantitative measures of circulating antibodies were available, the history of clinical disease was generally accepted as the measure of immunity and the number of clinical cases was considered synonomous with the number of infections. Subclinical infections were ignored or considered inconsequential. For measles during an epidemic, clinical disease was easily diagnosed and provided a useful measure for cases and infectors. Measles cases are considered infectious during the three day period before measles is diagnosed and the case removed from the group. History of clinical disease may be a reasonable measure of immunity but the converse that anyone without a history of disease is susceptible is a questionable measure of susceptibility.

Although these measures of C, I, and S are inaccurate, they have been used for the study of the pattern of spread of epidemic contagion. However, when the effective contact rate is computed from C/IS, the errors are magnified and a grossly inaccurate value is obtained. In contrast, equation 2, based on scientific principles, defines the effective contact rate in physical and physiologic terms, most of which can be independently determined. From this analysis it appears that r is a constantly changing rate which varies from moment to moment and person to person and does not remain constant during an entire generation of exposure.

A realistic epidemic model must simulate the varying activities and exposures for each susceptible individual in order to reproduce the observed pattern of disease spread. Even in an elementary school, a relatively simple and controlled social setting, it is not likely that any two susceptibles will experience the same activities and exposures during an entire generation of spread of contagious disease.

Although the mathematical model should be equally applicable to all airborne disease, over the years, measles has been the most consistent and predictable of the childhood contagions and there are many reports in the medical literature of excellent measles studies. In 1970, when Dr. W. T. Stille and I were testing a model for the spread of airborne contagion, measles vaccination was a recent addition to the preschool immunization program and it appeared unlikely that epidemic measles would occur among vaccinated school populations. Therefore, to test the model we selected the measles data from a study by Perkins and a group from the New York State Health Department which was reported in the *American Journal of Public Health* in 1947.[1]

Ventilation information was not reported, but on visiting the schools I found that the original, thermostatically controlled, general ventilating systems were still in operation. From engineering specifications and meterologic reports for the Syracuse, New York, weather station I was able to compute quantitative values for ventilation during the 1945 measles epidemic in the Mexico Central School near Syracuse, New York. Using these values our model simulated the observed pattern quite well.

While we were still debugging the computer program, reports of measles outbreaks among highly immunized school populations began to appear in medical journals. Whenever possible, I visited the site of the reported outbreak to obtain the detailed ventilation and activity data needed to test the model. After investigating measles outbreak in elementary schools near Cincinnati, Ohio[2] and Mayfield, New York,[3] I learned of an ongoing measles outbreak in an elementary school near my home in suburban Rochester, New York. Although no epidemiologic study was planned, the excellent health and attendance records from the school nurse and the detailed ventilation data from the architects and engineers provided the information needed to test the epidemic model. This study, reported in the May, 1978, issue of the *American Journal of Epidemiology*, illustrates the application of the model to an outbreak of measles.[4]

In this modern elementary school, kindergarten through third grade, measles was first reported on April 25, 1974; by the end of May the epidemic was over after 60 children had come down with measles. This school was one of nine in a large suburban school district with a total enrollment of 8,100 and serving a community of 31,000 persons. Sporadic cases occurred in other schools but there were no sharp outbreaks of measles. The study population consisted of 868 elementary school children, 97 percent of whom had been vaccinated against measles. Each of the four grades was divided into nine classes for a total of 36 classes. The kindergarten children attended half-day sessions, four classes in the morning and five in the afternoon.

FIGURE 1 shows the pattern of epidemic spread throughout the entire school. The index case was a second grader from classroom 16 who became ill on April 25th. Before she became ill and was removed from school, 28 susceptibles were infected, two from the home room and 26 from 13 different classrooms. Since the index case walked to school, the secondaries almost certainly were infected in school and the 26 cases from 13 different classrooms probably resulted from infectious particles in the air recirculated by the general ventilating system in the main building.

FIGURE 2 shows the general plan of the school building. The main school building, built in 1961 is shown in bold outline. It provided 25 classrooms and was ventilated by a large, 36,000 cubic feet per minute (cfm) general ventilating system with recirculation thermostatically controlled. In 1971 a new wing shown in right lower quadrant was added which provided seven additional classrooms, five for kindergarten and two for the third grade. The new wing utilized a similar but separate ventilating system with a capacity of 15,000 cfm. The utility rooms shown as F-1 and F-2 housed the ventilating equipment for the main building and the new wing. In both systems the amount of outside make-up air was thermostatically controlled and varied with the outside temperature as indicated by FIGURE 3. There was no recirculation when the outside temperature was above 60°F. The air supply for both buildings was filtered before it was distributed to the classrooms; the filters in the main ventilation system removed 12 percent of respirable particles, less than 5 microns, whereas the filters in the new wing removed 30 percent. The volume of make-up air and the effect of filtration of the

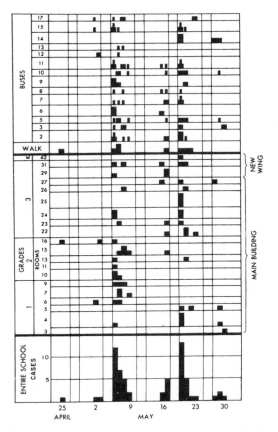

FIGURE 1. Distribution of measles cases in an upstate New York elementary school in spring, 1974, by calendar date of first day of school missed on account of measles. Vertical bars identify Saturdays and Sundays. From below up, separated by heavy horizontal lines, cases in the entire school; cases by grades and rooms; cases by means of transportation (walk or bus). Cases who travelled one way by bus are shown by narrow vertical bars. On the right the ventilating systems supplying rooms where measles occurred are identified.

recirculated air were taken into consideration in determining Q, the dilution with germ-free air.

Although the index case walked to school, 52 of the 60 measles cases travelled to and from school by bus and the possibility of infectious contact during bus rides could not be ignored. The identity of the occupants of each bus and the approximate duration of exposure was determined from the bus schedules but no information on dilution with outside air was available from either the bus companies or engineering literature. In order to establish a realistic dilution ventilation value, special studies were carried out with the common 60 passenger school bus. During a special bus run, complete with stops but no children on board, a gaseous tracer was released and the dilution rate determined from the washout. This test indicated a dilution rate of about 250 cubic feet per minute (cfm). Although the school district operated a large fleet of school buses, most were the 60 passenger model used for the test run and a dilution rate of 250 cfm was used in determining bus exposures.

From a careful study of the daily curricula of infectious cases and susceptible subjects and the type and amount of ventilation, three important exposure sites were characterized quantitatively: 1. Classroom(s) with infector(s); 2. other classrooms served by the same ventilating system; and 3. school buses with infector(s).

Although there were no general assemblies, there were casual contacts in the hallways and cafeteria and at social functions outside the school. These could not be quantified and were not included in the analysis.

When quantitative values for the effective contact rate, the number of infectors and the number of exposed susceptibles are used in a valid mathematical model, computations should simulate the observed epidemic pattern. For this study the number of reported cases was considered an adequate measure of the number infected. Although subclinical infections may have occurred, they could not be identified and have not been considered in this analysis. Each case was considered infectious for three days prior to the first day's absence from school with clinical measles; and this criterion was used to determine the number of infectors. Identification of susceptibles among a ninety-seven percent vaccinated school population presented a serious problem since history of clinical disease

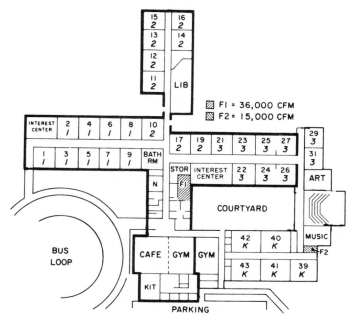

FIGURE 2. Floor plan of the upstate New York elementary school which experienced a measles epidemic in spring, 1974. The main building, constructed in 1961, is shown in bold outline. The main ventilating system (36,000 cfm) was located at F-1. The 1971 addition, lower right, was supplied by a smaller 15,000 cfm ventilating system located at F-2. On the plan, room number appears above and grade below.

was meaningless and no antibody titres were obtained either before or after the outbreak. However, from the dynamics of this explosive outbreak, it has been shown that it is extremely unlikely that any exposed susceptible could have escaped infection by the end of the outbreak. It is therefore reasonable to assume that all susceptibles were infected and that the total number of reported cases was a valid measure of the susceptible population at the start of the outbreak.

The Reed-Frost model considers the probability of an individual susceptible becoming infected from a known exposure:

$$P = 1 - e^{-Ir} \tag{3}$$

Statisticians have shown that if the chance of becoming infected is $1 - e^{-Ir}$, the chance of escaping infection is e^{-Ir}. It has also been shown that the chance of

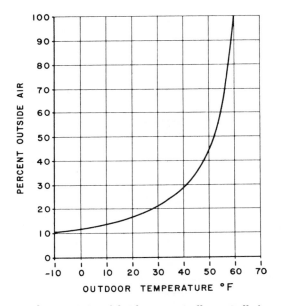

FIGURE 3. Response characteristics of the thermostatically-controlled ventilating systems in the upstate New York elementary school during the 1974 measles outbreak. This curve is specific for a room temperature of 68°F.

escaping infection from two independent exposures is equal to the product of the two chances, $e^{-I_1 r_1} \cdot e^{-I_2 r_2}$ which is the same as $e^{-(I_1 r_1 + I_2 r_2)}$. Where there are more than two independent exposures this expression can be expanded into the general expression $P = e^{-(I_1 r_1 + I_2 r_2 + \dots I_n r_n)}$. Thus the chance of an individual becoming infected from several independent exposures becomes

$$P = 1 - e^{-(I_1 r_1 + I_2 r_2 + \dots I_n r_n)} \tag{4}$$

The probable number of cases in the next generation is equal to the sum of the chances of all susceptibles from all their exposures. This expanded form of the

Reed-Frost model becomes

$$C = \sum_{1-i}^{S} [1 - e^{(I_1 r_1 + I_2 r_2 + \ldots I_n r_n)}] \quad \text{OR}$$

$$C = S - \sum_{i-1}^{S} e^{-Ir} total_i$$

(5)

This equation is simply the mathematical expression for the sum of all the individual susceptibles' chances of infection as determined from equation 4. Knowledge of the identity and whereabouts of all infectors and exposed susceptibles is needed to solve equation 5. As previously noted, probably all exposed susceptibles became infected during the outbreak and were infectious for three days prior to the diagnosis of measles. In retrospect it was possible to determine the whereabouts of all infectors and susceptibles during exposure periods and compute the probablilty of infection; the sum of the individual probabilities should approximate the number of observed cases.

Three major exposure sites: 1. Classroom(s) with infector(s), 2. other classrooms served by the same ventilating system; and 3. school buses with infector(s) were quantitatively evaluated. These sites provided the greatest opportunity for infection and together probably determined the observed epidemic pattern. The effective contact rates were determined from equation 2, $r = pqt/Q$. Reasonable values for every component except the dissemination rate, q, were known so r was expressed in terms of q, the unknown dissemination rate. For each susceptible child and each day of exposure, $I_1 r_1$, $I_2 r_2$ and $I_3 r_3$ were calculated and the daily values added together to give a total Ir for each susceptible for one generation. The equation expressed in terms of the unknown, q, was then solved by trial and error. By successive approximations a value of q was found which satisfied the mathematical model and was consistent with the epidemic pattern.

The single index case, a second grader in classroom 16 who walked to school, infected 28 susceptible children during the three days she attended class during the infectious period. Two cases resulted from home room contacts but 26 secondaries occurred in 13 different classrooms served by the large general ventilating system for the main school building. Since the single index case walked to school, there were no bus exposures during the first generation. In order to produce the reported number of cases among the exposed susceptible population, the index case is calculated to have disseminated 93 quanta of measles virus per minute.

If the 28 cases in the second generation had disseminated infection at the rate of 93 quanta per minute, calculations indicate less than one chance in ten thousand of a susceptible escaping infection and the epidemic would have ended with the third generation. However, the pattern suggests that the last four cases may represent a fourth generation; in that case, a dissemination rate of 8 or 9 quanta per minute would have been adequate to simulate the observed pattern. From these calculations it appears that dissemination rates may vary from 8 to 93 quanta per minute and still permit airborne spread of measles. The 93 quanta per minute is the highest rate so far calculated for any measles epidemic and it is apparent that the index case disseminated airborne measles virus at an exceptionally high rate.

Calculations such as these are possible only when quantitative values for the factors indicated in the mathematical model are available. From quantitative antibody measurements epidemiologists can identify susceptibles and measure changes in level of immunity; this should provide a better measure of the population at risk and make possible identification of subclinical infections as well as clinical disease. On the other hand, quantitative values for two of the components of the effective contact rate, the dilution ventilation rate and the dissemination rate, are not readily available. Professor Wells was well aware of the role of ventilation in the spread of airborne disease and used the term "equivalent sanitary ventilation"[5] to describe any mechanism which reduced the concentration of organisms at the same rate as dilution with germ-free air. This can be achieved by fresh makeup air, filtration of recirculated air or ultraviolet irradiation of upper room air. For buildings with mechanical ventilation, dilution with disease-free air can generally be determined but is seldom reported. Use of the equivalent sanitary ventilation rate in equation 2 to compute the effective contact rate can produce valid results only when steady state conditions and good mixing are present within the space or ventilating system.

Although dilution ventilation rates can generally be determined, there is currently no way to measure the dissemination rate directly. The definition of a quantum of infection as "that dose, whatever it may be in terms of number of organisms, required to produce infection in susceptible members of the species"[6] makes the dissemination rate in quanta per minute an indirect measurement based on the number of susceptibles infected. In this analysis the dissemination rate is considered unknown and the effective contact rate expressed in terms of the unknown q.

From careful studies of ventilation systems in elementary and secondary schools where well-documented measles outbreaks have occurred, I have determined the dissemination rates necessary to produce the observed pattern of spread. Even though the number of observations is too few to be statistically significant and the values are widely scattered, a pattern is beginning to appear. From the limited available data it is apparent that the distribution is not linear and that the geometric or log normal distribution describes the computed values reasonably well. When the logarithm of the dissemination rate is plotted against the relative cumulative frequency on probability paper, a geometric normal distribution generates a straight line as shown in FIGURE 4. The values so far computed for the dissemination rate range from one to 93 quanta per minute and this curve covers the entire rante. The computed dissemination rates from studies of elementary school measles epidemics often fall between 4 and 16 quanta per minute but values have covered a wide range. The curve shows a median value of 10 quanta per minute and indicates that 68 percent of observations, plus or minus one geometric standard deviation, would be expected to fall between 4— and 26+ quanta per minute. Similarly 95 percent of observations would be expected between 1.5— and 70— quanta per minute, plus or minus two geometric standard deviations. This indicates that the value 93 quanta per minute would be expected only about one time in one hundred observations.

The suggested distribution of individual dissemination rates was deduced from the study of several measles epidemics among school children. The values should be considered approximate and subject to revision as more data from studies of measles and other airborne diseases become available. The concept of a quantum of airborne infection deduced from the pattern of disease spread may seem nebulous and its meaning questioned. Wells has pointed out that airborne infection results from very small particles or droplet nuclei which remain airborne until breathed by an exposed subject, are vented from the system or die. The settling rate for these tiny airborne infectious particles is so slow relative to the room air currents that the effect is negligible. The number of infectious

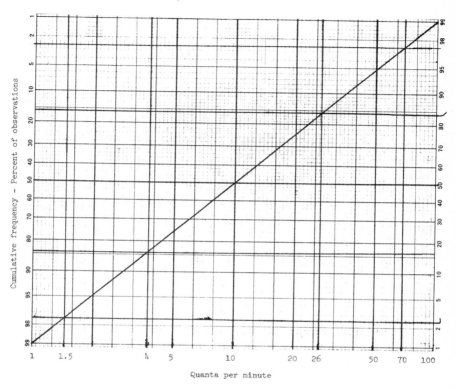

FIGURE 4. Proposed distribution for dissemination rates of measles cases during the infectious (3 day) prodromal period. Dissemination rates (quanta/minute) when plotted against cumulative relative frequency on logarithmic-probability paper should approximate a straight line if the geometric normal distribution is appropriate.

particles in one quantum of airborne infection has not been definitely established; observations indicate that it may be as small as one or perhaps several airborne infectious particles. For this discussion the exact composition of a quantum of infection is less important than a quantitative value for the dissemination rate. This indirect measurement provides a quantitative dissemination rate. This indirect measurement provides a quantitative dissemination rate that has been used to explain observed epidemic patterns and may be used to predict the likelihood of airborne infection under known environmental conditions.

This mechanistic model for a complex environmental and biological phenomenon identifies specific factors and provides a concept of airborne spread which can be tested by future investigators. Even though it may never be possible to measure accurately all the basic factors for all possible exposures of all susceptible subjects, without quantitative values for these factors it is impossible to test hypotheses or predict the risk of infection. The equations appear deterministic but the model can accept all quantifiable risks of infection and provide a rational basis for stochastic computer simulations of patterns of airborne contagion.

REFERENCES

1. PERKINS, J. E., A. M. BAHLKE & H. F. SILVERMAN. 1947. Effect of ultraviolet irradiation of classrooms on the spread of measles in large rural central schools. Am. J. Pub. Health 37: 529–537.
2. LINNEMAN, C. C. JR., T. C. ROTTE, G. M. SCHIFF & J. L. YOUTSEY. 1972. A seroepidemiologic study of a measles epidemic in a highly immunized population. Am. J. Epidemiol. 95: 238–246.
3. N. Y. STATE DEPARTMENT OF HEALTH. 1973. Communicable Disease Newsletter 4: 1–2.
4. RILEY, E. C., G. MURPHY & R. L. RILEY. 1978. Airborne spread of measles in a suburban elementary school. Am. J. Epidemiol. 107: 421–432.
5. WELLS, W. F., 1955. Airborne Contagion and Air Hygiene: 157, 176. Harvard University Press. Cambridge, Mass.
6. RILEY, R. L. & F. O'GRADY. 1961. Airborne infection: 76. The Macmillan Company, New York, N.Y.

CHANGING CONCEPTS OF AIRBORNE INFECTION OF ACUTE CONTAGIOUS DISEASES: A RECONSIDERATION OF CLASSIC EPIDEMIOLOGIC THEORIES

Alexander D. Langmuir*

Abel's Hill
Chilmark, Massachusetts 02535

INTRODUCTION

During the past 15 years, major programs have been launched against three so-called contagious diseases: smallpox, measles, and rubella. The results in terms of achievement of expected goals have varied in the extreme. The global eradication of smallpox within a decade rivals President Kennedy's inaugural boast in 1960, "We will go to the moon in ten years." The decline in measles incidence in the U.S.A. has been substantial but the stated goal of early eradication remains elusive. The rubella program was born in controversy and remains subject to constant reevaluation.

The "best and the brightest" epidemiologists participated in the decisions to embark on these programs and have continued to carry them out. Their successes, failures, and haunting uncertainties can clearly be ascribed to the adequacy, or perhaps more correctly the inadequacy, of their understanding of the epidemiology of these diseases. More specifically successes can be attributed to flexibility to accept new information making preconceived attitudes obsolete. Central to the control of all three diseases is the understanding of the theory of contact and airborne infection and its corollary: herd immunity.

In the present paper I will endeavor 1. To recall the prevailing attitudes among epidemiologists at the time these programs were started; 2. to reexamine the scientific validity of some of the theories that we so blithely accepted at the time; and 3. to appraise what we think we have learned from our vivid experiences during the past 15 years.

Prevailing Attitudes in Early 1960s

From the mid 1930s to 1960s our knowledge and attitudes toward the relative importance of contact and airborne routes of infection had been in a state of flux. Prior to 1935, contact, including direct droplet spread, was universally accepted as the only mode of spread of contagious diseases. The views of Charles V. Chapin, carefully constructed and forcefully expounded, were not questioned.[1]

In 1935, however, William Firth Wells, an engineer at Harvard, challenged Chapin.[2] He argued, presumably from an intuitive base, that measles was spread by droplet nuclei and he introduced ultraviolet lights into schools to test his hypothesis. One early success was followed by less impressive subsequent trials.[3] O. H. Robertson[4] in Chicago also challenged the dominance of the contact theory

*Formerly Chief Epidemiologist, Center for Disease Control, U.S. Department of Health, Education and Welfare, Atlanta, Ga. 30333.

35

by developing disinfectant vapors, propylene and later triethylene glycol for the potential control of streptococcal and other respiratory infections in hospitals and military barracks.

During the late 1930s and throughout the 1940s a series of field trials were undertaken to test these engineering methods. Practical field trials appeared to be the only way to test the airborne hypothesis.

In November, 1946, a Committee to Evaluate the Effectiveness of Methods to Control Airborne Infection reported at the annual meeting of the American Public Health Association.[5] James E. Perkins was chairman. I served as secretary and prepared the first and second draft reports. William Firth Wells and O. H. Robertson were active and articulate members. The final report represented a consensus to which all members concurred. I will quote one sentence over which we struggled for a long time:

> "Conclusive evidence is not available at present that the airborne mode of transmission of infection is predominant for any particular disease."

The gist of the report was simply that knowledge was not yet sufficient to warrant installation of ultraviolet irradiation or disinfectant vapor dispensers in schools, barracks, or other places of public congregation. During the next 15 years extensive research was carried out that led to a far greater understanding of the mode of spread of contagious diseases. This included:

1. The creation, behavior, and measurement of aerosols of pathogenic agents.
2. The physiology of the respiratory tract, particularly the deposition and retention of aerosol particles of varying size through the respiratory tract.
3. Experimental airborne infection in animals and man with a variety of pathogens.
4. The epidemiology of naturally occurring and laboratory acquired infections.

All of this provided the stuff on which a substantive theory of airborne infection could be based. As a result, the rapid advance of progress led to the sponsorship by the National Academy of Sciences of a large conference held in Miami in December 1960[6] that provides a substantive base of information of the status of knowledge of airborne infections to that date.

A large number of human diseases had become generally recognized as airborne. These included: psittacosis, Q fever, brucellosis, the pneumonic forms of tularemia and plague, the pulmonary mycoses, inhalation anthrax, and particularly, primary pulmonary tuberculosis. Each of these diseases was recognized as having its own unique pathogenesis, immunology and epidemiology.

Interestingly, smallpox and rubella do not appear in the index of the proceedings of this conference. Measles is discussed briefly by Dr. Riley in a paper primarily devoted to his brilliant studies with Wells on airborne tuberculous infection in the Baltimore Veterans Hospital. Clearly, the organizers of the conference, and I was one of them, did not consider these three diseases as airborne infections. The views of Chapin were still dominant. Perkins, Wells, and Riley were notable and far-sighted dissenters from this majority view.

Herd Immunity

Herd immunity is a concept that has evolved over the past half century or longer. It has its roots both in theoretical analysis and practical experience.

Hamer, in 1907 in London, stated the broad outline clearly. The basic concept assumes spread by contact. Each individual in a population has a certain probability, or contact rate, of making effective contact sufficient to spread a contagious disease, were he infected, with a limited number of other individuals in the population within a given time period. The contact rate will vary with crowding, the degree of intermixing, the infectiousness of the agent, with season, and other environmental factors.

The number of new cases that any particular case will cause within the next incubation period will be a direct function of the proportion of susceptibles in the population. For those contagious diseases that have existed for long periods of time, obviously some fluctuating ecological balance has been achieved known as the balance of immunes and susceptibles. This concept of Hamer has been expressed mathematically by Soper and Greenwood in London, by Reed and Frost at Johns Hopkins, and extended by E. B. Wilson at Harvard.[7]

Intrinsic to this theoretical approach to herd immunity is the assumption that a threshold of immunity exists above which the infection cannot be sustained. One new case encounters such a proportion of immunes and so few susceptibles that on the average it gives rise to less than one new case. Incidence thus declines to a very low level or extinction until the accretion of new births increases the number of susceptibles to the point where epidemic spread can recur.

Although the concepts of epidemic theory can be generalized without limit, the mathematical expressions of the theory had to be extremely simplified in order to be workable for the average student. A key assumption was that contagious diseases were spread by contact, that the contact rate of each case or carrier was reasonably constant under any given set of conditions, and that the major factors leading to variation in epidemic patterns were determined by environmental circumstances, particularly crowding, and by the proportion of susceptibles in the population. The studies of Chapin and many others of the high secondary attack rates among susceptible household contacts of many contagious diseases, particularly measles, supported these views. The Epidemic Theory, as expounded in the 1930s and 40s, left no room for airborne infection and ignored the concept of the occurrence of the occasional dangerous carrier or "super-spreader" that is now clearly recognized in many diseases.

Godfrey[9] applied the principle of herd immunity in New York State in the early 1930s during an intensive diphtheria immunization campaign. He set the goal based on past observation of 35 percent immunization of preschool children. He claimed that this threshold would prevent a diphtheria epidemic. He was notably successful in spite of the fact that he was also keenly aware that mild nasal cases of diphtheria were classic dangerous spreaders.

A classic demonstration is the study of Hedrich (FIGURE 1) in Baltimore.[10] He counted the monthly incidence of measles, corrected for under reporting, and matched his figures with new births. From these simple sums he could estimate the proportion of the population under 15 years of age susceptible to measles. The epidemics of measles are shown in the bottom line, and the fluctuating level of susceptibles on the upper line. Note that the proportion of susceptibles varied within the range of 30 to 50 percent.

A practical extension of such data, that appealed to me through most of my career, was the simplistic notion that were one able to raise the level of immunity by artificial means well above the threshold where epidemics can occur, then epidemics could be prevented. Measles could no longer survive. If the immunity were steadily maintained at such a high level, no measles epidemic could arise. An introduction from outside would possibly lead to a sputtering outbreak for a few generations but an epidemic could not ensue. Intrinsic in my personal thinking was the mistaken belief that once measles was eliminated from a community its reintroduction and beginning spread would lead to a spontaneous community response to immunize all susceptibles in the immediate vicinity and thus promptly snuff out the disease. This community reaction I call "the typical smallpox reaction." In practice, this did not occur. Instead there was to me an amazing apathy on the part of both citizens and health authorities rather than alert "fire fighting." Changing this apathy to prompt response when measles occurs is essential if the disease is to be eradicated.

Smallpox

In spite of the availability of Jennerian vaccination for almost 200 years, large areas of the world remained plagued with smallpox. In 1965 this scourge was

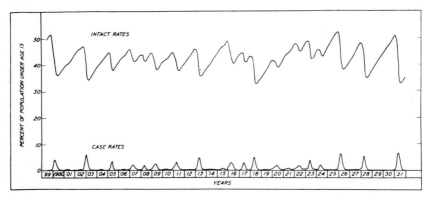

FIGURE 1. Estimated complete monthly attack rate from measles and intact ratios (proportions not previously attacked) for the population under age 15, Old Baltimore, Maryland, July, 1899 to December, 1931. (From Hedrich.[10])

endemic in Brazil, in Subsahara Africa, in South Asia, and Indonesia. Beginning first in 1959 on a small scale and then in 1965 on a grand scale, the World Health Organization mounted a program for the global eradication of smallpox. A ten year goal was set. The plan was to stress mass vaccination using newly improved freeze-dried stable vaccine, and modern methods of immunization, first the jet injector gun, and soon thereafter the simple bifurcated needle. From the beginning, the program incorporated a continuing surveillance, field investigation of outbreaks, and constant evaluation of results.

Faith in the broad applicability of mass immunization was high. The mode of spread of infection was confidently believed to be face-to-face contact. The program began with enthusiasm and progress seemed good, but thanks to the constant surveillance it was soon learned that in some areas residual outbreaks smouldered among small isolated enclaves of persons who opposed vaccination on religious or other grounds, and who maintained close contacts with each other often over some distances. Such smouldering outbreaks continued even when immune levels of the area were high. Conversely when vaccine supplies were temporarily short and conservation was forced on the workers, the containment of outbreaks was stressed by intensive case finding, contact tracing, and ring vaccination. These efforts were conspicuously successful even in areas where immunization levels were low.[11] Repeated experiences of these types led to a major reemphasis of approach with conspicuous success.

During the course of this program, a truly remarkable and profoundly disturbing event took place.[12] On December 31, 1969 a 20-year-old German electrician flew from Karachi to his home in Meschede, Germany. Ten days later he was admitted to a small general hospital with fever. Because he was known to be convalescing from hepatitis and was suspected of having typhoid fever he was placed in a separate room in the isolation wing of the hospital under the sole care of two trained nursing sisters. Strict isolation techniques were enforced.

On January 14, his fourth hospital day, he developed a rash. On January 15, smallpox was suspected; on January 16 this diagnosis was confirmed and the patient was transferred in a special plastic bag, to prevent cross infection, to a smallpox hospital.

From January 22 to 31, a total of 17 cases of smallpox with three deaths developed among 13 patients, 3 nurses, and one visitor. These cases were distributed equally on three floors of the hospital, their onsets all fell within a spread of a single incubation period assuming exposure between the 13th and the 16th of January.

A smoke generator placed in the patient's room revealed air current patterns of spread both out of the door of his room up a stairway well to the other floors as well as out of his window and upwards in a flat band of warm air into the windows above his room.

It is difficult to explain this outbreak by any mode of spread other than the airborne route. Interestingly and no doubt significantly, the patient had lesions within his mouth and was described as "coughing frequently," a somewhat unusual symptom of smallpox but one that might well have produced infectious aerosols.

This epidemic occurring at the very middle of the ten year eradication program cast serious doubt on the theoretical soundness of the whole program. If airborne infection from a single case could produce 17 cases among noncontacts at the far corners of a hospital building, how could a program based on the theory of face-to-face contact spread succeed?

Fortunately those in charge of the program persisted in the faith that their previous five years of experience had been successful and that the Meschede incident must have been a truly exceptional event, as indeed it turned out to be.

The rest of the smallpox story is familiar to all. Surveillance was conducted and containment was applied with devotion and intensity to Indonesia and progressively to the countries of South Asia. The last case of variola major occured in Bangladesh in October 1975, and the eradication of variola minor from the horn of Africa followed soon thereafter.

Thus the brilliant success of global eradication of smallpox vindicated Chapin's view of the predominant importance of face-to-face contact in the spread of the disease but, at the same time, cast grave doubt on practical validity of the concept of herd immunity. Furthermore, it established the existence but extreme rarity of airborne infection and of the dangerous spreader in this specific infection.

Measles

With the isolation of the measles virus by Enders in the mid 1950s it was widely recognized that within a short time an effective vaccine could become available.[13] The first commercial vaccine required concurrent injections of a small amount of gamma globulin to modify the reactions of the partially attenuated Edmonston B strain. This was a procedure sufficiently expensive and cumbersome to be applicable in private pediatricians' offices but not as a general public health practice. With the development of the further attenuated strain of measles vaccine virus a national campaign for measles eradication was launched. The Center for Disease Control (CDC) led in mounting the program with a formal paper at the American Public Health Association annual meeting in Miami in the fall of 1966. Two colleagues and I wrote the "official statement" which outlined in detail unqualified statements about the epidemiology of measles and made an unqualified prediction. My third position in the authorship of this paper did not adequately reflect my contribution to the work.[14] I will make but two quotes:

1. "The infection spreads by direct contact from person to person, and by the airborne route among susceptibles congregated in enclosed spaces." (Obviously the ideas of Perkins and Wells had penetrated my consciousness but not sufficiently to influence my judgment). 2. "Effective use of (measles) vaccines during the coming winter and spring should insure the eradication of measles from the United States in 1967." Such was my faith in the broad acceptance of the vaccine by the public and the health professions and in the infallibility of herd immunity.

The results of this prediction are well known. The reported incidence of the disease dropped from a level of 400,000-500,000 cases a year during 1960-1964, to 250,000 in 1965 and 200,000 in 1966. This clearly reflected the use of the early-type vaccines in private practice. Incidence further dropped to 50,000 in 1967 and to 25,000 in 1968 but since then has continued a fluctuating course.[15] The variability can be related to the degree of the total national effort, and the availability of federal funds to defray vaccine costs. Eradication remains elusive although intensification of effort during the past 12 months appears to have brought incidence to a lower point, near 12,000 cases.

There are many reasons and explanations for this rather egregious blunder in prediction. The simple truth is that the prediction was based on confidence in the Reed-Frost epidemic theory, in the applicability of herd immunity on a general basis, and that measles cases were uniformly infectious. I am sure I extended the teachings of my preceptors beyond the limits that they had intended during my student days.

In the relentless light of the well-focussed retrospectiscope, the real failure was our neglect of conducting continuous and sufficiently sophisticated epidemiological field studies of measles. We accepted the doctrines imbued into us as students without maintaining the eternal skepticism of the true scientist. This blithe overconfidence is now slowly changing. Many intensive epidemiological studies of the residual measles problem have been revealing and they show the following useful facts:[15]

1. Vaccine failures have occurred but constitute but a trivial factor. Measles vaccines now in use are safe and effective and seem to confer truly lasting immunity.

2. Unimmunized population groups notably preschool children in the inner city and neglected rural areas have been main foci of continuing cases.
3. A progressive shift in age incidence of cases has been observed. Formerly measles peaked in the three- to six-years-of-age group. In 1976 the highest attack rate occurred in the 10–14 year age group, followed by high incidences among junior high and high school students as well as military recruits.

As the years pass we can confidently expect more cases in adults over 20. Sharp outbreaks of short duration, one or two incubation periods, pick out the few remaining susceptibles in a large group of immunes. By classical theory this implies an astronomical contact rate. Clearly we must revise our theory and recognize that these outbreaks must be airborne in character involving exposure to aerosols presumably created by the rare super-spreader who contaminates a large populated enclosed space such as a school auditorium or gymnasium. These have happened sufficiently often to prove the far sightedness of Perkins and Wells when the rest of us were smugly secure in our epidemic theories, our traditional faith in contact infection and herd immunity.

It is far from clear to me yet whether measles is solely an airborne infection, as I think Wells believed, or whether contact and airborne routes both play roles in different circumstances. It is clear however that airborne infection is sufficiently common and important to be a determining factor in the continuance of measles at the present time. It must receive due respect and weight in planning the future steps necessary for eradication.

Rubella

The rubella program was undertaken not for the control of the disease itself but to reduce, if not eliminate, the occurrence of congenital rubella syndrome in babies born to mothers infected during pregnancy. It was not deemed safe to immunize all women or even women at the time of marriage because of fear of possible damage to the fetus from the live virus in the vaccine.

Therefore by direct analogy with measles, one of the most dangerous traits of epidemiologists, the program in this country stressed immunization of children from 1 to 12 years of age on the assumptions that rubella spreads primarily through schools by person-to-person contact, that herd immunity would apply, and that adults became infected from their children coming home from school.[16] The critical evidence to support these assumptions was nonexistent. Almost no simple descriptive epidemiological studies of rubella had been reported. In fact, the more recent studies of Schoenbaum et al.[17] contradicted this view. They showed that infection rates in primiparas were as high or higher than multiparas suggesting that women who were out of the home in jobs, travelling on public transport, etc., were more likely to acquire rubella than mothers at home with their families. At any rate, a national program of rubella immunization of children was launched and continues.

Actually the epidemiology of rubella is but poorly understood. Reporting is poor and inconstant and hard to improve. Trends must be interpreted with caution. Infection occurs largely in childhood but for some as yet unknown reason, a higher proportion of adults remain susceptible to rubella than to other contagious diseases. This disease is widely endemic at a low level of incidence but again quite inexplicably epidemics, one might even say pandemics of great intensity and amazingly short duration, occur from time to time, as in 1935, 1943, 1963–64. There is hope on a very flimsy foundation that the childhood immunization program will prevent future massive epidemics with their accompanying thousands of cases of congenital rubella syndrome, but the epidemiology of the disease is not sufficiently understood to make such a conclusion confident.

At the root of this insecurity is the slowly developing recognition that rubella is probably primarily an airborne infection. The basis for this statement is the reappraisal of the known epidemiology plus recent experience.

Epidemics of rubella occurring in the English so-called "public" schools[18] were extraordinarily explosive with high attack rates. Some lasted no more than three incubation period generations, indicating exhaustion of susceptibles. By classical Reed Frost Epidemic Theory, the contact rates to account for such epidemics would be even more astronomical than those mentioned previously

TABLE 1

GERMAN MEASLES ADMISSIONS FROM FIELD ARTILLERY REPLACEMENT TRAINING CENTER, FORT BRAGG, N.C.—DISTRIBUTION OF BATTERIES ACCORDING TO NUMBERS OF CASES OBSERVED AND EXPECTED*, MARCH–APRIL, 1943

| | Number of Batteries | |
Cases per Battery	Observed	Expected
0–1	—	.01
2–3	3	1.71
4–5	7	5.67
6–7	7	8.78
8–9	6	7.78
10–11	4	4.47
12–13	—	1.80
14–15	4	.50
16+	—	.12
Total	31	31.0

*Calculated from Poisson exponential, 237 cases among 31 × 250 men, attack rate equals 3.06 percent.

for recent measles epidemics. Such rates are not compatible with the concept of direct face-to-face contact. Therefore, again looking through the retrospectiscope, airborne spread must have dominated.

In 1943 at Fort Bragg, N.C., I had the opportunity to study a large epidemic of rubella as a side issue, a hobby of my main responsibility. A wave of the disease moved through a large replacement training center in a two month period centering in March of 1943. Data was readily available by training batteries (250 men each). There were 31 such batteries in training during the rubella wave. A distribution of batteries by numbers of cases in each is shown in TABLE 1 along with the expected number as calculated by Poisson Exponential. There is no deviation from randomness. The interpretation of such finding rather disturbed me at the time. In my notes is the comment: "Difficult to account for such a distribution on the basis of contact person-to-person spread. Only logical explanation would be random distribution of susceptibles with exhaustion at the end of epidemic. Airborne infection?"

The concepts of exhaustion of susceptibles, let alone of airborne infection, were too radical for a young Hopkins-trained epidemiologist to contemplate further at that time. In fact I wonder whether a manuscript reporting this epidemic with such a conclusion would have been accepted by an accredited epidemiological journal. Hence the data have lain dormant. Now, however, the studies of Horstmann at Fort Ord,[19] of Evans, Niederman, et al. at Yale,[20] and any of several issues of the Morbidity-Mortality Weekly Report during any recent year report rubella epidemics that seem to me can be accounted for only on the basis of airborne infection.

CONCLUSION

In conclusion, a review of three modern large scale control programs against smallpox, measles, and rubella have revealed deep insights into the relative roles of contact and airborne infection in natural settings and forced upon most of us, reconsideration of our long held and fondly cherished views of contact and airborne infection, epidemic theory, the balance of immunes and susceptibles and its corollary, the doctrine of herd immunity.

The smallpox success reaffirms the long held view that the mode of spread is by close face-to-face contact. Although airborne spread has been documented, it is so rare that global eradication based on the contact hypothesis succeeded. The doctrine of herd immunity was inconstant.

The measles eradication program faltered at least in part from our confidence in contact being the predominant mode of spread and herd immunity being the accepted doctrine. Clearly measles can often be airborne, how often is still to be appraised. It must be given far more respect and attention if effective means of eradication are to be developed.

Rubella remains a constant worry. The validity of the theory justifying the present program, namely immunizing children, both boys and girls, has seemed to some of us to be tenuous. The alternate program, as followed in Britain, of immunizing adolescent girls, and thus interfering to a minimal degree in the normal ecological balance, has simplicity and a certain elemental logic; but unless essentially 100 percent of adolescent girls are given a vaccine with duration of effectiveness of 30 years or more, one wonders what this program will achieve and how long it will take to eliminate Congenital Rubella Syndrome, if ever.

I have a lurking fear that Congenital Rubella Syndrome will continue to occur and may appear again in truly epidemic proportions sooner or later. Alertness to its occurrence in pregnant women and the prompt availability of abortions for those willing to accept this procedure should greatly reduce but cannot eliminate the problem.

More intensive, imaginative, critical and continuous epidemiological field studies, surveillance and investigations will be necessary for both measles and rubella if solutions are to be found. Furthermore, the epidemiologists of the future should clearly practice their profession with a greater humility and skepticism of their past teachings than some, at least one, epidemiologist of my close personal acquaintance.

REFERENCES

1. CHAPIN, C. V. 1912. Sources and Modes of Infection. 2nd Edit. John Wiley and Sons. New York.

2. WELLS, W. F. 1948. Sanitary ventilation. Am. J. Public Health **38**: 775–780.
3. PERKINS, J. W., A. M. BAHLKE, & H. SILVERMAN. 1947. Effect of ultraviolet irradiation of classrooms on spread of measles in large central schools. Am. J. Public Health **37**: 529–537.
4. ROBERTSON, O. H. 1943. Air-borne infection. Science **97**: 495–502.
5. Subcommittee for the Evaluation of Methods of Control Airborne Infections. 1947. Present status of the control of airborne infections. Am. J. Public Health **37**: 13–22.
6. Conference on Airborne Infection. Dec. 7–10, 1960. Division of Medical Sciences. National Academy of Sciences, Miami Beach, Florida. Bacteriol. Rev. 1961. **25**: 173–382.
7. SARTWELL, P. E. 1976. Memoir on the Reed-Frost epidemic theory. Am. J. Epidemiol **103**: 138–140.
8. FOX, J. P., L. ELVEBACK et al. 1971. Herd immunity: Basic concept and relevance to public health immunization practices. Am. J. Epidemiol **94**: 179–189.
9. GODFREY, E. S. 1933. Practical uses of diphtheria immunization records. Am. J. Public Health **23**: 809–812.
10. HEDRICH, A. W. 1933. Monthly estimates of the child population "susceptible" to measles, 1900–1931, Baltimore, Maryland. Am. J. Hygiene **17**: 613–636.
11. FOEGE, W. H., J. D. MILLAR & D. A. HENDERSON. 1975. Smallpox eradication in West and Central Africa. Bull. World Health Organization **52**: 209–222.
12. WEHRLE, P. F., J. POSCH, K. H. RICHTER & D. A. HENDERSON. 1970. An airborne outbreak of smallpox in a German hospital and its significance with respect to other recent outbreaks in Europe. Bull. World Health Organization **43**: 669–679.
13. Symposium on Live Measles Virus Vaccine. 1962. Recent Clinical, Laboratory and Epidemiologic Findings. Am. J. Public Health Part 2 **52**: 1–64.
14. SENCER, D. J., H. B. DULL & A. D. LANGMUIR. 1967. Epidemiologic basis for eradication of measles. Public Health Reports **82**: 253–256.
15. CONRAD, J. L., R. WALLACE & J. J. WITTE. 1971. The epidemiologic rationale for the failure to eradicate measles in the United States. Am. J. Public Health **61**: 2304–2310.
16. Proceedings of the International Conference on Rubella Immunization. 1969. Amer. J. Dis. Child. **118**: 1–410.
17. SCHOENBAUM, S. C., S. BIANO & T. MACK. 1975. Epidemiology of congenital rubella syndrome. The role of maternal parity. J. Am. Med. Assoc. **233**: 151–155.
18. Medical Research Council. 1938. Special Report No 227: Epidemics in Schools H.M. Stationery Office. London.
19. HORSTMANN, D. M. 1971. Rubella: the challenge of its control. J. Infect. Dis. **123**: 640–654.
20. EVANS, A. S., J. C. NIEDERMAN et al. 1971. Prospective studies of a group of Yale University freshmen. II The occurrence of acute respiratory infections and rubella. J. Infect. Dis. **123**: 271–278.

THE EPIDEMIOLOGY OF INFLUENZA IN HUMANS

Michael B. Gregg

Bureau of Epidemiology
Center for Disease Control
Atlanta, Georgia 30333

The epidemiology of influenza infection has been extensively studied—particularly since 1933, when the virus was first isolated. In this presentation I will summarize briefly what has been observed and concluded to be true about its epidemiology, touch upon a few of the more perplexing aspects of the spread of influenza, and then recount some unusual epidemics, particularly a recent extraordinary influenza outbreak that may shed some light on the still unanswered questions concerning the transmission of influenza.*

Although influenza remains one of the major uncontrollable epidemic communicable diseases still affecting the world, our measurements of its extent and impact are imprecise and often indirect. Reporting of influenza cases in the United States is not required because the illness can be difficult to diagnose, and many who are sick do not seek medical care. Virus isolation or serologic test results can often confirm the diagnosis, but neither patient nor physician materially benefits from such information. Therefore, health officials and epidemiologists have relied upon either unique, specialized, community-based studies from which broad conclusions are applied regionwide or countrywide or upon indirect assessments of influenza-related mortality as indicators of the frequency and distribution of influenza A.[1] Despite these limitations, yearly and secular trends of the illness do reflect the overall character and distribution of influenza infection.

In general, influenza occurs in three relatively distinct epidemiologic forms: 1. worldwide pandemics, 2. regional or nationwide epidemics, and 3. local, sporadic outbreaks.[2] Worldwide or pandemic influenza appeared in 1889, 1917–18, 1957–58, and 1968–69, usually coincident with major antigenic changes in the influenza virus. Such epidemics may begin at any time, extend for many months, affect 20% to 40% of the population, and seem to arise from a single focus of infection which often can be followed within countries and from continent to continent. Larger regional or nationwide epidemics have occurred fairly regularly every two to three years during winter months, have affected perhaps 5% to 10% of the population, have usually been associated with minor antigenic changes in the virus, and have appeared nearly simultaneously in communities throughout large regions of the country. In the United States and elsewhere, sharply localized, sporadic outbreaks occur nearly every respiratory season and affect small, separate, and discrete populations. Characteristic of all three epidemic forms of influenza are their short-lived duration in the community—they usually last two to four weeks or eight to ten weeks for the entire United States during interpandemic times—and the remarkable similarity of disease from epidemic to epidemic.

---

*This discussion will cover influenza A infection only. Influenza due to type B influenza virus occurs much less often, impacts less on the public's health, and possesses different epidemiologic characteristics. Infection from influenza virus type C is very rare: its public health importance is negligible.

0077-8923/80/0353-0045 $01.75/0 © 1980, NYAS

Influenza is primarily a disease of children, affecting predominantly the 5- to 15-year-old age group. However, age-specific attack rates vary considerably from epidemic to epidemic and probably depend in large part on previous exposure to closely related viruses. Virtually no age group is totally spared. In localized or closed community-type settings morbidity may be very high, affecting 40% to 50% or more of the population,[3,4] and when major epidemics appear, excess mortality is a predictable result of influenza A infection.[5] The influenza virus resides in the respiratory tract of humans and can be cultured from respiratory secretions for up to five to seven days after onset of febrile illness.

Transmission of influenza virus has been generally accepted to occur predominantly from person-to-person by direct contact with virus-laden respiratory secretions, either by physical contact or by droplets spread from coughing or sneezing. Multiple observations of naturally occurring infection and experimentally produced disease have established an incubation period of one to three days.[6]

However accepted and true the foregoing statements may be, some fundamental aspects of the epidemiology of influenza remain obscure and controversial. Such broad questions as why the virus changes, where it resides during nonepidemic times, and what specific forces direct the appearance and disappearance of epidemics still challenge virologists and epidemiologists alike.[7] Moreover, at the most basic community, school, or family level of observation, even the simple dynamics of virus introduction, appearance, dissemination, and particularly transmission vary from epidemic to epidemic, locale to locale, seemingly unmindful of traditional infectious disease behavioral patterns. As Stuart-Harris so aptly put it, "The simple view that epidemics result from a breakdown of community resistance to infection may appear applicable to a disease such as measles whose virus appears to be antigenically stable. But when the virus varies so widely, as does influenza virus A, other explanations need to be considered."[8] Certainly implied is the fact that both the human host and the environment also play key but still ill-defined roles.

For instance, during the pandemics of 1957–58 and 1968–69, multiple documented introductions of infection into communities and families failed to produce further community spread until weeks or months later when entire communities then became rapidly involved.[9,10] This so-called "seeding" of viruses may actually reflect person-to-person transmission of undetectable virus without clinical disease until some as-yet-unknown fortuitous environmental or host factors trigger the appearance of influenza throughout the community.[11] Equally perplexing during interpandemic occurrence of influenza are the community-wide epidemics that erupt simultaneously throughout large geographic regions without obvious earlier introductions of virus or other measurable environmental events, again suggesting previous widespread dissemination of virus without clinical disease or evidence of virus carriage.[12-14]

Frequent observations have documented the importance of children in the early recognition and widespread dissemination of influenza viruses within the community, and particularly in the introduction of infection into the family.[11,15] However, this is not invariably true, and even more important, as illustrated by Hope-Simpson, in some epidemics the household does not appear to be an important setting for influenza spread nor do all susceptibles become ill.[16,17] Cases that do occur within the family may have been more likely acquired in the community rather than from other family members, as judged by prolonged incubation periods between index and subsequent cases. Some observers have even interpreted these data to mean that longer incubation periods of five to seven days for different family members reflect nasal contact with the virus rather than lower respiratory tract invasion.[18]

Nevertheless, repeated observations of influenza epidemics, particularly in the military, in schools, or in other closed populations, have led to the firm conclusion that increasing the density of the population, or overcrowding, materially increases attack rates—to levels well above 50% and 60% in certain instances.[4,19] Often coincident with these high attack rates are extraordinarily rapid increases in the number of cases spanning very short periods of time followed by subsequent rapid decreases. Transmission presumably occurs more readily in these settings because of closer and more frequent person-to-person contact. However, several reports have shown that in the "closed" family unit, a larger family unit does not necessarily have increased attack rates.[18] Moreover,

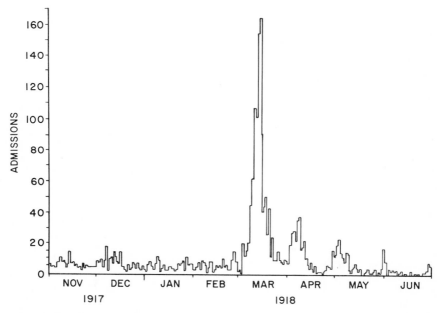

FIGURE 1. Admissions to base hospital for influenza by day, Camp Funston, Kansas, November 1, 1917 to July 1, 1918. (From Opie et al.[20])

not all susceptibles in other closed populations experience these explosive outbreaks regularly during influenza epidemics. It is these kinds of outbreaks that I wish to call your attention to, not only as examples of the variability of influenza occurrence, but as examples of modes of spread possibly different from the classically accepted person-to-person transmission of influenza.

The first example comes from the extensive studies of Opie et al. concerning the etiology of pneumonia in the Army at Camp Funston, Kansas, in late 1917 and early 1918.[20] In early March 1918 a "disease which has been diagnosed as influenza ... within a few days swept as a great epidemic through Camp Funston." Soldiers had temperatures of 99° to 102° or 103°F and complained of severe headache and myalgias. Few patients had coryza, and cough was unusual.

In most cases after 24–48 hours temperatures fell and improvement was noted. A total of 1,127 men from Camp Funston (which contained 29,000) were hospitalized for influenza between March 4 and March 29, 1918 (FIGURE 1). Many more were seen at the infirmaries of the camp. The truly remarkable features of this epidemic were its explosive onset and rapid disappearance, spanning slightly more than three weeks. While person-to-person spread certainly must have played a role in the transmission of the virus, the multiple contacts necessary to disseminate infection so rapidly are somewhat hard to imagine.

In 1943, again in the military, a sudden epidemic of influenza occurred at Pope Field, Fort Bragg, North Carolina, among Army glider mechanics. On November 27, 1943, 13 soldiers with acute respiratory disease were hospitalized.[21] Serologic test results confirmed influenza A in 12. Eleven men were members of a temporary detachment of 146 glider mechanics who had arrived early that morning by train from a camp in Kentucky. All 146 men were confined to two barracks designed for 63 men each. Within a week 38 more men were hospitalized for influenza (FIGURE 2), for a total attack rate of 35%. By contrast, an epidemic of influenza also occurred among men at the 92nd Air Base who were housed in barracks adjacent to the mechanics' barracks but the groups had no contact. The epidemic also shown on FIGURE 2 occurred among 650 men, extended over a month, involved only 5% of the men, and was quite comparable with other epidemics observed among many other units at Fort Bragg during that influenza epidemic. The apparent explosiveness of the outbreak among glider mechanics resulted in part from an accumulation of cases spanning several days while men were enroute to Pope Field and in part possibly from early hospitalization. However, as the Commission on Respiratory Diseases reported, "It is doubtful . . . that such a high attack rate . . . can be wholly accounted for on this basis."[21] Rather, it was asserted, more likely crowding aboard the train and in the barracks plus a week of quarantine "presented an unusually favorable opportunity for the dissemination of virus." Again, person-to-person transmission must have played an important role, but it does not explain why this group of men was uniquely affected relative to other units during that winter influenza season. Were there highly efficient shedders or spreaders of the virus, was the seeding phenomenon playing a role, were the viruses different, or could the virus have been disseminated in aerosols?

Probably the most remarkable documented outbreak of influenza that suggests transmission other than the classic person-to-person mode is that of an epidemic of influenza among passengers and crew of commercial jet airliner which Moser, Bender et al. investigated in 1977.[22] While many details of this epidemic were presented in their recent paper, many will be emphasized here, and further information will be added to complete the description.[24]

On Monday, March 14, 1977, a Boeing 737 began its scheduled flight from Anchorage to Homer and then to Kodiak, Alaska, carrying 5 crew and 24 passengers. The aircraft had a large cargo space in the front of the plane and seats for 56 passengers in the rear (FIGURE 3). After landing in Homer, 6 persons deplaned and 31 additional passengers boarded the aircraft, for a total of 49 passengers. During the takeoff to Kodiak, the jet's left engine failed, and there was a 4½ hour delay at the Homer airport. Subsequently, a second plane took most of the passengers to Kodiak, returned to Homer, and carried 15 remaining passengers and 5 crew back to Anchorage. Monday night, a third aircraft flew the 15 passengers directly to Kodiak. On Tuesday, 7 passengers in Kodiak had sudden onset of fever, headache, chills, myalgia, and severe nonproductive

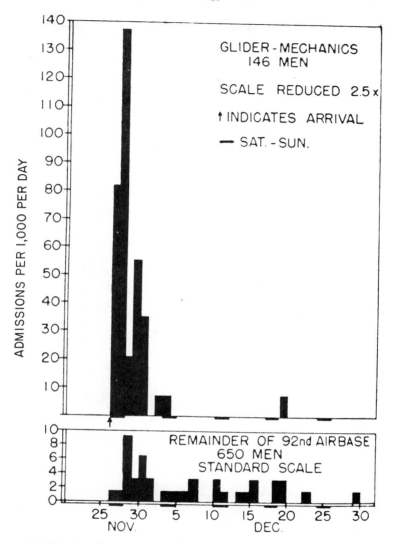

FIGURE 2. Epidemic influenza A at the 92nd Air Base, United States Air Force, 1943. (From the Commission on Acute Respiratory Diseases.[21])

cough. Two crew members were hospitalized in Anchorage with similar symptoms 60 hours after the flight. Ultimately, investigation revealed that of the 53 passengers and crew on the disabled jet, 37 (72%) became ill with typical flu-like signs and symptoms (FIGURE 4). Twenty of 22 patients had a fourfold or greater rise to A/Texas/1/77. Eight of 31 patients for whom cultures were done were positive for influenza. A virus similar to the A/Texas strain. The extraordinary

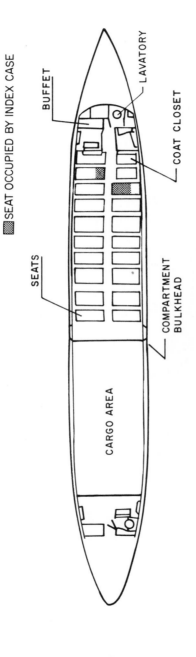

SEAT OCCUPIED BY INDEX CASE

BUFFET

LAVATORY

COAT CLOSET

SEATS

COMPARTMENT
BULKHEAD

CARGO AREA

OVERHEAD VIEW

FIGURE 3. Schematic of a Boeing 737 aircraft.

explosiveness of the outbreak suggested a common source of exposure, and the following facts were uncovered.

Among the 31 who boarded the 737 in Homer on Monday was a 21-year-old woman who became acutely ill with fever, chills, and a severe cough 15 minutes after boarding the plane. During the attempted takeoff she sat in the rear of the plane, and for the remaining 4½-hour delay, she lay across two seats coughing, too ill to move about or to leave the plane (FIGURE 3). She later boarded the second plane to Kodiak. She was seen by the investigators on Wednesday, still suffering from severe spasms of coughing described by one of the physicians as dry and brassy. Her acute- and convalescent-phase sera later showed an eightfold rise to A/Texas influenza virus.

Twenty-nine other passengers also remained on board the 737 during the entire 4½-hour delay in Homer, and 23 others left and boarded the jet periodical-

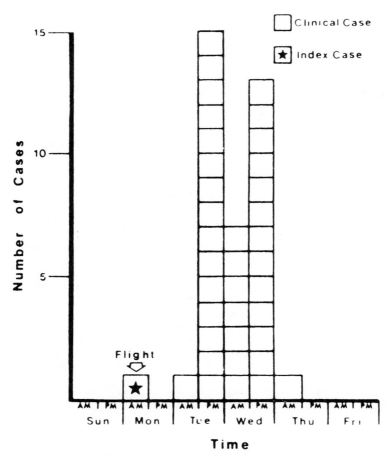

FIGURE 4. Onset of clinical influenza among 37 persons following exposure to an index case aboard a delayed airliner, Homer, Alaska, March 1977. (From Moser et al.[22])

ly. The passengers moved freely about the cabin; some visited the cockpit at the crew's invitation, although there was no reported direct contact between passengers or crew and the ill woman. Furthermore, following the engine failure, the main air ventilation system of the airplane was turned off for two to three hours, and even though the front cargo door and rear passenger doors were open, most passengers considered the air comfortable or warm and stale. Eventually, the auxiliary power unit was turned on to supply and move air normally.

Epidemiologic analysis showed increased attack rates for passengers who remained longest in the 737 cabin. Moreover, attack rates were higher for passengers seated five or fewer rows from the ill woman than for those located six or more rows distant—76% versus 50%—although the difference is not statistically significant.

The situation in which this epidemic occurred is remarkably suggestive of a common-source outbreak of airborne influenza infection. Within 83 hours after being exposed to a person with documented influenza, 37 of 52 persons became ill with typical symptoms of influenza well documented by virus isolation and serologic results. Placed in a poorly ventilated, enclosed cabin of 800 cubic feet for up to 4½ hours, the passengers and crew were in close but generally indirect contact with an acutely ill adult with a severe, persistent, dry, brassy cough. For two to three hours no fresh air was actively circulating throughout the cabin, and probably the only significant air movement was that produced by passengers walking up and down the aisle excluding, of course, the index case, who remained lying down nearly the entire 4½ hours. Although virus-infected droplets from the index case may have spread disease to some passengers, her location and lack of direct contact with others minimize the likelihood of traditional person-to-person transmission. Furthermore, the explosiveness of the epidemic and its high attack rate coupled with a cough characteristic of producing aerosols strongly suggest airborne spread of influenza aboard the 737.

Many other reports in the literature document the very rapid buildup of cases of influenza in closed or semiclosed populations. The assumption has been that most, if not all, infection was transmitted from person to person in the traditional contact sense. True airborne transmission via droplet nuclei has rarely been mentioned, and more importantly, the necessary, painstaking, meticulous reconstruction of events surrounding influenza outbreaks has seldom if ever been applied in an effort to discover how infection was transmitted.

As R.E.O. Williams wrote, "The epidemiological method is at its most convincing in unraveling the spread of diseases in which many persons are infected from a common source, or where infections occur through contact with particular vectors and this contact can be decisively interrupted . . . (however) when individuals are in the position to infect one another through small airborne droplet nuclei, they are usually also able to transmit large droplets. . . ."[23] Surely, this is the case with influenza. However, the outbreak associated with the 737 jet and other epidemics in closed or semiclosed populations suggest that true airborne transmission of influenza appears likely and clearly merits greater investigative attention in the future.

ACKNOWLEDGMENTS

The author gratefully acknowledges Dr. Alexander D. Langmuir for his advice and suggestions and Drs. Michael R. Moser, Thomas R. Bender, and

Harold S. Margolis who provided further information on the outbreak of influenza aboard the 737 jetliner.

REFERENCES

1. DOWDLE, W. R., M. T. COLEMAN & M. B. GREGG. 1974. Natural history of influenza type A in the United States, 1957–1972. Progr. Med. Virol. **17:** 91–135.
2. LANGMUIR, A. D. 1971. Influenza: Its epidemiology. Hospital Practice Sept.: 103–108.
3. STALLONES, R. A. & E. H. LENNETTE. 1959. Epidemiologic observations of an outbreak of Asian-strain influenza in a closed population. Am. J. Public Health **49:** 656–667.
4. BELL, J. A., J. E. CRAIGHEAD, R. G. JAMES & D. WONG. 1961. Epidemiologic observations on two outbreaks of Asian influenza in a children's institution. Am. J. Hyg. **73:** 84–89.
5. ASSAAD, F., W. C. COCKBURN & T. K. SUNDARESAN. 1973. Use of excess mortality from respiratory diseases in the study of influenza. Bull. WHO **49:** 219–233.
6. FRANCIS, T., JR., J. E. SALK, H. E. PEARSON & P. N. BROWN. 1945. Protective effect of vaccination against induced influenza A. J. Clin. Invest. **24:** 536–546.
7. KILBOURNE, E. D. 1970. Influenza 1970: Unquestioned answers and unanswered questions. Arch. Environ. Health **21:** 286–292.
8. STUART-HARRIS, C. 1979. Epidemiology of influenza in man. Br. Med. Bull. **35(1):** 3–8.
9. ANDREWS, C. H. 1959. Asian influenza: A challenge to epidemiology. In Perspectives in Virology. Morris Pollard, Ed.: 184–196. John Wiley & Sons. New York, N.Y.
10. SHARRAR, R. G. 1969. National influenza experience in the USA, 1968–69. Bull. WHO **41:** 361–366.
11. JORDAN, W. S., JR. 1961. The mechanism of spread of Asian influenza. Am. Rev. Respir. Dis. **83(2):**29–40.
12. CENTER FOR DISEASE CONTROL. 1968. Influenza-Respiratory Disease Surveillance. Report No. 84. Issued September 15, 1968.
13. CENTER FOR DISEASE CONTROL. 1974. Influenza-Respiratory Disease Surveillance, 1972–1973. Report No. 89. Issued February 1974.
14. CENTER FOR DISEASE CONTROL. 1977. Influenza Surveillance, 1975–1976. Report No. 91. Issued July 1977.
15. PHILIP, R. N., J. A. BELL, D. J. DAVIS, M. O. BEEM, P. M. BEIGELMAN, J. I. ENGLER, G. W. MELLIN, J. H. JOHNSON & A. M. LERNER. 1961. Epidemiologic studies on influenza in familial and general population groups, 1951–1956. Am. J. Hyg. **73(2):**123–137.
16. DAVIS, L. E., G. G. CALDWELL, R. E. LYNCH, R. E. BAILEY & T. D. Y. CHIN. 1970. Hong Kong influenza: The epidemiologic features of a high school family study analyzed and compared with a similar study during the 1957 Asian influenza epidemic. Am. J. Epidemiol. **92(4):**240–247.
17. HOPE-SIMPSON, R. E. 1951. Discussion: Influenza 1951. Proc. R. Soc. Med. **44:** 789–801.
18. FOX, J. P. & E. D. KILBOURNE. 1973. NIH News. Epidemiology of influenza–summary of Influenza Workshop IV. J. Infect. Dis. **128(3):**361–386.
19. HOPE-SIMPSON, R. E. 1970. First outbreak of Hong Kong influenza in a general practice population in Great Britain. A field and laboratory study. Br. Med. J. **3:** 74–77.
20. OPIE, E. L., A. W. FREEMAN, F. G. BLAKE, J. C. SMALL & T. M. RIVERS. 1919. Pneumonia at Camp Funston. J. Am. Med. Assoc. **72(2):**108–116.
21. THE COMMISSION ON ACUTE RESPIRATORY DISEASES. 1948. Studies of the 1943 epidemic of influenza A. VI. Epidemiological characteristics in varied types of military units and comparison with undifferentiated acute respiratory disease. Am. J. Hyg. **48:** 305–323.
22. MOSER, M. R., T. R. BENDER, H. S. MARGOLIS, G. R. NOBLE, A. P. KENDAL & D. G. RITTER. 1979. An outbreak of influenza aboard a commercial airliner. Am. J. Epidemiol. **110(1):** 1–6.
23. WILLIAMS, R. E. O. 1960. Intramural spread of bacteria and viruses in human populations. Ann. Rev. Microbiol. **14:** 43–64.
24. MOSER, M. R., T. R. BENDER & H. S. MARGOLIS. Personal communication.

EPIDEMIOLOGY OF THE COMMON COLD

Jack M. Gwaltney, Jr.

Division of Epidemiology and Virology
University of Virginia School of Medicine
Charlottesville, Virginia 22908

The problem of studying the common cold is complicated by the many viruses involved that do not behave in the same way. This review will mainly consider the rhinoviruses which cause the largest percentage of diagnosed colds ($\approx 30\%$) and have received the most study. A considerable amount of information is available on the background epidemiology of these viruses. Field studies have established that rhinoviruses spread best in the home[1-3] and at school.[4] The principle reservoir is the nose of the school child. The most typical patterns of spread are from child-to-child in the classroom or at some other location in school and from child-to-child and from child-to-parent in the home. Also, transmission between husband and wife may be relatively common. Spread of rhinovirus colds among persons at work does not appear to be as important as it is in the school or at home.[3] Thus, observations made in the natural setting suggest that close, if not intimate, contact is necessary for optimal rhinovirus transmission.

Moving on to studies of rhinovirus infection in volunteers, attempts to transfer infection from an infected to a susceptible (antibody-free) subject have been consistently successful only under two conditions of exposure. One of these conditions is that of married couples living in their own home. In this study, D'Alesio *et al.* infected one partner of 24 childless married couples by instilling virus in the nose. They then observed the couples while they continued their normal activities.[5] The infected partner transmitted the infection to the susceptible spouse in nine instances (37.5%). Transmission took place in association with the following conditions: the infected partner had $\geq 10^3$ $TCID_{50}$ of virus in the nasal wash, had virus on the hands and in the saliva, was at least moderately symptomatic, and spent at least 122 hours with the susceptible partner during a seven-day period.

The amount of time spent together during the first three days of the donor's illness may have been more important than time together over the entire seven days. With most couples, the conditions associated with spread of infection occurred only on the second and third days after inoculation of the donor. Also, the most common interval between inoculation of the donor and recovery of virus from the partner was five days. With a one-day incubation period for each partner included in this five-day period, the indication is that transmission occurred most often on the third day. The findings of this volunteer experiment support the conclusions drawn from studies of natural colds that rhinovirus spread depends on close, and perhaps prolonged, contact. Furthermore, it appears that the person who transmits the infection must be shedding significant amounts of *detectable* virus.

The second condition under which successful transfer of rhinovirus was achieved was in volunteer studies done in Charlottesville.[6] We compared the efficiencies of three different routes of transmission: hand contact/self-inoculation, exposure by air across a double wire partition ("small particle aerosol") and

0077-8923/80/0353-0054 $01.75/0 © 1980, NYAS

exposure by air around a small table ("large particle aerosol"). The conditions for all three types of exposure were designed to produce a situation that would favor transmission. With the hand route, the infected donor deliberately contaminated the hands immediately prior to hand-to-hand contact with the recipient. The recipient then deliberately touched the conjunctival and nasal mucosa with their fingers. With the wire partition exposure, the donors and recipients were continuously together in the same air space for 72 hours. For the exposure around the table, infected donors deliberately tried to shower recipients with respiratory secretions by coughing, singing, and other means. The same infected donors were used to expose recipients by all three methods. Under these conditions, hand contact was a very reliable way to transmit infection, 11 of 15 volunteers were infected by this route. Also, the hand route was decidedly more efficient than either the wire barrier exposure (0 of 10 infected) or exposure around the table (1 of 10 infected).

Other attempts to transmit rhinovirus infection using volunteers have not met with similar success. In an earlier unpublished study, done by Couch et al.,[7] 20 susceptible recipients were exposed to infected donors across a double wire barrier. No recipients became infected. In a study done by D'Allesio et al.,[8] four susceptible recipients escaped infection after confinement in a small room with infected donors who sang, coughed and sneezed. In two additional experiments by the D'Alesio group, susceptible recipients were exposed to infected donors by having them share dormitory sleeping quarters for three consecutive nights or by having an exposure by means of kissing.[5,8,9] Only two of 22 susceptible recipients were infected, one by each type of exposure.

Thus, the results of volunteer studies suggest that rhinoviruses do not spread well through the air, at least under experimental conditions. Whether these findings are representative of what happens under natural conditions is still not clear. To approach this question, one can examine the reasons why the air transmission exposures may have failed. Air transmission will not occur if there is: 1. Failure of the host to produce sufficient quantities of virus aerosol, 2. failure of virus to survive in the aerosol, or 3. failure of the aerosol to reach a portal of entry of the susceptible host.

An infectious aerosol will not be produced if the activity that creates the aerosol does not occur with the disease or if the virus is not present at the site where the aerosol is produced and, thus, is not incorporated into the aerosol. Coughing, sneezing, and blowing the nose have been shown to produce the largest quantities of aerosol from the respiratory tract, and, thus, are considered the most important activities in airborne spread. Buckland and Tyrrell,[10] using bacterial spores or bacteriophage tracers, found that sneezing and blowing the nose were over a thousandfold more efficient in producing infectious aerosols from nasal secretions than coughing. On the other hand, Couch et al.,[11] who collected coughs and sneezes from Coxsackie A21 virus infected volunteers in weather balloons, found that sneezing produced more total virus containing particles (that is, more virus was recovered from both the walls of the balloon and in the air sample than coughing). However, coughing produced more infectious particles in the air sample alone. Furthermore, the presence of Coxsackie A21 virus in air samples of the cough correlated with recovery of virus from room air samples. Also, coughing was noted to be frequently present in infected volunteers at times when sneezing was not. Buckland et al.,[12] also working with volunteers experimentally infected with Coxsackie A21 virus, found that blowing the nose resulted in viral contamination of the handkerchief and of the walls but not the air sample of a plastic collecting bag. In summary, these studies of aerosol production suggest that sneezing and nose blowing produce more large particle aerosols, and coughing more small particle aerosols.

How do these findings relate to rhinovirus infections? With natural rhinovirus colds, approximately half of persons reported sneezing on the first and second days of illness and 40% on the third day.[13] Coughing was reported by a third of persons on day one and 40% on days two and three. Also, cough and sneeze counts have been made by tape recorder during experimental rhinovirus infection.[6] The frequency of coughing (for five volunteers) ranged from 2–143 (mean 69) on the first day of illness, 3–214 (mean 89) on the second day, and 4–171 (mean 51) on the third day. Sneezing frequency ranged from 0–17 on day one (mean 5), 0–6 day two (mean 2), and 0–6 day three (mean 1). The actual numbers of sneezes per day were surprisingly low with these experimental colds but coughing, as an aerosol producing activity, was relatively common.

Perhaps a more critical question is, is rhinovirus present at the sites of aerosol production and, thus, available for incorporation into the aerosol? The major sites that have been proposed for aerosol production are the anterior mouth, which contains the anterior pool of saliva, and areas in the pharynx and lower respiratory tract. The anterior oral pool of saliva has been said to be the primary source of aerosols created by sneezing. Some authors have pointed out that with some sneezes, there may be a significant contribution from secretions in the nose.[14] Aerosols associated with coughing are presumably produced in the pharynx and in large airways in the lower respiratory tract where air velocity is sufficient to create an aerosol.

Rhinovirus has been found in two of these locations where aerosols are produced; the pharynx and the mouth, although with less frequency and at lower titers than found in the nose (TABLE 1). Rhinovirus is uniformly present in nasal secretions where the estimated geometric mean titer (GMT) is 300 and concentrations have ranged from $1-\geq16,000$ $TCID_{50}/ml$.[5,6,11,15,16] It has been suggested that rhinovirus replication takes place primarily or exclusively in nasal cells and that virus found in the pharynx and oral secretions may represent contamination. In the pharyngeal secretions and in saliva, GMT's are 30 and 10, respectively, with ranges of 1–3000 and 1–5000. The question of how often, if ever, rhinovirus infects the lower respiratory tract where the temperature (37°C) is restrictive for rhinovirus has not been answered. Rhinovirus has been recovered from the sputum of children with asthma[17] and sputum of adults with chronic bronchitis[18] but whether these specimens were contaminated with virus from other sources is not clear. Samples from the lower respiratory tract, which have not passed through the pharynx, have not been available for testing.

Attempts to recover rhinovirus in respiratory aerosols have met with limited success. Couch et al.[7] using a large volume air sampler could not detect rhinovirus in the air of a dormitory housing experimentally infected volunteers. During periods of sampling, it was estimated that 82% of the air in the room was tested. The room had a volume of 70,000 liters.[19] The air sampling device averaged an 11% efficiency when tested with artificial viral aerosols of known concentrations.[11]

We used a method of having 25 naturally infected volunteers simulate multiple coughs or sneezes, which were directed onto a 15 cm diameter glass petri dish containing viral collecting broth and held approximately 10 cm from the face.[15] Virus was recovered from sneezes of only one of 13 persons and from cough specimens of one of 12. The virus may have been in large particles of respiratory secretions, since the attempt to recover airborne virus, discussed above, was unsuccessful. Virus was present in the saliva of half of this group (8 of 16 who had all of the testing done), although no virus was recovered from their simulated cough or sneeze specimens.

In evaluating our low yield of virus recovery, we questioned if the simulated coughs and sneezes were similar enough to natural coughs and sneezes to provide valid results. To examine this question and to test the sensitivity of the petri dish sampling technique, we put increasing concentrations of rhinovirus ($10^{1.5}$, $10^{2.5}$, and $10^{3.5}$ TCID$_{50}$/ml) in the anterior oral pool of uninfected volunteers and collected simulated cough and sneeze specimens from them by the petri dish method.[15] At viral concentrations instilled into the mouth of $10^{2.5}$ and $10^{3.5}$ TCID$_{50}$/ml, we consistently recovered virus. With a viral concentration of $10^{1.5}$ TCID$_{50}$/ml, one-third of specimens were positive. Thus, it appeared that simu-

TABLE 1

ESTIMATED FREQUENCY OF RHINOVIRUS SHEDDING OR CONTAMINATION ON THE THIRD DAY OF INFECTION*

Source/Site	Frequency†	GMT‡ (Range)
Nasal secretions (wash or swab)	>90%	300 (1–≥16,000)
Pharyngeal secretions (gargle and swab)	70%	30 (1–3,000)
Saliva (expectoration)	50%	10 (1–5,000)
Lower respiratory tract (transtracheal aspiration)	ND	ND
Aerosol (large volume air sampler, cough/sneeze plate)	0 and 8%	ND
Hands	50%	10 (1–≥16,000)
Environment	10%	1

*Based on reported studies.[5,6,11,16,17]
†Percent of time virus recovered.
‡Geometric mean titer TCID$_{50}$/ml.

lated coughs and sneezes would produce an infectious aerosol if sufficient virus was present in the salivary pool. Also, the petri dish method appeared to be sensitive for recovering aerosolized rhinovirus.

To further look for rhinovirus in natural sneezes, we left petri dishes (with collecting broth) in the rooms of three experimentally infected volunteers, instructing them to collect natural sneeze specimens.[6] One specimen was collected from each volunteer on each of three days. The entire 10 ml sample was inoculated into 7 to 16 WI-38 cell culture tubes. No virus was recovered from nine specimens of natural sneezes. In summary, the data from these three studies suggest that aerosolization of rhinovirus is not a common event. This may be because of the infrequency of sneezing with rhinovirus colds (discussed earlier) or because of the relative scarcity of virus in the pharynx and salivary pool (and also possibly because of a scarcity of virus in the lower respiratory tract).

Based on the sampling with the petri dish method discussed above, it was found that only one of 12 or roughly 10% of coughs contained detectable rhinovirus. If this 10% figure is applied to the average number of coughs on the first three days of a rhinovirus cold (as measured by tape recorder, which was 70, 90, and 50), then the number of coughs per day expected to contain virus would be 7, 9, and 5, respectively. Whether an average of five to nine coughs per day containing rhinovirus is an accurate reflection of the amount of infectious aerosol produced with natural rhinovirus colds remains to be seen. Also, whether this amount of aerosolization, if it is representative, would sustain rhinovirus spread in nature is another interesting question.*

To proceed to the second possibility, was aerosol transmission impaired because rhinovirus is too fragile to survive well in an aerosol, or were there unfavorable environmental conditions which inactivated the virus? Rhinovirus has been incorporated into aerosols generated by a Collison atomizer which produced particle sizes ranging from 0.2 to 3.0 microns in diameter.[20] In this experiment, by Cate, et al.,[20] several 19 liter samples of the experimental aerosols were sampled in Shipe impingers. The samples consistently yielded rhinovirus, even after freezing at $-70°C$, indicating that rhinovirus does survive aerosolization. Also, volunteers became infected after challenge with 16 to 66 $TCID_{50}$ of virus, showing that the virus can infect the respiratory tract after transport in an aerosol. In another study in which volunteers were challenged with aerosolized rhinovirus, the HID_{50} for the aerosolized virus was substantially greater than that for the same virus given by nasal drops.[11] With nasal instillation, concentrations as low as 1 and 3 $TCID_{50}$ of rhinovirus have consistently infected volunteers.

In regard to the effect of environmental conditions on virus survival, rhinovirus, like other picornaviruses, is inactivated relatively quickly at humidities below 50%.[21,22] The Charlottesville volunteer studies were done during periods of both high and low relative humidity (November, January, March, and April) with similar results. Thus, there is nothing to suggest that airborne transmission failed because of either inherent fragility of the virus or because environmental conditions were unfavorable.

The third question, whether infectious aerosol failed to reach the susceptible volunteers because of dilution or sedimentation of the aerosol is an important one. The room used for the Charlottesville experiment was large, containing 285,000 liters of air. Assuming a ventilation rate of 10 liters per minute for susceptible subjects (which is probably high, since most subjects did not engage in even moderate exercise) and assuming no rebreathing or air exchange (through opened doors and around windows, etc.) each recipient would have inhaled only 15% (4,320 liters) of the air in the room during the 72-hour exposure. Since there were two recipients in each room, together they would have sampled a maximum of 30% of the air. In Couch's study,[7,11,23] the room volume was 580,000 liters. During the first three days each recipient sampled 7% of the air. All 20 recipients would have inhaled 140% of the air (assuming no rebreathing or air exchange).

In summary, the route or routes of natural rhinovirus spread are still unknown. Of the possibilities considered to explain the failure of aerosol transmission of rhinovirus, and assuming sensitivity of the aerosol sampling methods used, it appears that either lack of incorporation of rhinovirus into an aerosol and/or the dilution of any infectious aerosol that was produced seem most likely. However, it must be recognized that periods of aerosol production may be very transient, occurring only when rhinovirus is present in the anterior mouth or other critical sites in unusually high concentrations. These periods, which might have been missed in sampling, may be all that is necessary to lead to efficient dissemination of the virus through the air.

It is also possible that aerosol production might occur in only a few persons

---

*Two other sources of rhinovirus which might play a role in hand/self inoculation transmission are the hands and objects in the environment of persons with rhinovirus colds.

who were particularly effective disseminators of infection. However, results of family studies suggest this is not the case. After introduction of a rhinovirus into the home, secondary spread occurred in 54% of households.[3] This relatively high rate of secondary spread suggests that at least half of infected persons are efficient disseminators of virus at some time in their illness.

Further studies are needed of the mechanics of aerosol production in the infected host and of the sensitivity of methods for detecting the different respiratory viruses in aerosols. Also, ways to interrupt natural cold transmission by the various proposed routes should be tested. Advances in air purification and in viral diagnosis should permit the design of improved studies for the interruption of airborne (droplet nucleus) spread along the lines of the early ultraviolet light trials.[24,25] Currently, we are attempting to interrupt spread of natural rhinovirus colds by the hand contamination/self-inoculation route, using a method of treatment of the hands with a virucidal substance. It may also be possible to design ways to investigate the effect of blocking large particle transmission under natural conditions. Although field studies of this type are difficult to do, they provide direct information on the importance of the different proposed routes of spread and they may also lead to practical methods for control.

References

1. DICK, E. C., C. R. BLUMER & A. S. EVANS. 1967. Epidemiology of infections with rhinovirus types 43 and 55 in a group of Wisconsin student families. Am J. Epidemiol. **86**: 386.
2. MONTO, A. S. 1968. A community study of respiratory infections in the tropics. III. Introduction and transmission of infections within families. Am. J. Epidemiol. **88**: 69.
3. HENDLEY, J. O., J. M. GWALTNEY, JR. & W. S. JORDAN, JR. 1969. Rhinovirus infections in an industrial population. IV. Infections within families of employees during two fall peaks of respiratory illness. Am. J. Epidemiol. **89**: 184.
4. BEEM, M. O. 1969. Acute respiratory illness in nursery school children. A longitudinal study of the occurrence of illness and respiratory viruses. Am. J. Epidemiol. **90**: 30.
5. D'ALESSIO, D. J., J. A. PETERSON, C. R. DICK & E. C. DICK. 1976. Transmission of experimental rhinovirus colds in volunteer married couples. J. Infect. Dis. **133**: 28.
6. GWALTNEY, J. M. JR., P. B. MOSKALSKI & J. O. HENDLEY. 1978. Hand-to-hand transmission of rhinovirus colds. Ann. Int. Med. **88**: 463.
7. COUCH, R. B. Personal communication.
8. D'ALESSIO, D. J., C. R. DICK, & E. C. DICK. 1972. Transmission of rhinovirus type 55 in human volunteers. In Second International Congress for Virology. J. L. Melnick, Ed.: 115. S. Karger. Basel.
9. PETERSON, J. A., D. J. D'ALESSIO & E. C. DICK. 1973. Studies on the failure of direct oral contact to transmit rhinovirus infection between human volunteers. In Abstracts of the Annual Meeting of the American Society for Microbiology: 213. Miami, Fla.
10. BUCKLAND, F. E. & D. A. J. TYRRELL 1962. Loss of infectivity on drying various viruses. Nature (London) **195**: 1063.
11. COUCH, R. B., T. R. CATE, G. DOUGLAS, JR., et al. 1966. Effect of route of inoculation on experimental respiratory viral disease in volunteers and evidence for airborne transmission. Bacteriol. Rev. **30**: 517.
12. BUCKLAND, F. E., M. L. BYNOE & D. A. J. TYRRELL. 1965. Experiments on the spread of colds. II. Studies in volunteers with Coxsackie A21. J. Hyg. (Camb.) **63**: 327.
13. GWALTNEY, J. M. JR., J. O. HENDLEY, G. SIMON, et al. 1967. Rhinovirus infections in an industrial population. II. Characteristics of illness and antibody response. J. Am. Med. Assoc. **202**: 494.

14. BOURDILLON, R. B. & O. M. LIDWELL, 1941. Sneezing and the spread of infection. Lancet **2**: 365.
15. HENDLEY, J. O., R. P. WENZEL & J. M. GWALTNEY, JR. 1973. Transmission of rhinovirus colds by self-inoculation. N. Engl. J. Med. **288**: 1361.
16. REED, S. E. 1975. An investigation of the possible transmission of rhinovirus colds through indirect contact. J. Hyg. (Camb.) **75**: 249.
17. HORN, M. E. C., S. E. REED & P. TAYLOR. 1979. The role of viruses and bacteria in acute wheezy bronchitis in childhood: A study of sputum. Arch. Dis. Child. **54**: 587.
18. LAMBERT, H. P. & H. STERN. 1972. Infective factors in exacerbations of bronchitis and asthma. Brit. Med. J. **3**: 323.
19. GERONE, P. J., R. B. COUCH, G. V. KEEFER, et al. 1966. Assessment of experimental and natural viral aerosols. Bacteriol. Rev. **30**: 576.
20. CATE, T. R., R. B. COUCH, W. F. FLEET, et al. 1965. Production of tracheobronchitis in volunteers with rhinovirus in a small particle aerosol. Am. J. Epidemiol. **81**: 95.
21. HATCH, M. T., M. J. HOLMES, J. A. DEIG, et al. 1967. Stability of airborne rhinovirus type 2 under atmospheric and physiological conditions. Abstracts of the Annual Meeting of the American Society of Microbiology: 193, Q 18.
22. DEJONG, J. C., M. HARMSEN & T. TROUBORST. 1975. Factors in the inactivation of encephalomyocarditis virus in aerosols. Infect. Immun. **12**: 29.
23. COUCH, R. B., R. G. DOUGLAS, K. M. LINDGREN, et al. 1970. Airborne transmission of respiratory infection with Coxsackie virus A type 21. Am. J. Epidemiol. **91**: 78.
24. WELLS, W. F. 1955. Airborne contagion and air hygiene. An ecological study of droplet infections: 249. Harvard University Press. Cambridge.
25. ANDREWES, C. 1965. The Common Cold. W. W. Norton. New York.

LEGIONELLOSIS: EVIDENCE OF AIRBORNE TRANSMISSION

David W. Fraser

Bureau of Epidemiology
Center for Disease Control
Atlanta, Georgia 30333

INTRODUCTION

Legionella pneumophila is a fastidious gram-negative bacterium that was first identified as a cause of human disease in 1976,[1] although the organism had been isolated as early as 1947.[2] Numerous outbreaks of legionellosis have been recognized in the last few years, as have hundreds of sporadic cases. Outbreaks have been of two clinical and epidemiologic patterns. Legionnaires' disease—as it occurred among American Legion conventioneers in Philadelphia in 1976—is characterized by an incubation period of 2–10 days, an attack rate of 0.1%–5.0%, the occurrence of pneumonia in 90% of cases, and when no specific therapy is given, a case-fatality ratio of 15%–20%.[3] Pontiac fever has been seen in two outbreaks and is typified by an incubation period usually of 24–48 hours, an attack rate of ≥95%, and an influenza-like syndrome without pneumonia or death.[4]

Evidence of Airborne Spread

Of all outbreaks of legionellosis studied, the explosive 1968 outbreak of Pontiac fever[4] had the most convincing evidence of airborne spread. Beginning on Monday, July 1, at the Pontiac office of the Oakland County Health Department 1 employee became ill; 66 became ill on July 2; and 22, on July 3. In all, 95 of 100 employees were ill. In addition, the illness affected 49 of 170 visitors to the building in July and the first week of August. The attack rate increased with increasing duration of exposure. Among visitors exposed for <1 hour the attack rate was 9%, for visitors exposed >6 hours it was 59%, and for employees exposed >6 hours it was 95%. Early in the investigation, airborne spread was suspected because of the high attack rate and lack of other discernible common exposure, especially among the visitors. Furthermore, although the incubation period for most persons ranged from 24 to 48 hours, three visiting epidemiologists who first entered the building on Saturday, July 6, when the building's air-conditioning system was turned off, did not become ill until Tuesday night, 1½ days after the air-conditioning system had been turned back on Monday morning. Attack rates were higher for persons exposed early in the morning than for those first exposed in the afternoon or evening, raising the possibility that there was increased risk associated with starting up the air-conditioning system, as occurred on weekday mornings. Experimental confirmation of airborne spread came from studies in which guinea pigs were exposed to air in the Pontiac building at the time of the outbreak; 9 years later *L. pneumophila* was recovered from lung tissue, frozen in the interim, of exposed guinea pigs. Examination of the air-conditioning system showed at least 2 defects. Air leaving the building's evaporative condenser, which was located in the basement, was exhausted on

61

0077-8923/80/0353–0061 $01.75/0 © 1980, NYAS

the roof, less than 2 meters from the fresh-air intake for the building. Furthermore, the exhaust duct from the evaporative condenser passed adjacent to one supply-air duct carrying cooled air from the air-conditioning unit; defects in their common walls had permitted droplets of water from the evaporative condenser exhaust to collect in a puddle in the supply-air duct. At the time of the initial investigation, it was hypothesized that the evaporative-condenser water was contaminated with the Pontiac fever agent even though the identity of the agent was not known at the time. This hypothesis was confirmed in 1977 when *L. pneumophila* was recovered from lung tissue of guinea pigs that had been experimentally exposed to aerosols of evaporative-condenser water collected during the 1968 outbreak.

Airborne spread in an outbreak of Legionnaires' disease was most clearly demonstrated in the 1978 outbreak in Memphis.[5] On August 8, a flash flood inactivated the cooling towers that usually served a large hospital, so an auxiliary cooling tower located on the second floor over the entrance of the hospital was put into service from August 8 to September 7, the first time it had been used in two years. Between August 11 and September 16, 39 cases of Legionnaires' disease occurred in persons who had been patients, staff, or visitors at the hospital or passersby in the 10 days prior to onset of illness. Risk of illness (cases per thousand) was estimated to be 1.7 for employees, 2.4 for patients, 3.4 for overnight visitors, and 0.2 for daytime visitors during the epidemic. The risk of nosocomial Legionnaire's disease depended on location within the hospital. Hospital patients whose rooms received air from 1 of 2 intakes located directly above the auxiliary cooling tower had a risk of pneumonia of 2.8 cases per 100 bed-months, whereas those in rooms that received air from intakes elsewhere had a risk that averaged 0.5 per 100 bed-months ($p < .01$). The abrupt beginning and end of the outbreak corresponded exactly with usage of the auxiliary cooling tower, assuming an incubation period of 2–10 days. Smoke studies showed that air in the vicinity of the auxiliary cooling tower could easily drift toward the nearby air intakes as well as to the street below, where several passersby apparently were exposed. *L. pneumophila* serogroup 1 was isolated from 2 samples of water taken from the cooling tower in early September.

Several other outbreaks contribute evidence that legionellosis is spread by the airborne route. On July 2–7, 1978, 8 golfers at an Atlanta country club developed "atypical" pneumonia.[6] The attack rate was 2.1% for all golfers. Three of the 8 had ≥4-fold rises in titer to *L. pneumophila* serogroup 1 by indirect immunofluorescence, and 3 others had convalescent-phase titers of ≥128, strongly suggesting that this tight cluster was of Legionnaires' disease. Seropositivity was more common among sick golfers than among well golfers, nongolfers, or employees. Specific activities within the clubhouse, on the golf course, or elsewhere in the country club were not associated with increased risk of illness or seropositivity, but the golfers with pneumonia had played considerably more golf in the period June 22–July 5 than had other golfers; the bulk of the difference in golfing had been in the period July 1–5 (39.4 holes vs 19.4 holes; $p < .004$). In the course of the investigation in August, many environmental specimens were cultured. Only from the clubhouse evaporative condenser was *L. pneumophila* serogroup 1 recovered. Further investigation indicated that the air from this evaporative condenser was exhausted horizontally from one wall of the clubhouse, but was directed toward the 10th and 16th tees, 160 and 100 feet away, respectively. It may be that golfers playing the "back nine" were exposed to airborne *L. pneumophila* disseminated from the evaporative condenser. Several features are unexplained, however, including why the outbreak started and why it stopped despite the fact that the evaporative condenser was still positive for *L. pneumophila* on August 23.

In the 1976 Philadelphia outbreak,[3] illness occurred most commonly among those American Legion conventioneers who stayed overnight at the Bellevue-Stratford hotel, the headquarters hotel, but 39 persons who never entered the hotel (but had been within one block of it) were affected. Risk of illness was directly associated with the time spent in the lobby of the hotel or on the sidewalk in front of it. Among convention delegates, for example, patients with Legionnaires' disease spent an average of 259 minutes in the lobby, whereas well controls spent an average of 133 minutes. The pattern of illness suggested airborne spread in the lobby and adjacent sidewalk area; however, the source of spread was not identified. Attempts to recover *L. pneumophila* from numerous environmental samples, including water from the rooftop cooling tower, were unsuccessful, in part perhaps because of the two-year storage of specimens prior to the development of successful methods for isolating *L. pneumophila* from environmental specimens.

Airborne spread from sites of soil excavation was suggested as the cause of an outbreak of Legionnaires' disease in 1965 at a psychiatric hospital in Washington, D.C., that had no central air-conditioning system.[7] In that outbreak, 81 cases were identified, with 14 deaths. Risk of illness was found to be highest for those permitted to walk around the campus of the hospital and for those whose rooms were next to windows. Attack rates were higher in buildings located within 20 feet of sites of excavation (for the purpose of installing a lawn-sprinkler system) than in buildings not near excavation (17.8 vs 1.7 per 1,000, respectively). The epidemic curve showed two peaks, each occurring five days after the filling in of excavation sites, suggesting that in the process of closing the excavation, *L. pneumophila* may have become airborne and infected patients nearby.

In 1973, on the James River in Virginia, 10 men who cleaned the inside of a steam turbine condenser with compressed air developed Pontiac fever. Whether *L. pneumophila* was spread by aerosol or contact or was airborne in that outbreak is uncertain, but the source was almost certainly the river water, silt, or other debris that had accumulated inside the cast iron condenser chamber.[8]

Several other outbreaks have occurred in patterns consistent with airborne spread, but the place of exposure and source of *L. pneumophila* were not identified. Notable examples are: the outbreak that affected one neighborhood in Kingsport, Tennessee, in 1977;[9] the citywide outbreak in Burlington, Vermont, in 1977;[10] and the continuing foci of Legionnaires' disease in and around the Indiana Memorial Union in Bloomington, Indiana,[11] and the Wadsworth Medical Center in Los Angeles, California.[12] The use of home air conditioning was associated with increased risk of community-acquired Legionnaires' disease in the Vermont outbreak, although such units have not been associated with increased risk in sporadic cases.[13]

Analysis of sporadic cases may be of some value in determining the mode(s) of spread of legionellosis, but the improbable vignette may also be misleading. Because unusual circumstances concerning a case of pneumonia may prompt the clinician to obtain specimens needed to confirm a case as legionellosis, confirmed sporadic cases, as a group, tend to be a bit odd. Only at the risk of circularity in argument can the odd circumstances surrounding a given case be inferred to be causally related to that case. For example, two of the earliest of the sporadic cases of Legionnaires' disease to be confirmed were in a physician who one week before onset had used a coat hanger to extract, piece by piece, a bird's nest (with embryos) from behind a grating in his attic; another in a merchant seaman whose only port of call in the 10 days prior to onset had been a guano-covered pier in southern California. These cases could not be used to implicate birds as a source of spread but could be (and were) used to suggest hypotheses to be tested in a systematic analysis of sporadic cases and controls. Storch et al. identified and attempted to obtain epidemiologic information about the first 100 community-acquired cases of confirmed Legionnaires' disease.[13] As clinical controls they chose 100 persons with negative serodiagnostic tests for Legionnaires' disease matched for age, sex, and state from which the specimens were submitted. It was felt that the clinical controls would be as likely as the persons with cases to suffer from the selection biases because clinicians had had to suspect the diagnosis of Legionnaires' disease and collect the appropriate specimens for them to be found to be seronegative. For each case and clinical control, an acquaintance control was chosen by the patient from persons residing in the same community and of the same age and sex. Legionnaires' disease patients were more likely than acquaintance controls (relative risk = 3.0, p < .05) and clinical controls (relative risk = 2.3, p < .05) to have lived near excavation sites. Also, they were more likely than clinical controls (relative risk = 2.7, p < .05) or acquaintance controls (relative risk = 1.7, p > .20) to have lived near construction sites. Clinical controls differed from their acquaintance controls in neither respect. The apparently specific association of sporadic Legionnaires' disease cases with excavation and construction sites suggests a situation parallel to that seen in the 1965 St. Elizabeth Hospital outbreak where windborne dust may have spread L. pneumophila.[7] Perhaps supporting this hypothesis was the observation from Storch's study that the only occupational group found to be statistically significantly at increased risk of Legionnaires' disease was that involved in construction work.

Search for Other Modes of Spread

No natural mode of spread of L. pneumophila other than airborne has been proven despite concerted efforts to do so. In the 1976 outbreak, evidence of person-to-person spread was sought by surveillance for illness among household contacts who had not traveled to Philadelphia but who had been exposed to a family member with Legionnaires' disease.[3] None of 193 household contacts developed illness that met the clinical criteria for Legionnaires' disease (fever and pneumonia, or temperature ≥ 102 F and cough) in the 24 days after the end of the American Legion convention. Roommates at the convention hotel were not found to be more likely to contract Legionnaires' disease. In the eight days after onset in the index case, 5 of 231 case contacts in the Pontiac fever outbreak in 1968 developed illness that included three or more of the following symptoms: fever or chills, generalized myalgia, malaise, and headache. None of these possibly secondary cases was confirmed by seroconversion and a control group of contacts of noncases was not surveyed in a similar manner to determine the background incidence of such illness.[4] Serosurveys of hospital workers in several outbreaks have not suggested they are at risk of acquiring legionellosis from patients with the disease,[9,10,12,14] although Saravolatz et al. found 9.3% of hospital workers on wards that had had a person with confirmed Legionnaires' disease and only 3.7% of workers on other wards had hemagglutination titers to L. pneumophila serogroup 1 of ≥ 128.[15] Seropositivity was not related to intensity of exposure to the index patient, however, and the specificity of the hemagglutination test is unproved so it is difficult to interpret this finding.

Among delegates to the 1976 American Legion convention, consumption of water at the headquarters hotel was more common for those with Legionnaires' disease (45 of 69) than for those without (469 of 976) (p < .01).[3] However, many cases occurred in people who had never even entered the hotel so airborne rather than waterborne spread seemed more likely. Because L. pneumophila can survive in tap water for many months,[16] the possibility of waterborne spread should not be rejected; subsequent outbreaks may suggest water plays some role in spread.

The possibility of foodborne spread was examined in the 1976 outbreak, but no supporting evidence was found.[3]

No evidence of spread from birds or mammals was found by questionnaire of patients or serosurvey of local rats and pigeons. The case-control study of sporadic Legionnaires' disease disclosed no increased risk associated with exposure to insects, birds, or bird roosts, other animals or fish aquariums.[13]

Needed Information

Legionnaires' disease and Pontiac fever are both spread through the air and, at least on some occasions, from similar sources, but the striking differences in attack rates, incubation periods, and clinical severity remain unexplained. Although differences as yet unidentified in the infecting organism as well as the susceptible host may be critical, the dose of organisms, particle size, and toxic or microbiologic cofactors may determine which syndrome occurs.

Study of airborne transmission of L. pneumophila would be helped by development of methods to recover the organism from air. The only method used successfully has been sentinel guinea pigs (in the 1968 Pontiac fever investigation),[4] but even that method was unsuccessful in investigations of Legionnaires' disease.[1,12] Air sampling by filtration has been attempted without success,[17] but studies of the ability of L. pneumophila to survive the drying that accompanies air filtration have not been reported. Impingement of air into a liquid medium may be more likely to permit recovery of L. pneumophila.

The effectiveness of ultraviolet irradiation or high-efficiency filtration of air in limiting spread of legionellosis should be studied. Such techniques might be expected to be of greatest use in ongoing outbreaks within a single building, such as the situation at Wadsworth Medical Center in which more than 100 cases of nosocomial disease have occurred over 2½ years but where the source has not been identified.[12]

Although cooling towers and evaporative condensers have been implicated as the sources of L. pneumophila, our understanding would be furthered by demonstration that risk of legionellosis is related to concentration of L. pneumophila in cooling tower or evaporative condenser water, rate of dissemination of the organisms in drift from such units, and intensity of exposure to that drift.[18]

REFERENCES

1. McDade, J. E., C. C. Shepard, D. W. Fraser, T. F. Tsai, M. Redus, W. R. Dowdle & Laboratory Investigation Team. 1977. Legionnaires' disease: isolation of a bacterium and demonstration of its role in other respiratory disease. New Engl. J. Med. **297** (22): 1197–1203.
2. McDade, J. E., D. J. Brenner & F. M. Bozeman. 1979. Legionnaires' disease bacterium isolated in 1947. Ann. Intern. Med. **90** (40): 659–661.

3. FRASER, D. W., T. F. TSAI, W. ORENSTEIN, W. E. PARKIN, H. J. BEECHAM, R. G. SHARRAR, J. HARRIS, G. F. MALLISON, S. M. MARTIN, J. E. MCDADE, C. C. SHEPARD, P. S. BRACHMAN & FIELD INVESTIGATION TEAM. 1977. Legionnaires' disease: description of an epidemic of pneumonia. New Engl. J. Med. **297** (22): 1189–1197.

4. GLICK, T. H., M. B. GREGG, B. BERMAN, G. MALLISON, W. W. RHODES, JR. & I. KASSANOFF. 1978. Pontiac fever: an epidemic of unknown etiology in a health department. I. Clinical and epidemiologic aspects. Am. J. Epidemiol. **107** (2): 149–160.

5. DONDERO, T. J. JR., R. C. RENDTORFF, G. F. MALLISON, R. M. WEEKS, J. LEVY, E. W. WONG & W. SCHAFFNER. 1980. Outbreak of Legionnaires' disease associated with a contaminated air conditioning cooling tower. New Engl. J. Med. **302**: 365–370.

6. CORDES, L. G., D. W. FRASER, P. SKALIY, C. A. PERLINO, W. R. ELSEA, G. F. MALLISON & P. S. HAYES. 1980. Legionnaires' disease outbreak at an Atlanta country club. Evidence for spread from an evaporative condenser. Am. J. Epidemiol. **11**[4]: 425–431.

7. THACKER, S. B., J. V. BENNETT, T. F. TSAI, D. W. FRASER, J. E. MCDADE, C. C. SHEPARD, K. H. WILLIAMS, JR., W. H. STUART, H. B. DULL & T. C. EICKHOFF. 1978. An outbreak in 1965 of severe respiratory illness caused by the Legionnaires' disease bacterium. J. Infect. Dis. **138** (4): 512–519.

8. FRASER, D. W., D. C. DEUBNER, D. L. HILL & D. K. GILLIAM. 1979. Nonpneumonic, short-incubation-period legionellosis (Pontiac fever) in men who cleaned a steam turbine condenser. Science **205** (4407): 691–692.

9. DONDERO, T. F., JR., H. W. CLEGG, T. F. TSAI, R. M. WEEKS, E. DUNCAN, J. STRICKLER, C. CHAPMAN, G. F. MALLISON, B. POLITI, M. E. POTTER & W. SCHAFFNER. 1979. Legionnaires' disease in Kingsport, Tennessee. Ann. Intern. Med. **90** (4): 569–573.

10. BROOME, C. V., S. A. J. GOINGS, S. B. THACKER, R. L. VOGT, H. N. BEATY, D. W. FRASER & FIELD INVESTIGATION TEAM. 1979. The Vermont epidemic of Legionnaires' disease. Ann. Intern. Med. **90** (4): 573–577.

11. POLITI, B. D., D. W. FRASER, G. F. MALLISON, J. V. MOHATT, G. K. MORRIS, C. M. PATTON, J. C. FEELEY, R. D. TELLE & J. V. BENNETT. 1979. A major focus of Legionnaires' disease in Bloomington, Indiana. Ann. Intern. Med. **90** (4): 587–591.

12. HALEY, C. E., M. L. COHEN, J. HALTER & R. D. MEYER. 1979. Nosocomial Legionnaires' disease: a continuing common-source epidemic at Wadsworth Medical Center. Ann. Intern. Med. **90** (4): 583–586.

13. STORCH, G., W. B. BAINE, D. W. FRASER, C. V. BROOME, H. W. CLEGG, II, M. L. COHEN, S. A. J. GOINGS, B. D. POLITI, W. A. TERRANOVA, T. F. TSAI, B. D. PLIKAYTIS, C. C. SHEPARD & J. V. BENNETT. 1979. Sporadic community-acquired Legionnaires' disease in the United States. Ann. Intern. Med. **90** (4): 596–600.

14. MARKS, J. S., T. F. TSAI, W. J. MARTONE, R. C. BARON, J. KENNICOTT, F. J. HOLTZHAUER, I. BAIRD, D. FAY, J. C. FEELEY, G. F. MALLISON, D. W. FRASER & T. J. HALPIN. 1979. Nosocomial Legionnaires' disease in Columbus, Ohio. Ann. Intern. Med. **90** (4): 565–569.

15. SARAVOLATZ, L., L. ARKING, B. WENTWORTH, E. QUINN. 1979. Prevalence of antibody to the Legionnaires' disease bacterium in hospital employees. Ann. Intern. Med. **90** (4): 601–603.

16. SKALIY, P. & W. V. MCEACHERN, 1979. Survival of the Legionnaires' disease bacterium in water. Ann. Intern. Med. **90** (4): 662–663.

17. CORDES, L. G., W. D. GOLDMAN, J. S. MARR, S. M. FRIEDMAN, J. D. BAND, E. O. ROTHCHILD, D. W. FRASER & FIELD INVESTIGATION TEAM. 1980. Legionnaires' disease, New York City, August–September 1978. Bull. N.Y. Acad. Med. In press.

18. MILLER, R. P. 1979. Cooling towers and evaporative condensers. Ann. Intern. Med. **90** (4): 667–670.

LEGIONELLOSIS: ENVIRONMENTAL ASPECTS

G. F. Mallison

Bacterial Diseases Division
Bureau of Epidemiology
Center for Disease Control
Atlanta, Georgia 30333

INTRODUCTION

Most cases of legionellosis are sporadic—not associated with known clusters or outbreaks. As indicated by Fraser,[1] there has been strong evidence for airborne spread of legionellosis in a number of the outbreaks investigated by the Center for Disease Control (CDC). Few data support person-to-person transmission of legionellosis for outbreaks or sporadic cases. Thus, the disease is apparently transmitted in air from a reservoir in the inanimate environment.[2]

Environmental Epidemiology

The seasonality of legionellosis in almost all the outbreaks that CDC has investigated in the United States coincides with the time most cooling towers and evaporative condensers in the country are operated, and at the highest temperatures. In this country, over 100,000 cooling towers and evaporative condensers are used in systems for cooling intramural air. In most of the United States, the level of use of these units is lowest in the winter and spring, when few recognized outbreaks of legionellosis have begun.

Several other outbreaks of legionellosis investigated by CDC, in addition to those discussed by Fraser,[1] also appear to have been spread by the airborne route. In these outbreaks, not only were contaminated cooling towers near people who acquired disease, but also patterns of air currents would have permitted contaminated aerosols from cooling towers to reach the areas where patients worked, lived, or visited.

Role of Cooling Towers

Large volumes of extramural air pass continuously through cooling towers or evaporative condensers (a type of cooling tower in which refrigerant gas is condensed in the tower rather than in a remotely located condenser to which cooled water circulates). The concomitant large amount of water sprayed through cooling towers makes them efficient scrubbers that transfer many types of particulate contaminants from the air to the water.[3] Thus, cooling towers (or water used to fill them) probably are not the natural reservoir of *Legionella*. Rather, these organisms may originally come from the soil and/or natural bodies of water, be spread by wind to cooling towers, be scrubbed out by water spray, and then grow and be disseminated by aerosols created by such units.

In a number of outbreaks in which contaminated cooling towers or evaporative condensers were strongly associated epidemiologically with legionellosis, or in outbreaks in which airborne spread was the highly likely but not proven route

67

0077-8923/80/0353-0067 $01.75/0 © 1980, NYAS

of transmission, the water-cooling units were operated at temperatures ranging from 35–45 C. *Legionella* survives at temperatures up to about 60 C.[4]

In most of the contaminated cooling towers that have been associated with outbreaks of legionellosis, the "wet-deck" or "slat" fill (the material in a cooling tower that is used as a contact surface for air and water during heat exchange) was porous wood rather than nonporous material such as plastic or metal. Microbial growth, including slime and algae, has been seen on the wood wet-deck of a number of contaminated cooling towers associated with disease outbreaks and provides evidence of an outstanding ecologic niche for continuing proliferation of microorganisms. Also, algal blooms were associated with slimes and scale (chemical deposits) on wet-deck surfaces of almost all cooling towers that CDC found to be contaminated with *Legionella*; we do not yet know whether this observation has any relevance to growth of *Legionella*.

Recently, *Legionella* was found in a large number of ponds or lakes in the southern United States.[5] Some of the organisms were viable, but most were not. This finding may indicate another possible environmental reservoir of the bacterium, although the possibility of significant aerosolization is probably very small from ponds and lakes.

Travel

A CDC case-control study showed that sporadic legionellosis was associated with travel.[6] A possible cause for this association is that the travelers were closer to cooling towers (or evaporative condensers) in temporary lodgings than they would have been at home or at work. I have no data to support this speculation, but I believe it likely to be the case. In addition, the case-control study showed that living near construction sites was more commonly associated with patients with legionellosis than with controls who did not have the disease, and significantly more patients than controls in the study were construction workers.[6] Travel might also be associated with greater proximity to construction sites. Transmission of sporadic cases may, in fact, be associated with soil, construction, travel, or cooling towers. All of these associations may be related to environmental reservoirs and/or to airborne transmission of the disease.

Potential of Airborne Spread of Disease by Contaminated Dust

Cases of legionellosis have occurred in at least two outbreaks in cool periods of the year when cooling towers were used little or not at all in the area. This observation leads to at least two speculations about airborne transmission of legionellosis.

Legionella is probably highly unlikely to grow in air-duct systems in buildings, because the water sprayed in air-duct systems used for heating buildings or cooling outside air is seldom as warm as 30 C. However, organisms that came originally from a contaminated cooling tower or extramural dust may lodge for a time in air ducts. Then later, possibly because of vibration or changing of filters, viable organisms may cause disease by being dislodged, made airborne, and distributed to be breathed by susceptible persons.

A second speculation is that legionellosis may sometimes be caused by dead *Legionella* organisms that accumulate in air ducts during the part of the year when they might have grown and been aerosolized from an extramural source, a cooling tower, or simply in extramural dust. Such organisms blown through ventilation systems and inhaled might cause legionellosis of endotoxic origin[7] in immunologically compromised persons.

Recommendations for Maintaining Water Cooling Systems

As discussed above, a number of outbreaks of legionellosis either have been, or may have been, associated with airborne spread of L. pneumophila from contaminated cooling towers or evaporative condensers that were reservoirs for the organism. For many years, it has been recommended that regular programs be set up to prevent bio-fouling of heat-exchange surfaces of cooling towers and evaporative condensers.[8] Preventive efforts have been directed toward reducing the rate at which the structure of the cooling tower or evaporative condenser deteriorates in order to increase the useful life of the equipment, to prevent or control corrosion or biological or chemical deposits, and to permit continuing effective heat exchange throughout the water-cooling system. For these purposes, cooling towers or evaporative condensers should be regularly treated with chemicals that prevent slime, algae, corrosion, scale, or high concentrations of bacteria in the cooling water. If chemicals that are biocidal for L. pneumophila are included in the recommended regimen of chemical treatment for the other purposes just mentioned, the likelihood of significant growth of L. pneumophila in water cooling units, and thus the likelihood that aerosols will cause disease, should be lowered.

A preliminary report of laboratory studies on environmental decontamination of Legionella by the CDC gives some guidance on what chemicals may or may not be effective in controlling Legionella in water.[9] The report shows that 50% didecyl dimethyl ammonium chloride was effective at all concentrations studied. The concentrations of calcium hypochlorite and 2, 2-dibromo-3-nitrilopropion-amide studied were less effective. Three other products (sodium pentachlorophe-nol, an isothiazolin, and a dithiocarbamate) showed little activity in inhibiting L. pneumophila in the laboratory tests. However, CDC does not wish to imply at this time that any type of chemical treatment of cooling towers or similar equipment is necessary to prevent legionellosis, nor do we yet have data proving that any chemical treatment is effective in preventing this disease. Appropriate studies are under way. Further, we hope that public or private research organizations, and perhaps the U. S. Environmental Protection Agency (EPA), will conduct studies under actual operating conditions to determine which chemicals will prevent growth of Legionella in cooling towers or evaporative condensers.

The U.S. EPA has authority in this country to register pesticidal chemicals sold in interstate commerce. Any product used for cooling tower chemical treatment should be registered by the EPA and used in a manner consistent with the directions on the EPA-approved label of the product.

Operation and Treatment of Cooling Towers

Water should be continuously drained from cooling towers or evaporative condensers to prevent the build-up of solids left behind when some of the water evaporates as it is sprayed and circulated to be cooled. As water is drained and replaced, whatever chemicals have been added in attempts to control microbial contamination (or physical deterioration) will be diluted because of the drainage (commonly known as "blowdown"). Thus, to maintain the desired chemical concentration due to dilution by blowdown, chemicals are added either continuously or regularly in "slug" doses. The general recommendations of most firms involved in supervising chemical treatments for water-cooling equipment are to add chemical biocide in a slug dose at least once a week. Sometimes another slug dose of the same or another chemical biocide, or a chemical to control scale or corrosion, is also added later each week. This once- or twice-a-week treatment regimen has been shown over the years to be practical and reasonable; it is suggested that any products used in studying the control of *Legionella* be added according to the same schedule.

Finally, a second potential disease risk, not related in any way to legionellosis, has been observed with many water-cooling systems. Unsatisfactory, submerged inlets for potable water make-up, connected to float valves, often have been found. Cooling towers are frequently placed on the top of buildings where potable-water pressure is the lowest in the building. An air gap vertically measuring two times the diameter of the water-supply pipe *above* the overflow rim of the water reservoir must be maintained to prevent any possibility of a health risk created by back-siphonage from the cooling tower should potable-water pressure drop to or near zero at the water-supply float valve for the cooling tower.

REFERENCES

1. FRASER, D. W. This annal.
2. SANFORD, J. P. 1979. Legionnaires' Disease: One person's perspective. Ann. Int. Med. **90:** 699–703.
3. MILLER, R. P. 1979. Cooling towers and evaporative condensers. Ann. Int. Med. **90:** 667–670.
4. FLIERMANS, C. B., 10/24/78. Personal communication.
5. FLIERMANS, C. B., W. B. Cheng, L. L. Orrison & L. Thacker. 1979. Isolation of *Legionella pneumophila* from nonepidemic related aquatic habitats. Appl. & Env. Micro. **37:** 1239–1242.
6. STORCH, G., et al. 1979. Sporadic community-acquired Legionnaires' Disease in the United States: A case-control study. Ann. Int. Med. **90:** 596–600.
7. FRASER, D. W., D. C. DEUBNER, D. L. HILL & D. K. GILLIAM. 1979. Nonpneumonic, short-incubation period Legionellosis (Pontiac Fever) in men who cleaned a steam turbine condenser. Science **205:** 690–691.
8. Handbook of Industrial Water Conditioning. 1976. 7th Edit. Betz Laboratories. Trevose, Pa. 19047
9. Preliminary studies on environmental decontamination of *Legionella pneumophila*. 1979. Morbidity and Mortality Weekly Report **24:** 286–287.

PHYSICS OF AIRBORNE PARTICLES AND THEIR DEPOSITION IN THE LUNG*

Paul E. Morrow

Departments of Radiation Biology and Biophysics, Pharmacology
and Toxicology
University of Rochester
School of Medicine and Dentistry
Rochester, New York 14642

INTRODUCTION

There have been a number of books and papers published on the physics of airborne particles[1-3] and a comparable number of expositions on particulate deposition in the airways and lungs of man.[4-6] There is a large difference in the sophistication of these efforts. Often papers in both categories are by the same authors since it is well known that the respiratory deposition of particles is, to a considerable extent, described by the physical laws of particle behavior in the airborne state. In fact, it was the realization of this relationship that prompted W. Findeisen to accomplish his masterful work in Hamburg during 1931-2 described in his paper "Über das Absetzen kleiner, in der Luft Suspendierter Teilchen in der Menschlichen Lunge bei der Atmung,"[7] which was the starting point of many of the subsequent modeling efforts. Despite this rich background of information, the organizers of this conference have asked me to speak on the topic of aerosol physics and particulate deposition in the lungs. It must follow that they want a description that is uncomplicated and directed as much as possible toward airborne contagion. These will be my objectives.

Particle Size-Deposition Relationships and the Underlying Aerosol Physics

Galileo Galilei's famous experiment with objects dropped from the Tower of Pisa could not have worked except for the fact that the objects were relatively massive and the distance dropped comparatively small. Of course, the experiment works quite well with objects in a vacuum irrespective of their mass, shape, or size or the distance dropped. Almost any object falling in air will fail to follow the behavior predicted by Newton of a constant gravitational acceleration toward the earth. On the contrary, the object's acceleration rather quickly goes to zero and the velocity of the object remains constant because of the resistive force of the air. For a free-falling human body, for example this occurs at around 220 miles per hour whether it falls from 75,000 feet or 7,500 feet.

It is not surprising, therefore, that the behavior of small particles suspended in air (aerosols) is largely governed by the resistive force of air, i.e., its viscous drag. For small particles, their falling, or sedimentation, due to gravity is characterized

*This paper is based, in part, on work performed under an intra-agency contract with the U.S. Environmental Protection Agency and the U.S. Department of Energy at the University of Rochester, Department of Radiation Biology and Biophysics and has been assigned Report No. UR 3490-1723.

71

by achieving a uniform velocity almost instantaneously so their entire descent in tranquil air is at a uniform velocity. Since this velocity is the terminal velocity of the particle, it is usually referred to as such.

Stokes mathematically described the resistive force of air (F_R) to a spherical particle as follows: $F_R = 3\pi d\eta v$, where $3\pi d$ is derived from the size and shape of the particle, η is the viscosity of air, and v is the relative velocity of the sphere with respect to the air. In the case of sedimentation, the force of gravity on the particle is described by

$$F_g = \frac{\pi}{6} d^3(\rho_p - \rho_a) \cdot g.$$

This is a restatement of the familiar force = mass × acceleration equation with $(\pi/6)d^3$ being the volume of the sphere, $(\rho_{particle} - \rho_{air})$ the effective density of the particle (their product, volume × density, is the particle's mass), and g is the acceleration of gravity. When the gravitational force on the particle is matched by the resistive force of the air, the particle achieves its terminal velocity:

$$V_T = \frac{(\pi/6)d^3\rho_{eff}}{3\pi d\eta} = \frac{\rho_{eff}d^2g}{18\eta}.$$

In most cases, the density of a particle is so much greater than the density of air that the correction for the difference is insignificant. When the equation is used to describe sedimentation in some other fluid than air, then the effective ρ may be quite different from the $\rho_{particle}$ and, of course, η will also differ.

Thus, gravitational setting of particles between 1 and 50 μm diameter in air is described by Stokes Law: $V_T = (\rho d^2 g)/18\eta$. When particles are much larger than 50 μm diameter, their persistance in air is severely limited and their behavior departs from Stokes Law because the resistive force of the air is not completely described by its viscous nature; some now is due to turbulence. This is not a major problem inasmuch as particles >50 μm diameter are extremely unstable as aerosols and they have a very low probability of entering the respiratory system as we shall see subsequently.

At the other end of the particle size spectrum, particles <1 μm diameter also deviate from Stokes Law when they sediment. Again this is due to the changing nature of the air's resistance to the particle. As the particle size approaches the mean free path of air molecules, the viscous resistance of air is much lower than Stokes Law predicts; the particle is said to "slip," therefore. A slip correction factor is required to describe particulate motion for all particles in this size range (≤ 0.1 μm) whether their motion is attributed to gravity or any other force, e.g., electrostatic. Several empirical relationships have been described for the slip correction.[3]

According to the sedimentation equation, the distance a particle will travel along a circular tube, such as bronchial airway, will be directly proportional to the velocity of the particle due to air flow ($\overline{U}$) and inversely proportional to the V_T, the particle's velocity due to gravity. Therefore, in a given configuration, sedimentation is proportional to $V_T/\overline{U}$ or $\rho d^2/\overline{U}$ (remember 18η is a constant). If, for example, a particle is moving into a bronchial airway at its cross-sectional midpoint and the radius of the bronchiole is 1 cm, the length of the airway is 5 cm, the mean velocity of air (and particle) flow along the airway is 5 cm sec^{-1} and V_T is 0.1 cm sec^{-1} then, obviously, the particle will move vertically only 0.1 cm during its transit time and remain airborne, whereas, it will have also moved 5 cm axially and passed now into a more distal airway where its vertical distance to the bronchiolar wall is reduced, the value of $\overline{U}$ is also decreased (due to expanding volume of bronchial tree with each generation of branching), but V_T remains the same. This will continue to occur until the particle encounters the epithelial surface. Sedimentation is the predominant deposition process in the mid- and peripheral airways and in the transitional region of the parenchyma. It is the dominant deposition factor for particles within the 0.1-4 μm size range although it affects the deposition of all particles >0.1 μm in diameter.

We should digress briefly here to define aerodynamic diameter, d_a. This term applies to the V_T of unit density, spherical particles. For example, the V_T of a 10 μm diameter unit density sphere is ~0.3 cm sec^{-1} in normal room air. Under the identical conditions, any particle manifesting the same V_T is deemed to have a 10 μm aerodynamic diameter. One can estimate d_a from ρd^2 if the observed diameter and density of the particle are known. This lets us note, for instance, that a 3.3 μm diameter sphere with a $\rho = 9$ would have a $d_a = 10$ μm. Aerodynamic diameter is a convenient way to consider particle size, because shape, density and other factors may be unknown whereas V_T can be measured and the effective size of the particle thereby deduced. In all of the preceding equations containing ρd^2, this term can be replaced by d_a^2, since $d_a \approx \sqrt{\rho d^2}$.

Besides sedimentation, particles in the 1-50 μm diameter range experience inertial deposition or impaction. This occurs when a moving aerosol stream encounters an obstacle or is forced to make a directional change as in a branching airway. Whether or not a particle will inertially impact is related to its mass and velocity, i.e., its momentum, and its hindrance by the viscous drag of air. In the simplest case, it is a question of whether or not the aerosol particle will conform to the airstream or whether its momentum will be sufficient to force it across the streamlines where it will inelastically collide with the directing surface. The momentum of the particle in a given bronchial airway will be proportional to its mass (ρD^3) and its velocity, $\overline{U}$, which is determined by the volumetric rate of breathing $\dot{Q}$. The particle's velocity (or momentum) will therefore be higher in the trachea than in a 3rd generation bronchus since the collective cross-sectional area of 3rd generation airways is larger than that of the trachea. In all cases, the inertial motion of the particle is retarded by the viscous resistance of air which is inversely proportional to the diameter of the particle, hence, inertial deposition in a given structure can be expressed by the product $d_a^2 \cdot \overline{U}$ or $d_a^2 \dot{Q}$.

Extensive use of this basic relationship has been made, but perhaps the most interesting examples are in studes of nasal[8,9] and tracheobronchial deposition,[10,11] (FIGURE 1).

These examples indicate that experimentally-determined deposition patterns as well as those deduced from aerosol physical theory can work conjointly to predict or explain deposition behavior of particles with a d_a of >5 μm.

Let us consider briefly the only remaining particulate deposition process of importance, diffusion. There are two aspects to diffusional deposition that should be appreciated. First of all, aerosols of particles <0.1 μm diameter can be thought of as poorly-diffusible gases in matters of their airborne transport to, penetration into, and mixing within, respiratory structures. The diffusion coefficient (D) of a 0.01 μm (100 Å) diameter particle is only ~5 $\times$ 10^{-4} cm^2 sec^{-1} whereas gases commonly have coefficients around 10^{-1} cm^2 sec^{-1}. The diffusional diplacement of particles can be estimated from the Einstein equation: $\overline{\Delta}_x = 2Dt$ where $\overline{\Delta}_x$ is the mean displacement along cartesian coordinate x occurring in time t. For a 0.01 μm particle $\overline{\Delta}_x$ would be approximately 3 $\times$ 10^{-2} cms (300 μm) in one second.

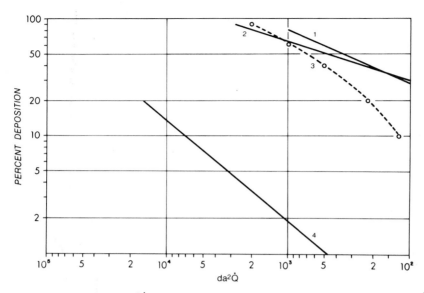

FIGURE 1. The use of $Da^2\dot{Q}$ in describing particle deposition. The parameter $Da^2\dot{Q}$ describes the inertial character of particles during breathing and correlates well with deposition in the upper airways. Curve 1, 2 and 3 describe nasal deposition and are derived from References 4, 5 and 9. Curve 4 is based on the relationship described by Lippmann and Albert[10] for particulate deposition at the level of the second generation of branching in the bronchial airways.

Secondly, both the force of, and resistance to, particle diffusion are derived from air molecules. The diffusion coefficient is described by the equation: $D = RT/N \cdot S_c/3\pi\eta d$. The term RT/N describes the kinetic energy of the air molecules responsible for the multiple interactions which cause the random movement (Brownian motion) of the particles. The term $S_c/3\pi\eta d$ describes the viscous resistance of the air to particle motion (Stokes Law) modified by the slip correction, S_c, discussed earlier. As the value of d becomes smaller, S_c becomes larger; with the resistive term diminishing, the value of D increases. Thus, diffusional deposition is important for submicroscopic particles, especially those below 0.01 μm diameter. In the size region around 0.1 μm diameter, particles are ineffectively deposited by diffusion; they are better regarded as a model of a nondiffusible gas. Particles between 0.1 and 0.5 μm are also too small to sediment appreciably or undergo inertial impaction, therefore these particles make the most stable aerosols and account for the fact that most aged aerosols, including those in the atmosphere, appear to have a median particle size in this range.

On the basis of the foregoing principles of aerosol behavior, extensions of the modeling approach pioneered by Findeisen, and experimentally obtained deposition data from human studies, a particle size-respiratory deposition relationship for man has emerged with the general form seen in FIGURE 2.

In FIGURE 2 relationship can be visualized as an estimate of the fraction of particles of each size which will be deposited in an average adult human during sedentary respiration through the nose. A recent experimental investigation by Heyder et al.[12] has provided an excellent perspective of particle deposition during mouth and nose breathing (FIGURE 3). Here the measurements are made of total deposition of particles of uniform size i.e., 0.2, 0.6, 1.0, 2.0 and 3.0 μm d_a. Although the tidal volume was constant at 1000 cm^3, the manner in which it was breathed was varied so as to produce distinctly different mean air flow rates of 125 cm^3 sec^{-1} and 1000 cm^3 sec^{-1} by changing the duration of respiratory cycle from 16 seconds to 2 seconds. The high nasal deposition efficiency for particles >2 μm and the increase in inertial deposition by higher air flows, are both noteworthy.

Airborne Microorganisms and the Implications of Deposition-Size Relationships

Experts agree that the airborne transmission of infection is a major basis for the dissemination of disease. With acute respiratory infections, for example, more than half the cases are attributable to airborne transmission.[13] The early work of Duguid[14] on the particle size of droplets generated by coughing, sneezing, and speaking showed that a wide range of droplet sizes (1–1000 μm diameter) was dispersed by each of these acts, but sneezing greatly exceeded the others in output.

Wells[15,16] also contributed much to the understanding of the airborne behavior of droplets and droplet nuclei, i.e., that which remains after partial or complete droplet evaporation. However, Wells erroneously believed that the Castelman Rayleigh theory of atomization predicts a water droplet size minimum of ~10 μm diameter, while in fact, the theory indicates this will be the approximate mean droplet size. He improperly inferred, therefore, that only by evaporation would

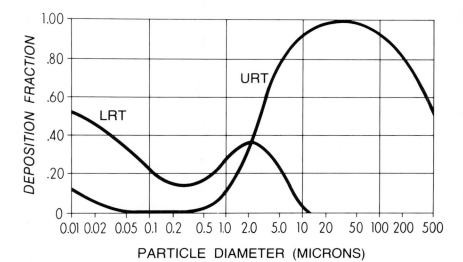

FIGURE 2. Particle size versus deposition. The URT curve describes deposition of particles in the airways above the epiglottis; LRT describes deposition in the tracheobronchial tree and alveoli. The curves are derived from theoretical and experimental sources. For particle size >1 μm diameter, the size axis is expressed as d_a.

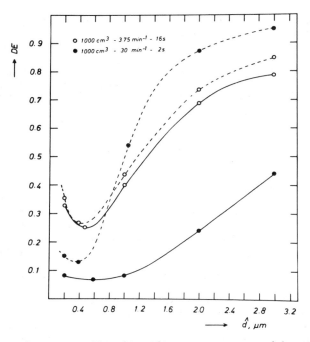

FIGURE 3. Mouth versus nasal breathing. This curve compares total deposition for nose breathing (dashed line) and mouth breathing (solid line) at a constant total volume (1000 cm³), but differing respiratory frequencies. (From Heyder et al.[12] By permission of Pergamon Press.)

spray droplets, from an atomizer, sneeze, etc., be formed that were <10 μm diameter.

Even in the 1930s, it was generally appreciated that small droplets of pure water (<5 μm diameter) evaporate in <1 sec even in water-saturated air. Saliva and respiratory secretions contain ~1 percent solute which causes droplet evaporation rate to be significantly slower than water. One can predict that the droplet nucleus from a 10 μm diameter droplet, containing one percent solute, will experience a volume reduction of $3\sqrt{100/1}$ or 4.64; therefore, 10/4.64 or 2.15 μm will be the predicted diameter of the resulting droplet nucleus (assuming a solute density $\rho = 1$). For common salts ($\rho = 2.3$), the diameter of the nuclei will be closer to 1 μm. The size of nuclei can be calculated rather precisely if the properties and concentration of the solute are known and the nuclei form compact, more-or-less spherical particles of the same ρ as the solute. It is a far more difficult task to predict how quickly and completely droplet evaporation will proceed. Rauoult's law is useful for estimating the evaporation rate of droplets of simple solutions, but if the droplets contain mixed salts and/or macromolecular species, e.g., proteins, and/or have appreciable surface charge, then theoretical estimations are hopelessly complex; one must study the droplet evaporation experimentally. We conclude that the final state of hydration of complex droplet nuclei can vary enormously; some will maintain a state of wetness, others will progressively dry and the temperature and humidity of the air will affect the outcome. This uncertain picture of droplet behavior associated with sneezing and coughing provides the basis for a controversy which continues today: Are droplets or droplet nuclei more important as vectors for airborne transmission of infection? This controversy, thereby impinges on the issues of airborne stability, particle size, and viability.

According to Duguid's analysis of sneeze droplets, the most common droplet or droplet nuclei diameter lies between 4 and 8 μm. This particle size, according to our size deposition relationship (FIGURE 2) is efficiently trapped by the nose. That the secretions of the nasal and tracheobronchial airways translocate in both directions seems established, so the efficiency of nasal deposition may not completely determine the ultimate loci of infection. Quite apart from this argument, there is a possibility that Duguid's assessment was faulty or incomplete. Certainly it was severely handicapped by the evaluation method used especially in quantifying the smallest droplets or droplet nuclei. Lidwell[17] showed (FIGURE 4), using Duguid's data, that sneezing produces large number of droplets (10^6) between 5 and 50 μm and these can be expected to form a nuclei distribution with roughly one-fifth the droplet diameters. Additionally, he showed that the number of viable units per milliliter of secretion was a good index of the number of airborne droplets produced; by nebulization of the

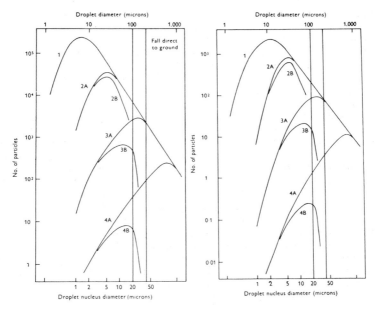

FIGURE 4. Droplet distributions expelled from the nose and mouth. These curves are taken from Lidwell.[17] The left set depicts the number and size of droplets emitted by an average sneeze (1); the size of droplets carrying one or more infective units (2A); the nuclei derived from aerosol 2A by evaporation (2B); and changes in the distributions associated with areal ventilation (3A, B and 4AB), these being irrelevant to the present discussion. The right set depicts the same information for droplets emitted by two coughs or speaking loudly 4000 words.

secretion; in other words, most of the droplets assayed had one or more infective units. With coughing and speaking, a similar picture of droplet size distribution is produced, but the total number of infective units expelled is less by a factor 10^{-2} to 10^{-3} (FIGURE 4).

Lidwell and coworkers also examined airborne streptococcus-carrying particles in clerical offices and found a dominance of droplets around 10 μm diameter. This corresponded quite closely to the streptococcal size distribution he obtained with normal saliva.[18]

An interesting study cited by Lidwell, performed by Eichenwald and coworkers, showed that the spread of staphylococcal infection in a nursery was mainly associated with particles less than 5 μm diameter.[19]

Davies and Nobel[20] examined airborne particles of desquamated skin and found the median aerodynamic size was ~8 μm. Common dust particles in the air have a broad size distribution with the greatest numerical frequency residing between 0.1 and 1 μm diameter. Whether these are also typical of dusts generated by shaking handkerchiefs or bedding, both highly effective methods of dispersing infective units, is not established although some evidence tends to suggest they are not. Rubbo et al.,[21] for instance, concluded the airborne units were associated with fiber nuclei, i.e., textile fiber particles that are much smaller than fibers. Information about the size and aerodynamic nature of these fiber nuclei is unknown.

From the foregoing account of the size of airborne infective units, one must conclude that nasal deposition will be especially important for bacteria, but there will always be airborne infective units which can penetrate the nose with a reasonable probability (10–30%); these droplets or nuclei will be mainly <5 μm aerodynamic diameter. They obviously cannot be smaller than the infective unit. This condition is underscored by studies of viral transmission where the droplet size is very much larger than the infective unit in contrast to bacteria and fungi where their intrinsic size range is comparable.

A number of interesting studies with viral aerosols show that particles below 2 μm d_a are especially prominent and important. Edward et al. indicated the mean size of airborne viral units was 1.3–2.3 μm diameter.[22] Couch et al.[23] and Akers,[24] using Jensen's data, deduced that more than ¾ of the airborne viral units had a d_a <3 μm using an Andersen impactor. Akers cited many additional studies of viruses with similar results, so a strong prima facie case is drawn that nasal penetration and broncho-alveolar deposition is greatly increased with airborne viruses compared to bacteria. The only problem with this conclusion is that it is based on studies of aerosolized solutions inoculated with different viruses: the chief determinants of the airborne particle size were probably the aerosol generation system and the solution composition, factors which seemingly made little imprint on the investigators interpretations. The solutions, used by the investigators, for example, contained gelatin, alantoic fluid, and buffers, as well as the viruses. Aerosol generators yield different droplet distributions and a given generator will produce different distributions as the operating conditions are varied. Dimmick[25] has discussed these relationships in the generation of infective aerosols and some of the dilemmas this creates for the investigator.

Clinical studies of the transmission of viral respiratory infections have not been helpful in establishing the size or nature of airborne viral units.[26] This is indeed unfortunate, so the suitability of the experimental models for viral transmission remains uncertain, notwithstanding their acceptability on intuitive grounds.

From the foregoing information on airborne microbes, it is evident that any model of respiratory deposition will predict that the nasal airways will be the dominant deposition site for virtually all airborne forms of bacteria and fungi. This may also be the case for the smaller infective units, e.g., viruses, phage, since most transmitter materials, sputum droplets, fibers, and desquamated skin, appear to be in a similar size range (4-10 μm d_a) and they control the sites of deposition.

Nevertheless, most studies show a broad distribution of droplet or droplet-nuclei sizes which extend well below 4 μm d_a. These aerosols and those particles that constitute the usual atmospheric aerosol, constitute a particulate population which can deposit throughout the respiratory system. How important this small-er-sized aerosol is compared to the larger is speculative as there are no definitive studies, and other factors, e.g., translocation of infective units from one respiratory site to another, the number of infective units per deposition site, and the number of infective units per transmission unit hinder any evaluation.

REFERENCES

1. GREEN, H. & W. R. LANE. 1964. Particulate Clouds, Dusts, Smokes and Mists. 2nd edit. E. and F. N. Spoor Ltd. London.
2. MERCER, T. T. 1973. Aerosol Technology in Hazard Evaluation. Academic Press, New York.
3. NATIONAL RESEARCH COUNCIL 1979. Airborne Particles. University Park Press, Baltimore, Md.
4. TASK GROUP ON LUNG DYNAMICS. 1966. Deposition and retention models for internal dosimetry of the human respiratory tract. Health Physics 12: 173-207.
5. LANDAHL, H. D., T. N. TRACEWELL & W. H. LASSEN. 1951. Retention of airborne particulates in the human lung: II. Am. Med. Assoc. Arch. Ind. Hyg. Occup. Med. 3: 359-366.
6. PALMES, E. D. & M. LIPPMANN. 1977. Influence of respiratory air space dimensions on aerosol deposition. In Inhaled Particles IV,359 W. H. Walton Ed.: 127-136. Pergamon Press. London.
7. FINDEISEN, W. 1935. Über das Absetzen kleiner in der Luft suspendierter Teichen in der menschlichen Lunge bei der Atmung. Pflüg. Arch. ges Physiol. 236: 367-379.
8. HOUNAM, R. F., A. BLACK & M. WALSH. 1971. The deposition of aerosol particles in the nasopharyngeal region of the human respiratory tract. J. Aerosol Sci. 2: 47-61.
9. LANDAHL, H. O. & T. N. TRACEWELL. 1949. Penetration of airborne particulates through the human nose. II. J. Ind. Hyg. Toxicol. 31: 55-59.
10. LIPPMANN, M. & R. E. ALBERT. 1969. The effect of particle size on the regional deposition of inhaled aerosols in the human respiratory tract. Amer. Ind. Hyg. Assoc. J. 30: 257-275.
11. JOHNSTON, J. R., K. D. ISLES & D. C. F. MUIR. 1977. Inertial deposition of particles in human branching airways. In Inhaled Particles, IV, Part 1. W. H. Walton, Ed. : 61-74. Pergamon Press. New York.
12. HEYDER, J., L. ARMRUSTER, J. GEBHART, E. GREIN & W. STAHLHOFEN. 1975. Total deposition of aerosol particles in the human respiratory tract for nose and mouth breathing. J. Aerosol Sci. 6: 311-328.
13. REILY, R. L. 1980. Airborne Infection In Pulmonary Diseases and Disorders. A.P. Fishman, Ed. Chap. 90. 1010-1014. McGraw-Hill. New York.
14. DUGUID, J. P. 1946. The size and the duration of air-carriage of respiratory droplets and droplet-nuclei. J. Hyg. 44: 471-479.
15. WELLS, W. F. 1934. On airborne infection. Study II. Droplets and droplet-nuclei. Amer. J. Hyg. 20: 611-618.
16. WELLS, W. F., Ed. 1955. Airborne Contagion and Air Hygiene. Harvard University Press. Cambridge, Mass.

17. LIDWELL, O. M. 1967. Take-off of bacteria and viruses. *In* Airborne Microbes. P. H. Gregory and J. L. Monteith, Eds.: 116–137. Cambridge University Press. London.
18. KINGSTON, D., O. M. LIDWELL & R. E. O. WILLIAMS. 1962. The epidemiology of the common cold. III. The effect of ventilation, air disinfection and room size. J. Hyg. **60:** 341–352.
19. EICHENWALD, H. F., O. KOTSEVALOV & L. A. FOSSO. 1960. The "cloud-baby"—an example of bacterial-viral interaction. Amer. J. Dis. Child. **100:** 161–170.
20. DAVIES, R. R. & W. C. NOBEL. 1962. Dispersal of bacteria on desquamated skin. Lancet **2:** 1295–1297.
21. RUBBO, S. D. & J. SAUNDERS. 1963. Liberation of organisms from contaminated textiles. J. Hyg. **61:** 507–513.
22. EDWARD, D. G., W. J. ELFORD & P. O. LAIDLAW. 1943. Studies on airborne virus infections. I. Experimental technique and preliminary observations on influenza and infectious ectromelia. J. Hyg. **43:** 1–10.
23. COUCH, R. B., P. J. GERONE, T. R. CATE, W. R. GRIFFETH, D. W. ALLING & V. KNIGHT. 1965. Preparation and properties of a small particle aerosol of coxsackie A_2. Proc. Soc. Exp. Biol. Med. **118:** 818–822.
24. AKERS, T. G. 1969. Survival of airborne virus, phage and other minute microbes. *In* An Introduction to Experimental Aerobiology. Chap. 12. R. L. Dimmick and A. G. Akers, Eds. Wiley-Interscience Publishers. New York.
25. DIMMICK, R. L. 1969. Mechanics of aerosols. *In* An Introduction to Experimental Aerobiology. Chap. 1. R. L. Dimmick and A. G. Akers, Eds. Wiley-Interscience Publishers. New York.
26. PAPPAGIANIS, D. 1969. Some characteristics of respiratory infection in man. *In* An Introduction to Experimental Aerobiology. Chap. 16. R. L. Dimmick and A. G. Akers, Eds. Wiley-Interscience Publishers. New York.

A TRIBUTE TO WILLIAM FIRTH WELLS

Edward C. Riley

Box 312 AA, Route 8
Fort Myers, Florida 33901

I first met Professor William F. Wells in 1933, shortly after Franklin Roosevelt had closed the banks but before repeal of the Volstead Act. I was studying sanitary engineering at Harvard but had run out of money. The dean, Gordon Fair, discovered an obscure trust fund established by a plumbers union for a fellowship in sanitary engineering. I was awarded the fellowship with Professor Wells as my tutor. The financial aid was welcome but I had no idea for a project and had not met Professor Wells.

Wells taught in both the School of Public Health and the Engineering College and his office in Pierce Hall was dingy and unimpressive. This slender, middle-aged man with black hair, dark eyes and a black mustache had a quizzical expression and a diffident manner. Puffing on the ever present briar pipe and gazing off into the distance, he was the picture of an absent-minded professor. He had recently developed an air centrifuge for sampling air for living organisms and suggested that I test the air around the Cambridge activated sludge sewage treatment plant for evidence of contamination by organisms from the human intestinal tract. Although not enthusiastic, I accepted his suggestion and this study provided not only material for my thesis but also an opportunity to work with a talented and dedicated investigator.

In 1934 a Harvard degree was no guarantee of a job and when Professor Wells asked me to join him in "An investigation of the air of textile mills with special reference to the influence of artificial humidification"[1] I was happy to accept the opportunity. This study of 14 textile mills in Lowell, Lawrence, Fall River and New Bedford was supported by the Massachusetts State Health Department as a follow-up to a similar study carried out by Clark and Gage in 1912.[2]

While there was legitimate concern for the health of workers exposed to airborne organisms from contaminated humidifying water, Wells saw the study as an opportunity to test his concepts and expand his understanding of airborne infection. At the time he was seeking an index, like the *E. Coli* index for contamination of drinking water, for human contamination of air in occupied spaces. In addition to the mill air samples he needed throat cultures from healthy subjects for comparison. For this he enlisted my brother, Dick, then a struggling and impecunious medical student. The textile mills study started an ongoing friendship and collaboration that continued through thick and thin until Wells' death in 1963 in the Baltimore VA Hospital, a span of nearly 30 years.

I have a few slides from this period which show the equipment used in the mill study and some of Wells' deductions. The first shows Professor Wells examining one of the tubes from the air centrifuge. Melted agar was poured into the tube and as it rotated in the centrifuge the agar formed a film over the inside of the glass tube and as air was drawn through the tube, centrifugal force deposited airborne particulates on the agar film. After an incubation period colonies of organisms became visible wherever an infectious particle had been deposited. The second slide shows the field equipment used in the mill study. The standard mill cart or dolly provided a convenient carrier for two Wells

81

0077-8923/80/0353-0081 $01.75/0 © 1980, NYAS

centrifuges and other equipment. If you look closely between the two centrifuges you can see a shelf supporting two Petri dishes. This arrangement permitted simultaneous collection of volume samples by centrifuge and settling samples on the Petri dishes. From the ratio of the settled sample count to the volume count, Wells determined settling velocities and equivalent diameters for airborne particles and refined his concepts of droplet nuclei. The last slide summarizes the inferences Wells drew from his studies up to the publication of the mill study in 1937.[1] The solid lines indicate geometric normal distributions; Wells deduced that the curve on the left with a median particle diameter of about 2.5 microns represented droplet nuclei from humidifying water and the middle one showing a median particle diameter of about 20 microns was comprised of bacteria-laden dust particles from raw material, either cotton or wool. The dotted lines indicate the mix of these two sources in various sections of the mills. The curve on the right represented coarse particles settled on outside samples in the vicinity of the mills.

I never knew what the Massachusetts State Department of Health did with that report but I know that through this study Dick and I acquired an appreciation of and a respect for Professor Wells as a person and as a researcher. His concepts of "airborne contagion and air hygiene"[3] initiated a reevaluation of mechanisms of dissemination of contagion which is still in progress. The variety of titles for papers at this conference on airborne contagion indicates the scope of this reevaluation.

INHALATION ANTHRAX

Philip S. Brachman

Bureau of Epidemiology
Center for Disease Control
Atlanta, Georgia 30333

Introduction

Inhalation anthrax, now primarily only of historical interest, remains an intriguing disease. When the rare case occurs, it raises epidemiologic questions that are difficult to answer.

At the Second International Conference on Aerobiology in 1966,[1] I reported in detail on a field experiment designed to study some of the clinical and epidemiologic features of this disease. In the study we exposed 91 cynomolgus monkeys (*Macaca fascicularis*) to naturally occurring aerosols containing *Bacillus anthracis* in a goat-hair processing mill; the resultant anthrax mortality rate was 25.3%. I discussed the pathologic findings and the dose-response relationships resulting from what in effect was chronic exposure to *B. anthracis*.

Today, I will briefly review the 18 cases of inhalation anthrax in humans that have been reported in the United States since 1900 and summarize a few of the more recent cases to point up some of the epidemiologic details of inhalation anthrax as currently seen in the United States.

Historical Aspects

The history of anthrax began in biblical times with one of the so-called great plagues, which is believed to have been anthrax. Inhalation anthrax was not specifically described, however, until the mid-1800s, when it was recognized as a significant problem among British woolsorters who worked in the textile industry, especially those employed in Bradford, England.[2] In 1837, mohair (a type of goat hair) from Asia Minor and alpaca from Peru were first introduced into the developing Bradford textile industry. Soon after, a mysterious and rapidly fatal illness began to occur among the sorters, who because they primarily sorted wool were known as wool sorters, and the disease was referred to as woolsorters' disease. However, the disease was the result of contact not with wool, but with goat hair or alpaca. A similar disease, though not as common, began to be seen in Germany in persons who handled rags, and the disease was known as ragpickers' disease.

From 1847 to 1877, as woolsorters' disease became more prominent, information accumulated concerning its clinical pattern, virulence and association with imported goat hair and alpaca. Workers became selective as to what batches of mohair they would sort.

In the late 1870s, Bell[3] studied inhalation anthrax among textile workers; he identified the organisms in blood which he used to transmit the disease by inoculation into mice and rabbits. To prevent the occurrence of the disease, Bell recommended that manufacturers wash potentially dangerous material before having it sorted, an action adopted by some manufacturers.

In 1880 a coroner's jury, having investigated one publicized death due to

83

0077-8923/80/0353-0083 $01.75/0 © 1980, NYAS

inhalation anthrax, recommended that bales of hair be steeped in salt water for not less than 12 hours and that they be washed at least twice in water at a temperature of 120° before being sorted.[2] They also made recommendations concerning ventilation and methods of cleaning work areas. These recommendations were put into effect in the early 1880's, which led to a decrease in the number of cases of woolsorters' disease.

An Anthrax Investigation Board for Bradford and District was formed in 1905[4] to further study the problem and make additional recommendations. A bacteriologist, F. W. Eurich, was appointed to classify materials according to the degree of risk of anthrax and to carry out experiments as to the practicality of lowering the risk of disease following manipulation of certain classes of wool and hair.

Over the past 20 years Eurich processed 200,000 cultures and bacteriologically analyzed more than 14,000 specimens of alpaca, mohair, and wool. His investigations demonstrated that the presence of B. anthracis was associated with the "general dirtiness" and blood contamination of the fibers. He classified goat hair from East India, Persia, and Turkey as the most heavily contaminated and evaluated the effectiveness of hot water, dry heat, formaldehyde, formalin gas, white wash, disinfectants, and several other compounds in killing spores. Eurich found that formaldehyde appeared to be the best disinfectant; in cooperation with an inspector of factories he developed a method of washing the fibers with an alkaline solution and formaldehyde. This destroyed anthrax spores in goat hair.

The Anthrax Prevention Act of 1919 stated that mohair, raw wool, and alpaca from specific areas could be imported into Great Britain but they had to be decontaminated at the government Wool Disinfection Station in Liverpool, which opened in 1921, before being processed.[2] Subsequently, inhalation anthrax was seen at a significantly lower rate among woolsorters; no cases have been reported since 1939.

Eurich also noted that there may be some relationship between woolsorters' disease and certain chronic health conditions, such as alcoholism, which I will comment on later.

One additional point of interest is that the Anthrax Investigation Board noted in 1918 that there was worldwide interest in inhalation anthrax and hoped "that the assistance of the United States in the war with anthrax would be as useful and effective as the aid had so effectively rendered to the Allied cause in the great conflict just ended."[5]

Clinical Aspects

Before reviewing the occurrence of inhalation anthrax in the United States, let me first briefly summarize its clinical aspects. The classic clinical picture is that of a biphasic disease. The initial stage consists of the insidious onset of mild fever, malaise, fatigue, myalgia, nonproductive cough, and at times a sensation of precordial oppression.[5] There are few objective findings aside from fever. Rhonchi may be heard on auscultation of the lungs. This initial phase typically lasts for several days, following which there may be some improvement in the clinical condition.

The second stage develops suddenly with the onset of acute dyspnea and subsequent cyanosis. The patient may appear moribund with accelerated pulse and respiration rate. The body temperature may be mildly elevated, or it may be subnormal because of shock. Stridor may occur perhaps as a result of partial extrinsic obstruction of the trachea by enlarged mediastinum nodes. Profuse perspiration is frequently present. Physical examination of the chest reveals moist, crepitant rales and signs of pleural effusion. Consciousness typically is maintained until death, but with meningeal involvement there may be disorientation, coma, and meningismus. A chest roentgenogram typically shows widening of the mediastinum. The average duration of the acute stage is less than 24 hours, which almost always ends in death.

Diagnosis of inhalation anthrax during the first stage is difficult since the signs and symptoms are that of a mild respiratory disease, and frequently the diagnosis is a "cold," influenza, or bronchitis. In the second stage the diagnosis is frequently cardiac failure or a cardiovascular accident. Though blood cultures may be positive in the acute phase, death usually ensues before the organism can be identified.

Pathogenesis

Historically, there were two theories on the pathogenesis of inhalation anthrax.[7] One was that the inhaled spores are phagocytosed by macrophages and transported through the alveoli to the mediastinum, where germination occurred and toxin was produced by the vegetative cells.[8] The other theory was "that the primary lesion was an erosion of the trachael bronchial mucosa—(similar to a cutaneous lesion) usually occurring near the point of bifurcation," and that pneumonia developed secondary to the initial point of entry.[9] Buchner[10] in 1888 infected rabbits, guinea pigs, and mice with clouds of B. anthracis spores and took sections of the lungs at intervals after exposure, but was unable to demonstrate the site of germination of the spores. In the 1940s Young, Zelle, and Lincoln[11] and Barnes[12] exposed animals to clouds of B. anthracis spores in the laboratory and determined that involvement of the pulmonary tissue was secondary to the systemic disease but were unable to determine the original site of invasion of the spores and the exact method by which they were transported. Druett, Henderson, Packman, and Peacock[13] exposed guinea pigs and monkeys to clouds of homogenous particles containing B. anthracis spores and surmised that infection of the animals occurred most effectively following inhalation of single spores of approximately 1 micron in diameter, though with particles up to a diameter of 5 microns there was only slightly less effectiveness. With particles larger than 5 microns there was a remarkedly rapid fall off in infectivity. Ross instilled liquid suspensions of B. anthracis spores intratracheally in guinea pigs and serially examined the tissues from these animals; he thus demonstrated that the spores were usually phagocytized within a matter of minutes by macrophages present in the alveoli, transported across the alveolor membrane and carried by the draining lymphatics, into the sinusoids of the lymph nodes where germination of the spores occurred with development of vegetative forms.[14] When the vegetative forms escaped from the macrophages, rapid multiplication occurred, and the bacilli were disseminated throughout the tissue. The toxin causes hemorrhage, edema, and necrosis. Since the organisms are initially localized in the mediastinal nodes, the initial and major site of involvement is the mediastinum; toxin causes massive hemorrhagic mediastinitis, which is typical of inhalation anthrax. Once a sufficient level of toxin has been reached, death almost invariably follows despite sterilization of the vascular system by antibiotics. It is clear that without preexisting pulmonary disease no true primary respiratory infection develops; secondary pneumonia has been reported.

Another acute-exposure study that added to our knowledge about inhalation anthrax was performed by Albrink and Goodlow,[15] who exposed chimpanzees to clouds of B. anthracis spores. When two animals were exposed to 35,000 spores, they had blood cultures positive for B. anthracis but no evidence of clinical disease. Two other chimpanzees were exposed to 40,000 and 65,000 spores respectively; both developed bacteremia on the first or second postexposure day and died on the sixth postexposure day. The animals appeared to be normal until approximately 4–7 hours before death and died on the eighth postexposure day. At autopsy, there was no evidence of pneumonia, but acute hemorrhagic mediastinitis with edema in the mediastinal area was present. The architecture of the tracheobronchial lymph nodes and others in the mediastinal area was obliterated by hemorrhage.

Inhalation Anthrax in the United States

In the United States, only 5% of anthrax cases are inhalation anthrax, the rest are cutaneous; gastrointestinal cases have never been reported here.[16] Eighteen cases of inhalation anthrax have been reported in the American literature since 1900. (TABLE 1) Sixteen were fatal. Ten of the cases occurred sporadically. Three of the cases that occurred over a 10-year span may have been associated with one tannery, and five of the cases that occurred over a 10-week period were part of an epidemic at one goat-hair-processing mill.[17] All of the inhalation cases were related to industrial sources of infection (except the two laboratory-associated cases); whereas 78% of the cutaneous cases were industry related and 22% agricultural.

Analysis of the type of industrial contact in the inhalation cases is shown also in TABLE 1; 10 patients had direct contact with the industrial source, and three had indirect contact (one patient was a home craftsman and two had laboratory contact). In two cases the source of infection was unknown. TABLE 2 compares the source of infection of inhalation and cutaneous industrial cases; the similarities can be seen.

Case Reports

To illustrate some of the clinical and epidemiologic features and protean aspects of inhalation anthrax, I will review a few of the cases that have been investigated.

The first case represents a patient who had no known predisposing ill health

TABLE 1

18 CASES OF INHALATION ANTHRAX, BY INDUSTRIAL CONTACT,
UNITED STATES 1900–1978

Industry (goat hair/skins or sheep wool/skins)	
Direct	10
Indirect	3
Home Craftsman	1
Laboratory	2
Unknown	2
Total	18

TABLE 2

INDUSTRIAL HUMAN ANTHRAX CASES, UNITED STATES
BY SOURCES OF INFECTIONS 1900–1978

Source of Infection	Inhalation 1900–1978		Total 1955–1978	
	Number	Percent	Number	Percent
Goat Hair	9	53	112	62
Goat Skins	2	12	16	9
Goat Hair or Skins	1	6	—	—
Wool	1	6	34	19
Tannery	1	6	—	—
Meat, Bones	—	—	8	4
Rugs	1	6	—	—
Laboratory	2	6	—	—
Unknown	1	6	11	6
Total	18	101	181	100

conditions and who had only brief exposure to contaminated aerosols. In 1961, a 51-year-old woman in good health reported weakness, chills, a nonproductive cough, and a dull chest pain, which eventually became constant, in her substernal area. Her physician diagnosed this as a viral illness. The following day her condition became worse, with generalized aches, abdominal pain, and temperature of 102°F, and she was hospitalized. On physical examination she had occasional bilateral wheezes over the lungs. Her white blood cell count was 13,100/mm^3. A chest roentgenogram revealed obliteration of the left hemidiaphragm and costophrenic angle with moderate prominence of the left hilar region. That evening she became cyanotic, and the following morning she went into shock and died.

At autopsy, she had pleural effusion, classic hemorrhagic edematous mediastinitis as seen in inhalation anthrax, and acute splenitis.

The textile mill where she worked processed imported goat hair. Prior to a company-wide vaccination program in 1957, the mill had reported one case of cutaneous anthrax per 100 mill employees per year and had never reported a case of inhalation anthrax. The patient had never been vaccinated against anthrax. She worked in an office next to an equipment storage area. She occasionally handled samples of the finished product but only infrequently handled samples of raw goat hair. Rarely did she walk into the mill, but on the day preceding the onset of her illness she did visit the carding room, a relatively dusty environment where raw hair is handled. An environmental sampling program after she died revealed gross contamination of the raw goat hair being processed as well as of the mill itself.

The most recent reported case of inhalation anthrax in the United States occurred in 1976 and involved a 32-year-old home craftsman.[18] Five days before being hospitalized he began complaining of fever and a sore throat. During the next five days his complaints included left-side chest pains, headaches, nausea, and anorexia. Physical examination at the time of admission revealed an acutely ill patient with decreased breath sounds over the left lower lung field. Neurologic examination demonstrated an inability to carry out simple commands, left upper and lower extremity spasticity, disconjugate gaze, and intact tendon reflexes.

X-ray examination of the chest displayed a moderate-size left pleural effusion and enlargement of the left pulmonary hilus. The cerebrospinal fluid protein was 220 mg/dl and glucose 65 mg/dl. Large gram-positive rods were seen in the spinal fluid and in the left pleural effusion fluid. The patient was treated with intravenous penicillin and intramuscular streptomycin, but died 28 hours after admission.

The autopsy revealed classic evidence of inhalation anthrax and, in addition, subarachnoid hemorrhage. A small chromophobe adenoma of the pituitary gland was present.

The patient was a self-employed artistic weaver who worked in his own home with yarn obtained from commercial sources. The yarn he was working with had been imported from Pakistan and contained various animal fibers. It was cultured and found to be positive for B. anthracis.

These two cases represent individuals with no known predisposing conditions as related to developing inhalation anthrax. Their exposures were brief and at least in the last case unusual.

This next case raises a question concerning the association between several potential predisposing health factors and inhalation anthrax in an individual with only sporadic exposure to B. anthracis.

The patient, a 53-year old man, had been employed in a biological laboratory as an electrician for six years before his terminal illness. His work took him into many buildings where various laboratory activities were in process. He had had some contact with beryllium but not in excess of that experienced by his coworkers. In 1957 laryngeal carcinoma in situ was noted and removed. In May 1958 two months before his terminal illness, a routine physical examination including a chest roentgenogram was negative. Two weeks before the onset of his terminal illness, he received yellow fever, tularemia, and smallpox vaccines and a brucellosis skin test. He had never received anthrax vaccine.

On June 29, 1958, he experienced the abrupt onset of fever, headache, and muscle aches, and on the following day was admitted to a hospital, where his rectal temperature was 103.6°F. He was not acutely ill. The white blood cell count was 8,100/mm^3 with 84% neutrophils. A chest film revealed symmetrical widening of the upper mediastinum, apical capping, and a focal area of consolidation in the right mid-lung field.

On the day after admission, his white count had risen to 15,000/mm^3 and repeat roentgenograms showed linear atelectasis in the left lower lobe and fluid in the left base. He was started on intravenous tetracycline, 2 grams a day.

During the following several days he developed a slight cough, bilateral pleural effusion, and tachycardia; his blood cultures were positive for B. anthracis. On the sixth day of his disease he was cyanotic and developed expiratory wheezes over the right lung; roentgenograms showed focal areas of density throughout the lung field, and bilateral pleural fluid; the mediastinal widening persisted. He became more restless and apprehensive; his breathing became labored and he expired on the same day.

A significant difference between this case and previous cases was the more graduate development of the acute phase without any evidence of improvement between the two phases of the disease.

At autopsy the principal pathologic findings were those of edematous, hemorrhagic mediastinitis as seen in inhalation anthrax. A hemorrhagic area in the middle lobe of the right lung was present, and beryllium was found in trace amounts in the same area. Old fibrotic and calcific changes in the pulmonary tissues associated with anthracosis were noted and were felt to be the cause of some lymphatic obstruction. Additionally, there were some minor anatomic abnormalities of the upper respiratory passage.

Environmental culturing in buildings in which he had worked during the two weeks prior to his terminal illness revealed B. anthracis organisms in small numbers in three of the eight buildings; organisms were recovered from the surface of his tool pouch.

It is hypothesized that he was exposed to B. anthracis spores while working in one of the buildings in which B. anthracis spores had previously been handled. He had inhaled the organisms through an upper respiratory tract with some minor anatomical abnormalities that may have reduced the effectiveness of the filtering mechanism. Because of the multiple immunization procedures two weeks prior to his illness, his resistance to a new infection may have been reduced. In addition to generalized toxemia, because of the defective pulmonary tissue (old fibrosis) and the focus of beryllium involvement in one lung, secondary pulmonary changes developed.

The next case portrays another individual with several compromising health conditions, but only peripheral and probably brief contact with B. anthracis.[19] The patient, a 46-year-old man with a history of alcoholism, recurrent pancreatitis, and diabetes, had worked in a metal fabricator shop for only three weeks when the plant closed for a 2-week summer vacation. Six days later he was found mildly intoxicated and complaining of fatigue. For the next two days he was tremulous, but this was attributed to his alcoholic indulgence. On the following day, or three days after onset of symptoms, he appeared to have improved, he was alert, and only a chronic cough persisted. One day later he fell out of bed and was noted by his wife to be confused, lethargic, and perspiring. His family physician found him to be unresponsive, perspiring, and cold, with shallow respirations. He was taken to a local hospital.

Pertinent physical findings included loud tracheal gurgling with bilateral basilar pulmonary rales. A chest roentgenogram revealed a paratracheal mass, basilar pneumonia, and pleural effusion on the right side. He had a hematocrit of 50 percent and a white blood cell count of $15,800/mm^3$ with 50 percent neutrophils and 41 percent band forms.

The patient was treated with insulin, intravenous fluid, chloramphenicol and penicillin. He became hypotensive, was refactory to pressor agents, and died six hours after admission.

At autopsy the mediastinum and mediastinal lymph nodes were hemorrhagic and edematous as seen in inhalation anthrax. There was 1500 cc of bloody right pleural effusion. The pulmonary parenchyma was congested, but there were no areas of consolidation. Microscopically, the brain was covered with diffuse hemorrhagic leptomeningitis, and the lungs were congested, with patchy areas of focal hemorrhage. Large gram-positive bacilli were seen in the mediastinal lymph nodes, meninges, and lungs. Bacillus anthracis was recovered from the hemorrhagic mediastinal lymph nodes.

The epidemiologic investigation revealed that the metal fabricating plant in which the patient and 35 other employees worked was located across a 60-foot alley from the building that housed the goat-hair-processing mill associated with the 1957 epidemic of inhalation anthrax. In the period from January 1941 to June 1957 the mill had reported 136 cases of cutaneous anthrax, or 8.2% cases per year. Following the epidemic of inhalation anthrax in 1957, all employees had been vaccinated. During the 10 years following vaccination, only four cases of cutaneous anthrax or 0.4 cases per year, had been reported. The source of goat hair remained unchanged. The dustiest operations involved in processing the imported goat hair were performed in the corner of the mill closest to the metal fabricating shop. This operation created heavy aerosols that could be discharged into the alley by means of 2 window exhaust fans and through open doors and windows facing the alley.

Six months after the case occurred, an environmental sampling program was conducted. In the mill, B. anthracis was recovered from 25% of the gross samples of hair obtained from unopened bales and from 70 (14.3%) of 489 surface swabs taken in the mill building. Twenty-five percent of the specimens obtained in the early-processing areas (those nearest the metal fabricating plant) were positive for B. anthracis, whereas only 6.2% of the swabs taken from the remaining processing areas were positive. In the picking area 1,190 liters of air were sampled, and three isolations of B. anthracis were made. Assuming a constant exposure, a worker breathing at a rate of 7 cubic meters per eight hours would inhale approximately 200 spores of B. anthracis particles less than 5 microns in size.

A total of 150 surface swabs were taken at the metal fabricating plant subsequent to renovation of the plant. Three of the swabs were positive for B. anthracis.

The epidemiologic and laboratory studies clearly revealed the opportunities for aerosol spread of B. anthracis from the mill into the alley and subsequently into the metal fabrication plant building. The workers confirmed that they often saw clouds of dust emanating from the open doors and windows of the picking and blending area of the mill. The patient worked in one end of the metal fabricating shop about 300 feet from the most contaminated area of the mill; however, on the last afternoon prior to vacation (six days before he became ill) the patient had worked for three to four hours in the alley directly opposite the picking and blending area. Weather records recorded temperatures in the 80s on this day with no rain showers during the work day. The windows and doors of the mill building would have been opened under these conditions.

The clinical course and pathologic findings confirmed the diagnosis of inhalation anthrax. The projected incubation period of six days resembled those of previous cases. We do not know whether chronic alcoholism, diabetes, and chronic pancreatitis could have predisposed the patient to inhalation anthrax.

The next case is that of a young man with a chronic disease, sarcoidosis, who developed inhalation anthrax. The patient was a 28-year-old-man with a 2½-year-old, biopsy-proven history of sarcoidosis.[20] In April 1957 he gave a one week history of increasing dyspnea, frequent coughing, and weight loss of seven pounds. Chest X-rays were similar to previous films. He was given prednisolone, 5 mg every four hours, of which he probably took two or three tablets that day. In the afternoon of the same day he had severe substernal chest pains, and shortness of breath, was anorectic, and became restless. He was given penicillin, but within the next several hours his restlessness and dyspnea increased, and he produced a cupful of pink-streaked sputum.

He was admitted to a hospital early the following day in acute distress, complaining of chest pains, hemoptysis, and severe dyspnea. On physical examination his respirations were 60 per minute, and he was cyanotic. Moist rales were heard over both lung fields. He was given morphine for sedation but subsequently coughed up bright red watery material, and died one hour after admission.

The pathologic findings were those of generalized sarcoidosis, inhalation anthrax, B. anthracis septicemia, and acute necrotizing pneumonia.

The one-week history of illness may have resulted from a recrudescence of sarcoidosis or a bacterial or viral pneumonia secondary to sarcoidosis. Either situation may have predisposed him to infection with B. anthracis. Possibly the week long illness represented inhalation anthrax, with its usual course retarded by the previous involvement with sarcoidosis. The development of acute necrotizing pneumonia may have been related to the impairment of the normal removal of B. anthracis organisms by sarcoidosis involvement of the lungs so that the retained organisms developed into the vegetative state within the alveoli cells resulting in focal, necrotizing pneumonitis. Additionally, pyogenic organisms may have been present initially but not revealed by postmortem cultures, so the autopsy findings may have resulted from the combined effects of sarcoidosis, B. anthracis, and septic pneumonia.

Gross examination as well as selected environmental culturing of a wooden furniture-frame manufacturing plant and a furniture store where he worked and his home revealed no sources of B. anthracis.

The most likely source of infection appeared to be the open receiving area of a tannery he walked past daily on his way to the bus stop where he caught a bus that took him home. He was never known to have gone inside the plant and had no acquaintances among the employees. Bacillus anthracis was isolated from 10 of 147 swabs (7%) obtained in the area of the tannery's receiving room six weeks after the patient's death. Three floor-sweeping specimens were positive for B. anthracis. No cases of inhalation anthrax had been reported among the employees of the plant, although a case of cutaneous anthrax had been reported in 1945. It was observed that air currents blew from the tannery receiving area onto the street in the specific area where he walked.

Of interest are two other cases of inhalation anthrax also possibly related to the same tannery. One case was in a 50-year-old woman who in December 1948 complained of a "slight cold."[20] The next day she was better, but on the following evening she vomited, and early the next morning, she complained of a headache and four hours later was found comatose. A physician diagnosed acute meningitis, administered penicillin, and hospitalized her. Physical examination revealed the woman to be cold and clammy and cyanotic with severe respiratory distress with a rectal temperature of 105°F. Noisy breathing obscured auscultation of the cardiac and pulmonary sounds. The neck was rigid and there was flaccid paralysis of the extremities with hyperactive deep tendon reflexes. The white blood count was $14,800/mm^3$ with 74% neutrophils, and the cerebrospinal fluid was bloody. She died six hours after admission. Subsequently, the cerebrospinal fluid cultures were reported positive for B. anthracis. Pathologic findings were of hemorrhagic mediastinitis and subarachnoid hemorrhage. Gram-positive bacilli were seen in the blood vessels of the brain in the area of the subarachnoid hemorrhage. This woman, who was a housewife, lived one and one-half blocks from the tannery; no epidemiologic investigations were conducted at the time of her illness.

The other case possibly related to the same tannery was in a 37-year-old housewife with inhalation anthrax in 1951.[20] She lived one and one-half miles from the tannery and also 200 yards from a plant that processed waste wool and hair. No epidemiologic studies were conducted, so the possible association with the tannery can only be speculative. It is hypothesized that all three individuals may have become infected by the airborne route from the tannery, which was shown to be contaminated with B. anthracis.

As we stated at the 1966 Second International Conference on Aerobiology, "It is not clear why more cases have not occurred in goat hair and woolen mills and in tanneries, especially among employees working in the dustiest areas where the most concentrated *Bacillus anthracis*-containing aerosols were created." We suggested that the reason may be related to the dose to which employees are exposed, that resistance might develop among the employees with chronic exposure, or that more cases may have occurred but not have been diagnosed. We also stated that "equally unusual has been the sporadic occurrence of cases in people with no industrial exposure. It may be that these individuals are unusually susceptible . . ."

Reviewing the 18 cases in the United States since 1900 does not add any new information that answers these questions. The various studies conducted over the past 25 years, both in the laboratory and of naturally occurring aerosols in industrial plants where imported goat hair is processed, confirmed that the experimental disease in primates is similar to the disease in humans naturally exposed to industrial aerosols. The critical question concerning the infective dose for humans remains difficult to answer, and inferences can only be speculative. Although the human industrial case may reflect an unusually large dose of organisms, the influence of other factors, such as the possible role of potentiating substances also contained within the aerosol, or a highly virulent strain of *B. anthracis* are unknown. A few of the strains recovered from these patients have been studied in the laboratory. However, they do not appear to have any characteristics significantly different from typical strains.

The other area of concern, the health status of the host, may be related to the development of inhalation anthrax in at least some of the sporadic cases. The influence of a chronic disease on the subsequent development of inhalation anthrax was first mentioned in the reports of the Anthrax Investigation Board in England.

In at least three of the cases reviewed above, the individuals had chronic disease conditions that could have influenced their susceptibility. One of these individuals had berylliosis and potentially a compromised immune system, in addition to anatomic abnormalities of the upper respiratory tract. Another had chronic alcoholism, diabetes, and chronic pancreatitis; the third had chronic sarcoidosis. In several of the other cases, information is not adequate to show whether a chronic disease may have influenced the development of inhalation anthrax.

The five epidemic cases are easier to explain in that each of the patients was exposed to aerosols created by one particular lot of imported goat hair as it was being processed. Investigation revealed that the hair in this particular lot was heavily contaminated with *B. anthracis* and thus could have represented a common source of infection as it was being processed. It is possible that this lot may have been heavily contaminated. Except for the possibility that three cases were related to a single tannery, none of the other cases are related to each other or to a common source.

As we stated in the 1966 conference, "More specific information about inhalation anthrax in man is currently difficult to obtain because almost all workers in high risk industries within the United States have been immunized." Additionally, during the past 13 years because of decreased importation and use of goat hair, the decrease in the number of persons working with the imported materials, the routine use of a human anthrax vaccine, and improvements in industrial hygiene, there has been a further reduction in the occurrence of this already rare disease. Thus, we should not look to additional field studies to provide new information that might answer the questions raised above. We can only assume that sporadic cases occur because individuals with greater susceptibility to infectious diseases are exposed to aerosols containing *B. anthracis* organisms, either in excessively high concentration or of unusual virulence.

REFERENCES

1. BRACHMAN, P. S., A. F. KAUFMANN & F. G. DALLDORF. 1966. Industrial Inhalation Anthrax. Bacteriological Reviews **30:** 646–657.
2. LAFORCE, L. M. 1978. Woolsorter's Disease in England. Bull. N.Y. Acad. Med. **54:** 956–963.
3. BELL, J. H. 1902. Anthrax: Its relation to the wool industry. *In* Dangerous trades. T. Oliver, Ed.: 634–643. Dutton. London.
4. ANTHRAX INVESTIGATION BOARD (Bradford & District). 1906. First Annual Report.: 3–4.
5. ANTHRAX INVESTIGATION BOARD (Bradford & District). 1918. 13th Annual Report.: 15.
6. PLOTKIN, S. A., P. S. BRACHMAN, M. UTELL, F. H. BUMFORD & M. M. ATCHINSON. 1960. An epidemic of inhalation anthrax, the first in the 20th century. I. Clinical features. Am. J. Med. **29:** 992–1001.
7. ALBRINK, W. S., 1961. Pathogenesis of inhalation anthrax. Bacteriol. Rev. **25:** 268–273.
8. EPPINGER, H. 1894. Die Hadernkrankheit, eine typische Inhalations-Milzbrandinfection beim Menschen unter besonderer Berucksichtigung inhrer pathologischen Anatomie and Pathogenesis auf Grund eigener Beobachtungen dargestellt.: 139–141. G. Fischer. Jena, Germany.
9. FRAENKEL, E. 1925. Uber Inhalationsmilzbrand. Virchows Arch. Pathol. Anat. Physiol. **254:** 363–378.
10. BUCHNER, H. 1888. Untersuchungen uber den Durchtritt von Infection serregern durch die Intacte lungenoberflache. Arch. Hyg. **8:** 145–245.
11. YOUNG, G. A., JR., M. R. ZELLE, and R. E. LINCOLN. 1946. Respiratory pathogenicity of *Bacillus anthracis* spores. I. Methods of study and observation on pathogenesis. J. Infect. Dis. **79:** 233–246.
12. BARNES, J. M. 1947. The development of anthrax following the administration of spores by inhalation. Brit. J. Exp. Pathol. **28:** 385–394.
13. DRUETT, H. A., D. W. HENDERSON, L. PACKMAN & S. PEACOCK, 1953. Studies of respiratory infection. I. The influence of particle size on respiratory infection with anthrax spores. J. Hyg. **51:** 359–371.
14. ROSS, J. M. 1957. The pathogenesis of anthrax following the administration of spores by the respiratory route. J. Pathol. Bacteriol. **73:** 485–494.
15. ALBRINK, W. S. & R. J. GOODLOW. 1959. Experimental inhalation anthrax in the chimpanzees. Am. J. Pathol. **35:** 1055–1065.
16. BRACHMAN, P. S. 1977. *In* Infectious diseases. P. D. Hoeprich, Ed. 807–812.
17. BRACHMAN, P. S., S. A. PLOTKIN, F. H. BUMFORD & M. M. ATCHINSON. 1960. An epidemic of inhalation anthrax: The first in the 20th century. II. Epidemiology. Am. J. Hyg. **72:** 6–23.
18. SUFFIN, S. C., W. H. CARNES & A. F. KAUFMANN. 1978. Inhalation anthrax in a home craftsman. Human Pathol. **9:** 594–597.
19. LAFORCE, F. M., F. H. BUMFORD, J. C. FEELEY, S. L. STOKES & D. B. SNOW. 1969. Epidemiologic study of a fatal case of inhalation anthrax. Arch. Environ Health. **18:** 798–805.
20. BRACHMAN, P. S., J. S. PAGANO & W. S. ALBRINK. 1961. Two cases of fatal inhalation anthrax, one associated with sarcoidosis. New Engl. J. Med. **265:** 203–208.

AEROSOL DISSEMINATION OF BACTERIAL PLANT PATHOGENS

Monty D. Harrison

Department of Botany and Plant Pathology
Colorado State University
Fort Collins, Colorado 80523

Transmission of bacterial plant pathogens by splashing rain, insect vectors and contact between diseased and healthy plant parts has been considered to be of major epidemiological importance in the spread of bacterial diseases of plants. The possible role of aerosols in the dissemination of phytopathogenic bacteria, which is widely recognized for human and animal pathogens, has only recently been considered a possibility by plant pathologists. Conceptually, the basic difficulty lay in appreciating how aerosols of phytopathogenic bacteria could be generated. Recent reports,[1-4] however, have shown that aerosols of phytopathogenic bacteria can be produced by natural processes and that bacterial cells can survive in the airborne state for sufficient time for viable cells to spread over a distance. This has introduced a new dimension to the investigation of the epidemiology of bacterial diseases of plants. The study of aerosol dissemination of phytopathogenic bacteria is in its infancy and the full significance of this means of spread remains to be fully elucidated. Several investigations, however, have already indicated that it may be highly important and expanding studies are likely to provide stimulating areas for further research. The significant aspects of the observations and research in this area of plant pathology to date are considered in this paper.

Aerosol Generation

At least three mechanisms have been implicated in the generation of aerosols of phytopathogenic bacteria: (1) impaction of raindrops on infected tissue, (2) impaction of water from overhead sprinkler irrigation, and (3) mechanical pulverization of plant (potato) stem tissue and foliage prior to harvest. All three mechanisms appear to generate aerosols naturally and thus provide a source of bacteria which may infect healthy plants in the field.

In controlled laboratory studies Graham and Harrison[3] showed that simulated raindrops striking potato stems infected with *Erwinia carotovora* var. *atroseptica* (van Hall) Dye generated large numbers of aerosolized *Erwinia* propagules (colony forming units, cfu) which remained suspended in still air for 60–90 minutes and moved readily with slow air streams. Water drops as small as 2 mm diameter falling at near terminal velocity possessed enough kinetic energy to generate detectable airborne cells but 4–5 mm diameter drops were more efficient.

Venette and Kennedy[4,6] detected *Pseudomonas glycinea* Coerper [*Pseudomonas syringae* van Hall] aerosols in a soybean crop infected by the pathogen during rain or sprinkler irrigation. Their data (TABLE 1) showed that an average of 1.51×10^{-1} cfu per liter of air were collected during rainfall periods but only 9.4×10^{-2} cfu/liter were detected when samples were taken during sprinkler

94

0077-8923/80/0353-0094 $01.75/0 © 1980, NYAS

irrigation. This suggests that, generally speaking, rain is superior to overhead sprinklers as an aerosol generator. Subsequent laboratory studies by Venette and Kennedy[5] showed that a single drop of water (0.02–0.15 ml) impacting infected soybean leaves could generate P. glycinea aerosols provided the leaves were premoistened for two–five minutes before impaction. Nonpremoistened leaves required the impaction of 20 drops before detectable aerosols were generated, presumably because sufficient pre-wetting was required to suspend bacterial cells on leaves and thus make them available for aerosolization.

Several studies[4,5,6] have shown that the predominant size range for aerosol particles generated by rainfall, sprinkler irrigation or simulated raindrops in the laboratory is 2.1–3.3 μm with a range from 0.65–7.0 μm. This indicates that the cfus probably consist largely of free bacterial cells.

In 1973 Perombelon and Lowe[1] reported that airborne cells of Erwina carotovora var. atroseptica (van Hall) Dye and Erwinia carotovora var. carotovora Dye could be detected in large numbers in areas where potato stems and foliage were being pulverized by mechanical vine beaters prior to harvest. Subsequent work[7,8] verified that mechanical destruction of symptomless or Erwinia-infected stems in the field or the laboratory generated large quantities of

TABLE 1

PROPAGULES OF AIRBORNE PSEUDOMONAS GLYCINEA IN AEROSOLS GENERATED BY RAINFALL AND SPRINKLER IRRIGATION OF INFECTED SOYBEANS IN THE FIELD*

	Viable Propagules per Liter of Air†
Sprinkler irrigation	9.4×10^{-2}
Rainfall	1.51×10^{-1}

*From Venette and Kennedy.[4]
†Mean of four experiments.

bacterial aerosols. Eighty percent of them were less than 7.0 μm in size and approximately 50%–55% of the particles were in the 2.1–4.7 μm size range.

Occurrence of Naturally Produced Bacterial Aerosols in the Field

The fact that aerosol generation can be demonstrated experimentally in the laboratory or in small field plots tells little about their possible significance under natural conditions in the field. Some studies have, therefore, already been undertaken to determine if aerosols occur naturally in areas where crops are grown. Much of the research by Perombelon et al.[1,7,8] involved field sampling for the presence of Erwinia carotovora aerosols in the vicinity of field plots where mechanical stem and foliage destruction was in progress. Their work has shown that Erwinia aerosols are generated in the field by vine destruction. Quinn et al.,[9] Graham and Harrison[3] and Harrison (unpublished) have sampled air extensively in Scotland and in Colorado, U.S.A. to determine if Erwinia carotovora aerosols are generated from potato crops by rainfall and overhead sprinklers. Graham and Harrison[3] reported in 1975 and Graham[10] in 1976 that airborne Erwinia cells were captured downwind from potato crops during rainfall or when overhead sprinklers were operating. During three cropping seasons, Harrison (unpublished) sampled air downwind from potato crops in Colorado during sprinkler irrigation. Small numbers of airborne *Erwinia carotovora* var. *carotovora* and *E. carotovora* var. *atroseptica* were detected during each of the three seasons although rainfall is very rare during the summer months. Viable *Erwinia* cells were detected only during the late evening, night or early morning hours, never during the daytime. *Erwinia* aerosols were usually not present until relatively late in the growing season (i.e., after August 10). The most extensive study on the presence of naturally occurring *Erwinia* aerosols is that of Quinn et al.[9] who collected frequent air samples using a high volume Casella bacteria sampler at numerous sites in Scotland from August, 1977 to October, 1979. Both *Erwinia carotovora* var. *carotovora* and *E. carotovora* var. *atroseptica* were detected regularly in the air near potato crops but also in locations where potato fields were not present in the immediate vicinity. *Erwinia* aerosols were not detected before mid-to late summer. Viable cells were not commonly present in detectable numbers before the beginning of August (although a few collections were made in July) and the highest numbers usually occurred in September and October. Of special interest is the fact that *Erwinia* aerosols were detected as late as December 23 in 1977, long after potato crops, presumably the major sources of the bacteria, had been harvested. The origin of these bacteria remain unknown but plant debris remaining in the field may prove to be the source.

Quinn et al.[9] failed to detect *Erwinia* aerosols in the absence of rainfall in the sampling area. This would be expected if raindrop impaction was responsible for aerosol generation. The numbers of airborne bacteria generally increased in proportion to the intensity of the rainfall and *Erwinia* population and also that of numerous other bacteria increased in the air as the rainfall intensity increased. This led to the conclusion that rain is a major generator of aerosols of many kinds of bacteria found in the open air. It is notable, however, that their studies also showed that rainfall is not the only means of aerosol generation. In a study of atmospheric bacterial populations over a 24 hr period in October, 1979, the bacterial count in the air rose during rainfall and fell as rainfall ceased. During a dry period beginning about 3–4 hours after the rainfall ceased, however, the counts of one organism (a species of *Micrococcus*, a widely distributed bacterium in nature) rose and fell between the hours of 8:45 P.M. and 9:30 A.M. The origin of the organism and the means of aerosolization is so far unknown.

Venette and Kennedy[4,6] showed that *Pseudomonas glycinea* aerosols are produced from infected soybean crops in the field by rain or overhead sprinkler irrigation.

Quantitative Aspects of Aerosol Generation

Comparatively little has been done to determine numbers of airborne cells of phytopathogenic bacteria generated by water impaction or by stem and leaf pulverization under laboratory or field conditions. In the case of *Erwinia carotovora*, however, two carefully controlled experiments have been completed. No such definitive experiments have been made with other plant pathogens. Graham et al.[11] performed experiments in which aerosols were generated by water drops from weighed quantities of potato stems infected with *Erwinia carotovora* var. *atroseptica*. The tissue was incubated for 48 hr after inoculation to produce the maximum numbers of viable bacterial cells. Tissue samples were bombarded with 3 mm or 5 mm water drops in an apparatus consisting of a chamber in which aerosols were generated and a short wind tunnel connected to the chamber through which humidified air could be moved.[3] Air samples were drawn isokinetically from the wind tunnel through a sampling tube connected to Casella bacteria samplers, and deposited on a suitable medium until no further airborne cells were detected in the system. Their results showed that from 5.6×10^3 to 2.99×10^4 aerosol propagules per gram of infected tissue were generated with an average of approximately 1.6×10^4 cfu per gram of tissue. Comparisons of the total number of cells in the tissue to the number of aerosol propagules generated showed that only about .003% of the available viable bacteria were aerosolized by the water drops. Slightly more airborne cells were generated by 5 mm than 3 mm drops, no doubt because of the higher kinetic energy of the larger drops.

Using these data Graham et al.[11] calculated the theoretical numbers of Erwinia propagules that could be released into the air by water impaction from a blackleg infected potato crop. The data (TABLE 2) showed that from a potato crop with 2% of the stems infected by Erwinia approximately 8.1×10^8 propagules/ha could be generated by 5 mm water drops and slightly fewer (2.6×10^8) by 3 mm drops. Proportionately more aerosol propagules would be expected with increasing amounts of infection in the field.

Perombelon et al.[7,8,12] used the same apparatus as Graham et al.[11] to study quantitatively the generation of Erwinia aerosols by simulated mechanical plant

TABLE 2

ESTIMATION OF ERWINIA CAROTOVORA/HA IN AEROSOLS GENERATED BY RAIN FROM A CROP WITH 2% BLACKLEG INCIDENCE* AND BY MECHANICAL STEM PULVERIZATION†

Rain		Stem Pulverization	
5 mm Drops	3 mm Drops	Blackleg-free Plants	Blackleg Plants‡
8.1×10^8	2.6×10^8	4.1×10^8	1.1×10^8

*From Graham et al.[11]
†From Perombelon et al.[7]
‡One infected stem per one plant in 100.

destruction. Known amounts of healthy or Erwinia-infected potato stem tissue were chopped with a small hammer mill and the number of Erwinia propagules released was determined by isokinetic sampling of the air in the wind tunnel. The results, when extrapolated to a field scale (TABLE 2), showed that an average of 4.1×10^8 (range = 5.7×10^7 to 1.1×10^9) aerosolized propagules could be produced by pulverization of 1 ha of nonblackleg-infected plants. About another 10^8 cells/ha would be generated if the field contained 1% blackleg-infected stems. The results also showed that 10^{12}–10^{13} bacterial cells/ha were not released from the tissue as aerosols in the pulverization process but remained in the plant debris on the ground where some might be aerosolized by subsequent rainfall.

Quantitative measurements in the field have generally shown low numbers of naturally generated bacterial aerosol propagules per unit volume in air samples collected from various locations and under different environmental conditions. Quinn et al.[9] reported populations of Erwinia carotovora ranging from 1.0×10^{-3} to 2.0×10^{-5} cfu/liter of air in air samples from the field during periods of rainfall in Scotland. Harrison (unpublished) found 3×10^{-4} cfu of Erwinia carotovora/liter of air downwind from potato crops irrigated by overhead sprinklers in

Colorado and 7.0×10^{-4} cfu/liter downwind from a potato crop being pulverized by a mechanical vine beater.

Venette and Kennedy[4,6] found as many as 4.2×10^{-1} cfu of *Pseudomonas glycinea*/liter of air near infected soybeans in Minnesota during rainfall but only up to 1.53×10^{-1} cfu/liter during sprinkler irrigation. This number is considerably higher than reported for *Erwinia carotovora* on potatoes and suggests that higher populations of airborne bacterial cells may be generated in the case of leaf infecting than for nonleaf infecting plant pathogens. More data will be required, however, before this can be proposed as a general principle. A major problem with field experiments is the fact that no apparatus presently exists to sample isokinetically in the open air. The data reported above represent more or less anisokinetic sampling and thus the actual numbers of organisms per unit volume of air can only be roughly determined.

Survival Dispersal and Deposition of Phytopathogenic Bacteria in Aerosols

It is obvious from the preceding evidence that aerosols of *Erwinia carotovora* and *Pseudomonas glycinea* can be generated by several mechanisms. One would conclude from this information that by analogy, aerosols of other plant pathogenic bacteria, especially foliar pathogens, are also likely to be produced by the same mechanisms. Definitive studies on these organisms remain to be done but recent work by Venette[13,14] and by Southey and Harper[2] suggests that aerosols of *Xanthomonas phaseoli* (Erw. Smith) Dowson, *Pseudomonas phaseolicola* (Burkholder) Dowson and *Erwinia amylovora* (Burrill) Winslow *et al.* may occur.

Once aerosol generation is known to occur, the next problem that arises concerns survival of bacterial cells in the aerosolized state in the open air, dispersal over a distance and deposition on healthy plants. These steps must be successfully accomplished for a bacterial aerosol to be of significance in the epidemiology of a bacterial disease. Research in this area of bacterial aerosols in relation to plant disease epidemics has only recently been attempted. However, a few good studies on survival, dispersal and deposition of a limited number of bacterial plant pathogens have been made and some observations on dispersal distances have been reported. Much still remains to be done in these areas.

Survival of Phytopathogenic Bacteria in Aerosols

In 1975, Graham and Harrison[3] generated aerosols of *Erwinia carotovora* var. *atroseptica* from infected potato stems with small water drops and found that viable airborne cells remained suspended in humid air inside a small wind tunnel for 60 to 90 minutes at $10.6°C$. Southey and Harper[2] studied the survival of *Erwinia amylovora* cells in the laboratory and in the open air. Cells of the organism were exposed to the air by depositing them on microthreads of spider webs wound on metal frames, according to the so-called "captive aerosol" method of May and Druett.[15] The cells generally survived well at relative humidities between 40% and 90% (up to three hours under the most favorable conditions in the laboratory). Greater loss in viability occurred in the open air but significant numbers were viable after two hours exposure.

An extensive study was conducted by Graham *et al.*[16] in which aerosols of strains of *Erwinia carotovora* var. *carotovora* and *E. carotovora* var. *atroseptica* were generated and loaded onto microthreads using a mobile Henderson apparatus described by Druett.[17] Microthreads holding bacterial cells were then exposed to a range of environments in the laboratory and in the open air. In a laboratory test at 20°C and 65% relative humidity (rh) the *Erwinia* strains studied were divided into two groups. The first group, which included all of the strains of *E. carotovora* var. *atroseptica* except one, survived poorly. No viable cells were detected after two hours exposure in most cases. In all cases less than 20% of the cells survived after five minutes, 10% after 15 minutes and 2% after 30 minutes exposure.

The second group, which included most strains of *E. carotovora* var. *carotovora* and only one strain of *E. carotovora* var. *atroseptica*, survived considerably longer than the organisms in the first group. In most cases, there was greater than 25% survival after 5 minutes, 5% after one hour and 2% after two hours exposure. Poorer survival of all strains of *Erwinia* was observed than for a reference strain of *Escherichia coli* (MRE 162), which was known to be an aerosol stable organism and to withstand exposure for long periods in a simulated airborne state.[2]

Results of experiments using a single, selected strain each of *E. carotovora* var. *carotovora* and *E. carotovora* var. *atroseptica* to determine survival over a range of conditions in the open air showed that the organisms survived poorly under warm, dry conditions (18–26°C and 43%–70% rh). No viable cells of either organism were present after 30 minutes. Under such stressful conditions the strain of *E. carotovora* var. *carotovora* survived slightly better than the strain of *E. carotovora* var. *atroseptica*. Cool-moist conditions (12–12.5°C and 86%–90% rh with rain falling) favored longer survival of both organisms and significant numbers of viable cells were detected after two hours. Approximately 10% of the original population of both organisms was viable after 60 minutes. The authors concluded that aerosolized cells of both organisms would survive long enough under favorable conditions (cool, moist environments) to easily spread from crop to crop over a considerable distance.

Perombelon[8,12] and Perombelon et al.[7] studied survival of "captive aerosols" of *Erwinia carotovora* var. *atroseptica* cells suspended in potato sap to simulate aerosols generated by plant pulverization. The cells were deposited on microthreads and exposed to 18°C and 65% rh. The number of viable cells decreased exponentially with time but 50% of the population survived for five-ten minutes and from 1%–15% survived for at least one hour under these conditions. The results were comparable to those of Graham et al.[16] and reinforce the conclusion that sufficient *Erwinia* cells probably survive long enough to be carried significant distances by air streams.

Venette and Kennedy[18] reported that detectable numbers of aerosolized cells of *Pseudomonas glycinea* survived up to 60 minutes in the air at 40%, 65% and 97% rh in a closed system in the laboratory.

Venette[14] studied survival of bacterial cells suspended in air in stirred settling chambers and reported that airborne *Pseudomonas phaseolicola* cells were still viable after 180 minutes at 22–24°C and 90% rh but that no viable cells were present after 35 minutes at 60% rh or 80 minutes at 35% rh. Subsequent work[25] showed that viable cells of this organism could be detected after 185 minutes at 23°C and 75% rh. Viable *Xanthomonas phaseoli* cells, however, were present after 180 minutes at 90%, 65% and 40% rh. In both cases, viable populations declined more rapidly as relative humidity decreased. Venette concluded that airborne cells of both pathogens could survive in excess of three hours under the proper environmental conditions.

Dispersal and Deposition of Aerosolized Phytopathogenic Bacteria

Several qualitative studies and observations have been made in which bacterial aerosols were sampled at various distances downwind from a presumed natural source (a crop) or an artificial aerosol generator to gain information on dispersal distances under certain conditions. Harrison (unpublished, 1975–1979) found that propagules of *Erwinia carotovora* can be captured from the air in Colorado up to ca 183 m downwind from where they are presumably generated from blackleg-infected potato crops by overhead sprinkler irrigation.

Quinn et al.[9] captured viable *Erwinia carotovora* cells from the air when presumed sources of the bacteria in Scotland (potato crops) were at least 500 m away from the sampling site. This suggests that the aerosols may be carried

TABLE 3

ESTIMATED NUMBERS OF *ERWINIA CAROTOVORA* PROPAGULES DEPOSITED DOWNWIND FROM AEROSOLS GENERATED BY 5 mm WATER DROPS FROM A CROP WITH 2% BLACKLEG INFECTION*

Source	Estimated Number of Propagules Deposited/m^2 at Various Distances (m) Downwind from the Source†			
	10	100	1,000	10,000
Area	9.5×10^{10}	2.3×10^{11}	1.8×10^{10}	1.0×10^9
Point	—	1.2×10^7	5.6×10^4	—

*From Graham et al.[11]
†The model of Gregory (1961) was used in the calculations.

considerable distances but the authors cautioned that it is possible that unknown sources of the organism(s) may have been present in the sampling areas nearer than was apparent.

Using an artificially generated point source of a rifampin-resistant strain of *Xanthomonas phaseoli*, Venette[13] studied the dispersal of aerosolized cells downwind from the inoculum source in North Dakota. Viable airborne cells were detected 3, 4.5, 6 and 7.5 m above the ground at a point 30.5 m from the source but the largest numbers were found in samples taken from the 3 and 7.5 m heights. By placing open plates of selective medium on the ground in a semicircle around the aerosol generator Venette demonstrated that at a distance of 30.5 m from the source the aerosol had diffused sufficiently that viable cells were deposited in a 120° arc around the source. No bacteria were detected upwind nor laterally from the generator.

Perhaps the most significant attempts to determine potential distances of travel and possible deposition of bacterial aerosols were made by Graham et al.[11] and by Perombelon et al.[7,8,12] Using the theoretical numbers of aerosolized *Erwinia carotovora* cells generated/unit area as determined in laboratory studies as the bacterial source strengths, these authors calculated theoretical deposition gradients downwind from the source using the atmospheric diffusion and deposition models of Gregory[19,20,21] Pasquill[22] and Chamberlain.[23] Calculations by Graham et al.[11] (TABLE 3) using Gregory's model[20] showed that as many as 1.0 × 10^9 bacterial cells/m^2 would theoretically be deposited as far as 10,000 m downwind from an area inoculum source on a cloudy day with a steady wind speed and a field width of 100 m. According to their calculations considerably

TABLE 4

THEORETICAL NUMBERS OF *ERWINIA CAROTOVORA* CELLS DEPOSITED PER m² DOWNWIND FROM A GROUND LEVEL SOURCE WITH A STRENGTH OF 10^8 CELLS*

Model	Assumed Atmospheric Condition	Number of Cells/m² Deposited			
		50 m	100 m	1,000 m	10,000 m
Gregory	Stable	—	4.37×10^5	6.68×10^3	1.41×10^2
Pasquill	Stable	—	3.24×10^2	4.80	0.07
	Unstable	—	2.80×10^1	3.92	0.02
Chamberlain	Stable	2.09×10^3	7.06×10^1	1.24	0.19

*From Perombelon.[7]

smaller numbers would theoretically be deposited from a point source with the same strength (only 1.2×10^7 and 5.6×10^4 cells/m² at 100 and 1,000 meters, downwind, respectively). The authors suggested that based on these data airborne *Erwinia* cells could play a significant role in the spread of the organism over distances of up to 1,000 m. They cautioned, however, that other models such as that of Pasquill[22] could give different estimates of the effective distance that significant numbers of bacterial cells could be carried.

Perombelon *et al.*[7,8,12] presented data from similar studies using theoretical source strengths derived from laboratory studies on aerosol generation from pulverized potato stems. They compared the models of Gregory,[19-21] Pasquill[22] and Chamberlain[23] to estimate the deposition of airborne *Erwinia carotovora* cells assuming 100% viability during dispersal. The results (TABLE 4) showed that the numbers derived from the Gregory model agreed reasonably well with those reported for a point source by Graham *et al.*[11] The Pasquill and Chamberlain models however predicted much smaller numbers.

Perombelon *et al.*[7,12] also studied the natural deposition of *Erwinia carotovora* in a hay field on three separate days in 1978. *Erwinia* aerosols were artificially generated 10 cm above a plant canopy in numbers approximately equal to the source strength used in their theoretical calculations. Viable cells deposited 50 and 100 m downwind from the source were collected on the surface of a semiselective medium contained in trays positioned 10 cm above the plant canopy.

The results (TABLE 5) agreed reasonably well with the theoretical deposition predicted by the Pasquill and Chamberlain models. Perombelon[12] concluded,

TABLE 5

THE DEPOSITION OF ARTIFICIALLY GENERATED AIRBORNE *ERWINIA CAROTOVORA* CELLS DOWNWIND FROM THE SOURCE IN THE FIELD*

Experiment	No. of Bacteria Generated at the Source	Atmospheric Conditions	Numbers of *E. carotovora* Deposited/m²	
			50 m	100 m
1	5.49×10^8	Stable	3×10^3	6×10^2
2	2.19×10^8	Intermediate	6×10^1	7
3	4.83×10^8	Unstable	1	0

*From Perombelon *et al.*[7] and Perombelon.[12]

based upon these experiments, that the chances for the deposition of significant numbers of *Erwinia* cells from aerosols would be small at distances >100 m but that deposition at distances <100 m could be high enough to be epidemiologically important.

Perombelon's data (TABLE 5) show, however, that in a stable atmosphere considerable numbers of cells (6 × $10^2/m^2$) can be deposited at least 100 m from the source. This suggests that under certain environmental conditions the deposition of significant numbers of cells at distances >100 m might be possible.

Discussion and Conclusions

Sufficient data have been generated during the past five years to allow one to conclude that aerosols of at least several phytopathogenic bacteria including *Erwinia carotovora, Pseudomonas phaseolicola* and *Xanthomonas phaseoli* are probably commonly generated by natural mechanisms, including rainfall and overhead sprinkler irrigation, in the field. Although data for other phytopathogenic bacteria are unavailable it seems prudent by analogy to conclude that aerosols of many important pathogens, especially the foliar infecting organisms, probably occur in nature. In fact, the probability is high that raindrops (or drops from overhead sprinklers) are responsible for a general production of airborne cells of both phytopathogenic and nonphytopathogenic bacteria as suggested by Quinn et al.[9] The deposition of cells from a general atmospheric bacterial aerosol may explain in part the widespread occurrence of many kinds of bacteria on the surface of many plants.

Survival studies have shown that populations of airborne phytopathogenic bacteria decline quite rapidly, especially under warm, dry conditions. Data, however, have shown that significant numbers of viable cells survive long enough (a few minutes to one–three hours) to be transported considerable distances by air movement. The limited data available suggest that some of the foliar or flower pathogens such as *Erwinia amylovora, Pseudomonas glycinea, Xanthomonas phaseoli* and *Pseudomonas phaseolicola* may survive more efficiently in aerosols than the nonfoliar infecting pathogens such as *Erwinia carotovora*. The foliar inhabiting pathogens are in a better position to become airborne and perhaps they also possess characteristics which favor their survival and dispersal through the air. Critical studies on survival, dispersal and deposition of these pathogens similar to those completed and in progress for *Erwinia carotovora* would be important, interesting and highly relevant to the epidemiological studies on the diseases they cause.

Data on dispersal and deposition of airborne *Erwinia carotovora* cells strongly suggest that they survive sufficiently long to be deposited in significant numbers on plants up to 100 m downwind from the source. In fact, data presented by Perombelon et al.[7] suggest that during stable atmospheric conditions several hundred viable cells/m^2 may be deposited at distances of at least 100 m or more. Since these studies were made under conditions which were not ideal for the survival of *Erwinia* in aerosols (15.8–18.3°C and 55%–82% rh), it appears possible, if not probable, that under cooler, more humid conditions which often occur at night (even in the arid areas of the western United States, such as Colorado) or during periods of rainfall, the successful distance of dispersal could be increased.

Available data suggest that successful aerosol generation and dispersal will probably occur in regions with frequent rainfall to generate aerosols, and cool, humid conditions to favor survival of aerosolized cells. Warm, dry, sunny areas such as Colorado and other western states are probably environments much less conducive to the successful spread of phytopathogenic bacteria in aerosols. It should be kept clearly in mind, however, that cool, humid conditions occur in many such arid areas at night. The use of overhead sprinkler irrigation systems during these periods may result in the generation and successful dispersal of bacterial aerosols and this could be an important epidemiological factor. Data from Colorado (Harrison, unpublished) which show that airborne *Erwinia carotovora* cells can be detected as much as 183 meters from overhead sprinklers at night or in early morning support this conclusion.

The full significance of aerosols of phytopathogenic bacteria in the epidemiology of bacterial diseases of plants remains to be determined. Sufficient evidence has been gathered, however, to allow one to predict that eventually they will prove to be highly significant even in drier, warmer regions.

Current observations and available research data already strongly suggest that airborne bacterial cells may be responsible for the recontamination of *Erwinia*-free potato crops grown in the field. When an aerosol of a known serotype of *Erwinia carotovora* var. *carotovora* was released upwind from a potato crop, Graham[10,16] reported that the same serotype was found to be present in tubers harvested from the crop even though no symptoms of *Erwinia* infection were observed in the field.

Data from Scotland[24] and Colorado (Harrison, unpublished) have shown that when *Erwinia carotovora* cells are deposited on potato foliage at least a few of them can survive for from 72 hours[24] to several (up to 10–15) days in the field (Harrison, unpublished). Perombelon[24] also found that *Erwinia* populations, especially on old senescent leaves, may increase under wet conditions. These results strengthen the view that *Erwinia carotovora* aerosols could play an important role in the recontamination of *Erwinia*-free potato crops (and possibly others) at a considerable distance from inoculum sources. Recent data suggest that sufficient numbers of cells could be deposited on potato foliage at distances between 50 and 100 m from an inoculum source to result in recontamination of the tubers. At greater distances, however, it appears that few viable cells would be deposited. If a few cells were introduced into a clean crop by this means, however, the increase of this inoculum on the foliage, redistribution to other plants by rain splash and subsequent wash down to the tubers could result in the establishment of reinfection in a crop located a considerable distance from an *Erwinia* source. This possibility has been suggested by Perombelon.[24] It is also conceivable that even very few cells deposited per plant could wash down to tubers and establish latent infection. Quinn *et al.*[26] have shown that as few as 20 cells of *Erwinia carotovora* var. *carotovora* deposited on the leaves of a potato plant can establish latent tuber infections. The same cycle, perhaps, could explain the widespread rapid outbreaks of foliar bacterial diseases.

Although much more research is needed to fully clarify the role of bacterial aerosols in plant pathology the current data strongly indicate a highly significant role of airborne bacterial cells in the epidemiology of plant diseases. This relatively new concept of bacterial dissemination poses problems to the plant pathologist and should provide a stimulus to look at plant disease epidemiology in a novel way.

REFERENCES

1. PEROMBELON, M. C. M. & R. LOWE. 1973. Bacterial soft rot and blackleg of potato. Rep. Scott. Hort. Res. Inst. for 1972: 52–53.

2. SOUTHEY, R. F. W. & G. J. HARPER. 1971. The survival of *Erwinia amylovora* in airborne particles: tests in the laboratory and in the open air. J. Appl. Bact. **34**: 547–556.
3. GRAHAM, D. C. & M. D. HARRISON. 1975. Potential spread of *Erwinia* spp. in aerosols. Phytopathology **65**: 739–741.
4. VENETTE, J. R. & B. W. KENNEDY. 1975. Naturally produced aerosols of *Pseudomonas glycinea*. Phytopathology **65**: 737–738.
5. VENETTE, J. R. & B. W. KENNEDY. 1976. Generation of *Pseudomonas glycinea* aerosols by simulated raindrops. (Abstr.) Proc. Amer. Phytopath. Soc. **3**: 256.
6. VENETTE, J. R. & B. W. KENNEDY. 1975. Naturally produced aerosols of *Pseudomonas glycinea*. (Abstr.) Proc. Amer. Phytopath. Soc. **2**: 91.
7. PEROMBELON, M. C. M., R. A. FOX & R. LOWE. 1979. Dispersion of *Erwinia carotovora* in aerosols produced by pulverization of potato haulm prior to harvest. Phytopath. Z. **94**: 249–260.
8. PEROMBELON, M. C. M. 1977. A preliminary assessment of the spread of the blackleg and soft rot bacteria by potato haulm pulverization. Proc. Symposium on Problems of Pest and Disease Control in Northern Britain. R. A. Fox, Ed.: 39–40. The Scottish Horticultural Research Institute, Invergowrie, Dundee, Scotland, March, 1977.
9. QUINN, C. E., I. ANN SELLS, & D. C. GRAHAM. 1980. Soft rot coliform bacteria in the atmospheric bacterial aerosol. In manuscript.
10. GRAHAM, D. C. 1976. Re-infection by *Erwinia carotovora* (Jones) Bergey *et al.* in potato stocks derived from stem cuttings. EPPO Bull. **6**(4): 243–245.
11. GRAHAM, D. C., C. E. QUINN & LYNNE F. BRADLEY. 1977. Quantitative studies on the generation of aerosols of *Erwinia carotovora* var. *atroseptica* by simulated raindrop impaction on blackleg-infected potato stems. J. Appl. Bact. **43**: 413–424.
12. PEROMBELON, M. C. M. 1978. Dispersion and deposition of air-borne *Erwinia carotovora*. Proc. IV Int. Conf. Plant Path. Bact. II. 749–752.
13. VENETTE, J. R. 1979. Detection of *Xanthomonas phaseoli* downwind from an aerosol generator. (Abstr. No. 223) IX International Congress of Plant Protection, Washington, D.C.
14. VENETTE, J. R. 1979. Survival of *Pseudomonas phaseolicola* and *Xanthomonas phaseoli* in a stirred settling chamber. Ann. Rept., Bean Improvement Coop. In press.
15. MAY, K. R. & H. A. DRUETT. 1968. A microthread technique for studying the viability of microbes in a simulated airborne state. J. Gen. Microbiol. **51**: 353–366.
16. GRAHAM, D. C., C. E. QUINN, I. ANN SELLS & M. D. HARRISON. 1979. Survival of strains of soft rot coliform bacteria on microthreads exposed in the laboratory and in the open air. J. Appl. Bact. **46**: 367–376.
17. DRUETT, H. A. 1969. A mobile form of the Henderson apparatus. J. Hyg. Camb. **67**: 437–448.
18. VENETTE, J. R. & B. W. KENNEDY. 1975. Aerosols of *Pseudomonas glycinea* generated during spray inoculation of soybeans. (Abstr.) Proc. Amer. Phytopath. Soc. **2**: 92.
19. GREGORY, P. H. 1945. The dispersion of air-borne spores. Trans. Brit. Mycol. Soc. **28**: 26–72.
20. GREGORY, P. H. 1961. The Microbiology of the Atmosphere. Leonard Hill Ltd., London.
21. GREGORY, P. H. 1973. The Microbiology of the Atmosphere, 2nd Edit. Leonard Hill. London.
22. PASQUILL, F. 1961. The estimation of the dispersion of windborne material. Met. Mag. **90**: 33–49.
23. CHAMBERLAIN, A. C. 1953. Aspects of travel and deposition of aerosol and vapour clouds. Atom. Energy Res. Estab. Rep. AERE/HP/R1261:1–28. London HMSO.
24. PEROMBELON, M. C. M. 1978. Contamination of potato crops by air-borne *Erwinia carotovora*. Proc. 4th. Int. Conf. Plant Path. Bact. II. pp. 563–565.
25. VENETTE, J. R. Personal communication.
26. QUINN, C. E. Personal communication.

AIRBORNE SPREAD OF BRUCELLOSIS

Arnold F. Kaufmann, Marshall D. Fox, John M. Boyce,
Daniel C. Anderson,
Morris E. Potter, William J. Martone, and Charlotte M. Patton

Bacterial Diseases Division
Bureau of Epidemiology
Center for Disease Control
Atlanta, Georgia 30333, U.S.A.

INTRODUCTION

Brucellosis is a zoonotic disease that is transmitted from its animal reservoirs to humans by three primary routes: skin and conjunctival contact, ingestion, and inhalation of infectious aerosols. The relative importance of each route varies with the epidemiologic setting. Our discussion focuses on the respiratory route.

In his classic 1897 monograph summarizing the history of brucellosis, Hughes claimed that most patients were infected from breathing air contaminated with the causative bacterium arising from fecally polluted soil.[1] His theory was probably based more on the ancient concept of miasmas than on scientific observation. The role of domestic livestock in the epidemiology of brucellosis was not discovered until almost a decade later.

In reviewing the occurrence of brucellosis among Naval personnel stationed on Malta, Dudley described a shipboard outbreak of a protracted pulmonary disease with low mortality.[2,3] He theorized that the disease was caused by *Brucella melitensis* adapted to growth in the human lung and transmitted person-to-person via aerosols in the ship's crowded living quarters. His hypothesis is interesting, but no convincing experimental or epidemiologic evidence for person-to-person transmission via aerosols has been subsequently developed to support it.

Aerosol transmission of brucellosis is widely accepted as a potential biohazard in laboratories.[4-6] The largest single laboratory-associated epidemic of 45 cases (one fatal) occurred in Michigan in the period December 1938–February 1939.[7] Most of the patients were students taking courses on the second and third floor of a building containing a brucellosis laboratory in the basement. All modes of transmission except airborne were ruled out by the investigators.

More recently, Hendricks *et al.* described a large brucellosis epidemic in an abattoir which apparently involved airborne transmission.[8] The disparate attack rates for workers doing comparable work on different floors were best explained by differences in exposure to aerosols generated in the kill department. *Brucella suis* was isolated from air in the kill department of this abattoir.[9]

Experimental studies with guinea pigs show that brucellosis can be readily transmitted by aerosols.[10,11] Only a few more brucella organisms are required to infect guinea pigs by respiratory challenge than by subcutaneous challenge. Although brucellae readily invade through the lung, the respiratory challenge does not result in a primary pneumonia. The lesions caused by respiratory and subcutaneous challenge of guinea pigs are comparable with two exceptions.[10] More pronounced cervical and mediastinal lymphadenopathy occurs and epididymitis is less frequent following respiratory challenge.

Although brucellosis can certainly be transmitted by aerosols, the respiratory

105

0077-8923/80/0353-0105 $01.75/0 © 1980, NYAS

route of infection has not been traditionally considered to be epidemiologically significant.[12,13] This interpretation is probably correct in countries where brucellosis is predominantly acquired through consumption of unpasteurized dairy products and on farms and ranches. In the United States, however, brucellosis is now most prevalent among abattoir workers.[14] We will present evidence from a series of abattoir-associated brucellosis outbreaks that airborne transmission is important for this occupational group.

Potential Routes of Infection for Abattoir Workers

Potential routes of infection for abattoir-associated brucellosis include: (1) Direct contact of the conjunctiva or broken skin with animals, tissues, or contaminated fomites, (2) inhalation of infectious aerosols with invasion occurring through the mucous membranes of the upper respiratory tract or the lung, and (3) ingestion of tissues or fluids containing brucella organisms.

Ingestion appears to be of minor importance for abattoir-associated brucellosis in the United States. Workers interviewed in multiple outbreak investigations have reported that fresh animal tissues from processing lines, whether raw or cooked, were not commonly eaten. Also, experimental studies with guinea pigs indicate that significantly higher challenge doses are required to produce infection by ingestion than by the skin contact or respiratory routes.[10,15] Experimental studies of adult men have also shown that humans are readily infected by exposing broken skin to brucella organisms but that infection is difficult to produce by oral challenge.[16]

Assessing the relative importance of the contact and the inhalation routes of infection is more difficult because abattoir workers would seem to be exposed by both routes. However, analysis of exposure potential by slaughter process stage shows that risk varies by job location.

Slaughtering and processing of animals can be divided into three stages (FIGURE 1). In the first stage, the animals are sequentially immobilized and bled out. Hair is removed from the carcasses of swine in this processing stage. Employees who immobilize and bleed animals have contact with live animals and may be splattered with blood. Those who dehair swine have contact only with the skin of the unopened carcass. While the dehairing process may result in the generation of aerosols, they should contain few brucellae.

In stage II, the carcasses are beheaded and eviscerated. The hide is normally removed in this processing stage from all animals except swine. At the end of this processing stage, the carcasses are split with a power saw and washed before being chilled. Persons involved in stage II processing have continuous contact with freshly opened animals. Their hands and forearms are often bathed continuously with blood, tissue fluids, and water. In addition, their faces are frequently splattered with these fluids. Numerous operations in stage II, such as removing viscera and sawing and washing opened carcasses, may generate aerosols containing brucellae. Thus, stage II processing employees have significant exposure to both the contact and airborne routes of infection.

In stage III, the chilled carcasses are processed into wholesale and retail cuts, sausage, and canned or smoked products. This stage also includes processing of viscera and other tissues that have been chilled or cooked. Employees involved in processing carcasses after chilling frequently have intimate tissue contact; however, the carcasses and tissues processed in stage III are relatively free of lymphatic tissues and free-flowing blood and tissue fluids, and they should be less hazardous to persons in contact with them. The potential for generating aerosols during stage III is generally minimal; therefore, the respiratory route of infection should be unimportant in this stage.

Thus, stage I workers should be at minimal risk of brucellosis, stage II workers are at risk of infection by both the airborne and contact routes, and stage III workers are primarily at risk of infection by the contact route. These differences in exposure potential are dependent on physical separation of each processing

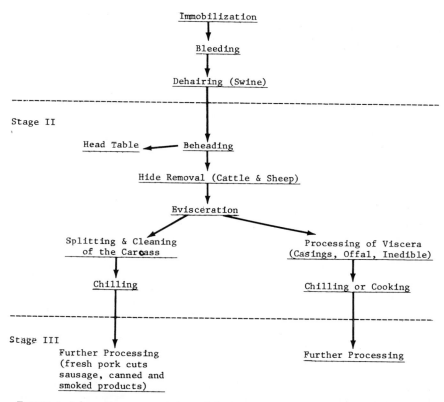

FIGURE 1. Schematic representation of the procedures followed in the slaughter of animals by processing stage.

stage. However, as we shall discuss, the relative separation of these stages varies in individual abattoirs.

Case Distribution in Abattoir-Associated Outbreaks

Six abattoir-associated brucellosis outbreaks investigated by the Center for Disease Control in collaboration with state health departments in the period

1960–1976 were selected for analysis on the basis of comparability of investigative approach. Four abattoirs slaughtered only swine, one slaughtered cattle and swine, and one slaughtered cattle, swine, and sheep. The slaughtering and processing procedures were similar at the abattoirs, although the physical separation of the various processing stages and the air flow patterns in the buildings differed. These variations resulted in a series of naturally occurring experiments on the importance of the respiratory route of infection for abattoir-associated brucellosis.

A total of 387 clinical cases of brucellosis occurred in the six outbreaks with attack rates ranging from approximately one to 11 percent. Case distribution by processing stage varied by abattoir (TABLE 1). The differences in case distribution correlated well with relative separation of processing stages and air flow patterns at the abattoirs (FIGURE 2).

Abattoir A

If contact exposure is the most important route of infection in the abattoir setting, the brucellosis attack rate should be similar for groups of employees with

TABLE 1

DISTRIBUTION OF BRUCELLOSIS CASES IN SIX ABATTOIRS BY PROCESSING STAGE

| Abattoir | Processing Stage* | | | | |
	I	II	III	Misc.†	Total
A	16 (13%)	73 (57%)	32 (25%)	7 (5%)	128
B	—	20 (38%)	23 (43%)	10 (19%)	53
C	3 (7%)	40 (89%)	1 (2%)	1 (2%)	45
D	—	8 (57%)	—	6 (43%)	14
E	16 (23%)	44 (62%)	6 (8%)	5 (7%)	71
F	8 (11%)	54 (71%)	9 (12%)	5 (7%)	76
Total	43 (11%)	234 (60%)	71 (18%)	39 (10%)	387

*Approximate distribution of workers by processing stage is: Stage I—4%, Stage II—15%, Stage III—57%, and Miscellaneous—24%.

†Includes maintenance, sanitation, management and other personnel who do not have primary meat or by-product processing duties.

comparable contact exposure, regardless of exposure to aerosols generated in the stage II processing area. However, the attack rate for employees who were exposed to aerosols from the stage II processing area at abattoir A was significantly higher than for unexposed control groups with similar contact exposure.[8]

At abattoir A, processing stages I and II were on the fourth floor of the building except that the head-trim department was located on the third floor. Stage III processing was conducted on both the third and fourth floors. Persons who worked on the fourth floor and had contact with carcasses and viscera before they were chilled (stages I and II) had a significantly higher ($p < 0.001$) attack rate of brucellosis than did head-trim department employees on the third floor (TABLE 2). If contact was the most important factor in the epidemiology of brucellosis in this setting, employees working in the head-trim department

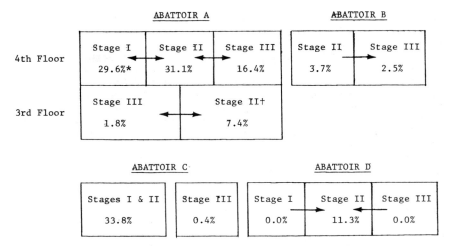

FIGURE 2. Schematic relationship of air-flow patterns and the brucellosis attack rates in selected employee groups at four abattoirs. Arrows indicate direction of air-flow, *is the percent attack rate and †, the head-table department.

should have had the highest attack rate because *B. suis* infections are frequently localized in the mandibular and retropharyngeal lymph nodes of swine.[17,18]

Stage I processing employees, as discussed earlier, should be at minimal risk of acquiring infection; yet this group, located on the fourth floor, also had a significantly higher attack rate ($p < 0.001$) than did employees in the head-trim department. The only adequate explanation is that head-trim department employees on the third floor were separated from aerosols generated in the stage II processing area on the fourth floor. The attack rate for the fourth floor stage I employees was comparable to that for stage II employees located on the same floor, again indicating that work location is more important than degree of contact exposure.

Equally striking was the comparison of attack rates for stage III employees who processed chilled carcasses. This processing was done on both the third and the fourth floors, and stage III employees on both floors had essentially similar contact exposure to chilled tissues; however, employees on the fourth floor who worked in an area adjacent to the stage II processing area and were exposed to

TABLE 2

BRUCELLOSIS ATTACK RATES IN PROCESSING STAGE I, II, AND III WORKERS BY FLOOR, ABATTOIR A

Floor	Processing Stage			Total
	I	II	III	
3rd Floor	—	4/54 (7.4%)*	3/159 (1.8%)	7/213 (3.3%)
4th Floor	16/54 (29.6%)	64/206 (31.1%)	27/161 (16.4%)	107/421 (25.4%)
Total	16/54 (29.6%)	68/260 (26.2%)	30/320 (9.4%)	114/634 (18.0%)

*No. brucellosis cases/no. workers at risk (%).

air from the stage II area had an attack rate of 16.4 percent, and employees on the third floor, who were not exposed to air from stage II, had a significantly lower attack rate of 1.8 percent ($p < 0.001$) (TABLE 2).

The various rooms of this plant were well-lighted, had high ceilings, and appeared to be well-ventilated. While the air-flow pattern was not confirmed with smoke candles, from on-site observations it appeared that the only air flow between floors was from the third to the fourth floor. The hot, humid air in the fourth floor stage II processing area could be seen rising and exiting through a large open skylight in the roof. The fourth floor also had exhaust fans, and the third floor did not. There was no active input of fresh air into the fourth floor. Also, the only direct connections between the floors were several chutes for conveying animal tissues. Brucellae were isolated from air in the fourth floor stage II processing area, and guinea pigs exposed to air exhausted from this area contracted brucellosis, confirming the presence of an etiologic agent in aerosols.[9]

Because the attack rate for employees exposed to aerosols from the fourth floor stage II processing area was significantly higher than for employees not exposed to stage II but with similar contact exposure, airborne transmission seemed a likely explanation of the case distribution in this epidemic.[8]

Abattoir B

If exposure to stage II aerosols is important in transmitting brucellosis to abattoir employees, forcing air from the stage II area into stage III processing areas should result in comparable attack rates in both areas. This distribution pattern occurred at abattoir B.

Abattoir B, which had approximately 2,700 employees, was composed of a complex series of directly adjoining processing buildings for the slaughter of swine, calves, cattle, and sheep. The stage II processing area for swine was maintained under positive air pressure relative to other areas in the plant. Air-flow studies with smoke candles showed that during normal plant operation, air was forced out of the swine kill floor (stage II) through various openings into many of the stage III processing areas and into the men's locker room.

In contrast to the other five epidemics, most employees involved in this outbreak worked in stage III processing on other floors and in buildings contiguous to the stage II swine processing area. The attack rates for the various stage III areas appeared to correlate with the amount of air they received from the swine kill floor (stage II).

A comparison of the attack rates for stage I and II swine processing employees (excluding casing, offal, and inedible departments) and for employees in the pork cut and boning departments (stage III) serves as an example. Fifteen of the 409 stage I and II employees (3.7 percent) had clinical brucellosis. The attack rate was comparable in the cut and boning departments, where 10 of 405 employees (2.5 percent) were affected. The cut and boning department employees were exposed to aerosols coming from the stage II area while working and while using the men's locker room.

Attempts to document the presence of airborne brucella organisms both by air sampling and by exposure of sentinel guinea pigs were unsuccessful at abattoir B. However, three patients had no contact with animal tissues and had not entered the kill area for many months to years before becoming ill. Two of these patients made cardboard boxes, and the third was a welder in the plant boiler room. All three were exposed to air being exhausted from the roof of the stage II processing area. A reasonable explanation for their brucellosis was exposure to airborne organisms.

Abattoir C

If the distribution of cases in an epidemic of abattoir-associated brucellosis correlates with exposure to air from the stage II processing area, putting stage II in a building separate from stage III processing areas should reduce the number of stage III workers who are infected. The epidemic at abattoir C supports this hypothesis.

Abattoir C, with about 400 employees for slaughtering cattle and swine, comprised several adjacent buildings. Processing stages I and II of both the cattle and swine slaughtering operations were done in the same building and involved about 130 employees. The other 270 employees, who were engaged in stage III processing and clerical operations, worked in other buildings.

In a 13 month period, 45 workers had brucellosis.[19] All but one worked in the building housing the stage I and II processing areas. *Brucella suis* was isolated from the air in this building on several occasions.

Abattoir D

If complete physical separation from the stage I and II processing areas virtually eliminates brucellosis among stage III workers, maintaining the stage II area under strong negative air pressure should have a similar effect. At abattoir D, the design of the plant resulted in such a situation.

Abattoir D consisted of a single large building. The stage II processing area at one end of the building was separated by a large cooling room from the stage III processing area. The stage II processing area was under negative air pressure that caused a strong in-flow of air from all surrounding areas. Air was exhausted from the stage II area through large roof fans and did not re-enter other areas of the building.

In the period 1970–1971, 14 of the 365 employees of this plant contracted brucellosis. Eleven of the 97 people working in the stage II processing area were sick. None of the 18 workers in the stage I area or the 110 workers in the cut department (stage III) where carcasses are processed immediately after chilling were affected ($p < 0.0004$).

The three patients who did not work in the stage II processing area were two clerks in the shipping department and a man who assembled cardboard boxes. None of these three patients handled animal products as part of their job but routinely walked through the stage II processing area to reach their work location.

Abattoirs E and F

The review of the first four abattoir-associated brucellosis epidemics shows that distribution of cases correlates to a large degree with distribution of air from the stage II processing area. Data from our next two naturally occurring epidemiologic experiments show that the same case distribution pattern applies to and is reproducible for endemic brucellosis.

Abattoirs E and F were virtually identical. They were located on adjacent premises, slaughtered only swine obtained from the same geographic area, and had similar sized work forces. The slaughtering and processing procedures at both plants were comparable. Also, the air from the kill department (stages I and II) at both plants was primarily exhausted through large ceiling fans over the stage I work area. Little air from the kill department entered stage III processing areas.

Brucellosis was endemic in the workers at both plants but did not occur in discrete epidemics. In the period 1968–1974, 71 cases occurred at abattoir E, whose average daily work force was 873, and 76 cases occurred at abattoir F, whose average work force was 997. Fifty-four of the 71 (82%) cases at abattoir E were among stage I and II workers, as were 62 of the 76 (82%) cases at abattoir F (TABLE 3).

TABLE 3

DISTRIBUTION OF BRUCELLOSIS CASES IN ABATTOIRS E AND F BY PROCESSING STAGE AND DEPARTMENT, 1968–1974

		Abattoir E			Abattoir F		
		Cases			Cases		
Stage	Department	Annual Mean	7-Year Total	Mean Daily Work Force	Annual Mean	7-Year Total	Mean Daily Work Force
I	Kill	2.3	16	41	1.1	8	34
II	Kill	5.4	38	114	6.9	48	108
	Inedible	0.3	2	8	0.6	4	10
	Lard	0.6	4	9	0.3	2	8
III	Cut	0.3	2	89	0.4	3	124
	Curing	0.1	1	45	0.3	2	41
	Fresh Pack	0.1	1	29	0.3	2	31
	Other	0.3	2	316	0.3	2	357
Misc.	Maintenance	0.3	2	61	0.3	2	63
	Other	0.4	3	161	0.6	3	221
Total		10.1	71	873	10.9	76	997

The attack rate for stage I and II workers was comparable at both plants. If tissue contact was of paramount importance, stage I workers who do not contact the deep raw tissues of the carcass should have had a lower attack rate. The fact that air from stage II moved past these workers enroute to the exhaust may explain the comparable attack rates. The incidence of brucellosis among stage III and nonprocessing workers was significantly lower. Extensive serosurveys of workers at these abattoirs confirmed these observations but did not provide any further epidemiologic insights.

DISCUSSION

The airborne route of infection clearly plays a role in abattoir-associated brucellosis. The distribution of cases in abattoirs correlates better with distribution of air from the stage II processing area than with degree of worker's skin contact to potentially infectious materials. Persons are also infected who are exposed to air from the stage II processing area but have no contact with animal tissues.

The kill department (stage II) of an abattoir is organized chaos centered on a rapidly moving carcass disassembly line. The splashing of viscera, hectic cutting operations, washing and carcass sawing generate aerosols at numerous points. Brucellae survive well in aerosols and resist drying.[20] Thus, their potential for transmission in this environment is great.

Brucellae have been isolated from the air in abattoir kill departments in three investigations. A single colony forming unit (CFU) of *B. suis* was isolated from 13,592 liters of air sampled over a 5 day period at abattoir A.[9] Four CFUs of *B. suis* were isolated from 84,664 liters of air sampled over a 30-day period at abattoir C.[19] In a third abattoir, air sampling was conducted while 136 swine from a brucellosis infected herd were being slaughtered.[12] Two CFUs of *B. suis* were isolated from 849 liters of air sampled over a 90-minute period.

The low yield of brucellae from kill department air and the evidence that airborne transmission of infection does occur suggest that the minimum infecting dose by the respiratory route is low for humans. The minimum oral infective dose of *B. abortus* and *B. suis* for guinea pigs is about 10^6 to 10^7 organisms;[15] experimental evidence suggests a comparable minimum oral infective dose for humans.[16] The minimum infecting dose by aerosol or subcutaneous injection of guinea pigs, however, is less than 100 organisms.[10] If a comparable disparity exists for humans, the minimum respiratory infecting dose may also be less than 100 organisms.

Controlling abattoir-associated brucellosis is difficult. Designing abattoirs to avoid spreading aerosols generated from stage II processing will reduce risk for workers in other departments but will not prevent the possibility of transmission by skin contact. Also, this approach will not affect risk for stage II processing workers, who already have the highest case incidence. The disease probably must be eradicated from domestic livestock or an effective human brucellosis vaccine must be developed in order to eliminate this occupational hazard.

SUMMARY

Review of epidemic and endemic brucellosis at six abattoirs demonstrates a correlation between case distribution and flow of air from the kill department (stage II) to other areas within an abattoir. Air from the kill department disseminated to nearby departments led to abnormally high brucellosis attack rates for persons who worked in these areas at two abattoirs. Complete physical separation or maintaining negative air pressure in the kill department was associated with reduced risk for workers in other areas at four abattoirs. Cases in persons who had exposure to kill department air but no contact with animal tissues provide strong evidence for airborne transmission of infection. Brucellosis is also contracted through skin contact with infectious animal tissues, but this route of transmission appears less important than formerly believed.

REFERENCES

1. HUGHES, M. L. 1897. Mediterranean, Malta or Undulant Fever. Macmillan and Co. London.
2. DUDLEY, S. F. 1931. Some lessons of distribution of infectious diseases in the Royal

Navy. Lecture III. The history of undulant fever in the Royal Navy. Lancet **1:** 683–691.

3. DUDLEY, S. F. 1935. On the biological approach to the study of epidemiology. President's address. Proc. R. Soc. Med. **29:** 1–14.
4. DALRYMPLE-CHAMPNEYS, W. 1960. Brucellosis Infection and Undulant Fever in Man. Oxford University Press. London.
5. MEYER, K. F. & B. EDDIE. 1941. Laboratory infections due to brucella. J. Infect. Dis. **68:** 24–32.
6. TREVER, R. W., L. E. CLUFF, R. N. PEELER & I. L. BENNETT. 1959. Brucellosis. I. Laboratory acquired acute infection. Am. Med. Assoc. Arch. Int. Med. **103:** 381–397.
7. HUDDLESON, I. F. & M. MUNGER. 1940. A study of an epidemic due to *Brucella melitensis.* Am. J. Public Health **30:** 944–954.
8. HENDRICKS, S. L., I. H. BORTS, R. H. HEEREN, W. J. HAUSLER & J. R. HELD. 1962. Brucellosis outbreak in an Iowa packing house. Am. J. Public Health **52:** 1166–1178.
9. HARRIS, M. M., S. L. HENDRICKS, G. W. GORMAN & J. R. HELD. 1962. Isolation of *Brucella suis* from air of slaughterhouse. Public Health Reports **77:** 602–604.
10. ELBERG, S. S. & D. W. HENDERSON. 1948. Respiratory pathogenicity of brucella. J. Infect. Dis. **45:** 271–282.
11. HENDERSON, D. W. 1960. Bacterial interference. Bact. Rev. **24:** 167–176.
12. BUCHANAN, T. M., S. L. HENDRICKS, C. M. PATTON & R. A. FELDMAN. 1974. Brucellosis in the United States, 1960–1972. An abattoir-associated disease. Part III. Epidemiology and evidence for acquired immunity. Medicine **53:** 427–439.
13. SPINK, W. W. 1956. The Nature of Brucellosis. The University of Minnesota Press. Minneapolis.
14. FOX, M. D. & A. F. KAUFMANN. 1977. Brucellosis in the United States, 1965–1974. J. Infect. Dis. **136:** 312–316.
15. HARDY, A. V., M. G. HUDSON & C. F. JORDAN. 1929. The skin as a portal of entry in B. *melitensis* infections. J. Infect. Dis. **45:** 271–282.
16. MORALES-OTERO, P. 1930. *Brucella abortus* in Porto Rico. Porto Rico J. Public Health Trop. Med. **6:** 3–88.
17. HUTCHINGS, L. M. 1950. Swine brucellosis. *In* Brucellosis Symposium. American Association for the Advancement of Science.: 188–198. Waverly Press. Washington, D.C.
18. MCCULLOUGH, N. B., C. W. EISELE & E. PAVELCHEK. 1951. Survey of brucellosis in slaughtered hogs. Public Health Reports **66:** 205–208.
19. WHITE, P. C., E. F. BAKER, A. J. ROTH, W. J. WILLIAMS & T. S. STEPHENS. 1974. Brucellosis in a Virginia meat-packing plant. Arch. Environ. Health **28:** 263–271.
20. ROSEBURY, T. 1947. Experimental Airborne Infection. Williams & Wilkins Co. Baltimore.

INTRODUCTION

Lloyd G. Herman

Environmental Microbiology, Safety Branch
National Institutes of Health
Bethesda, Maryland 20205

Just as our ancestors worshipped the four elements of nature, earth, fire, wind and water, we must also stand in awe of the effect that these elements have in our daily life. The earth as the soil and the home of all living matter, especially the microbes; the fire as the fever that these organisms can produce in man, animals and heaps of plant materials during decomposition or combustion; the wind as air currents that can carry dust and clouds of microbes released by man, plants and animals from community to community, into our homes, work areas, and hospitals; and, of course, the water as the element that supports all types of microbial plant and animal life as well as being its best transport mechanism. No wonder then, that they were worshipped as long as they were not understood— and little wonder then that even, today, few of us really appreciate or understand the effect of moisture and humidity in protecting all forms of life; heat, with temperatures from 0°C to 150°C for preserving or sterilizing our cultures, food and instruments; the role of wind, as air and various gases O_2, CO_2, N_2, which are useful for growing and preserving or sterilizing our microbial slaves; and last but not least, the soil or those parts of the earth that we must use to grow our plants as food for all living matter and which also becomes the pit into which we throw all of the residues, garbage and refuse we produce daily in blind faith that, somehow, the microbes will recycle them back into fertile soil.

If then, we depend on microbes to maintain the earth in an acceptable condition, we must also be aware of the deviates in the microbial world that are not satisfied to remain in the soil, but that have opted for a better life and so prefer to live on, in or with man, plants and animals. However, since none of these microorganisms are readily visible to the naked eye, even though their effects and efforts can be seen, smelled or tolerated in virtually every daily activity of nature and productive effort of man; hence, in order to survive, it behooves him to better learn to control these microbes and divert their energies, whenever possible, into more useful and less hazardous functions. With this background, let us then begin our session on "Fungi as Agents of Airborne Contagion."

AERIAL DISSEMINATION OF FUNGAL SPORES

Donald E. Aylor and Paul E. Waggoner

The Connecticut Agricultural Experiment Station
Box 1106
New Haven, Connecticut 06504

From the 9th Century and the St. Anthony's fire of ergot in the Rhine Valley on to the 19th Century and the Irish famine of potato blight on to 1970 and the disrupted markets of corn blight, fungal spores borne on the turbulent wind are the causes of pandemics of plant disease. Some pathogenic spores are injected into the wind and some are removed from sporophores by the wind itself. We shall examine how spores become airborne, how they fly and are diluted in the air and how they land to cause new lesions, contrasting spores that make their own way into the air and ones that are blown into the air by the wind itself.

We shall concentrate on the aerial dispersal of fungal spores that are liberated by wind. For concreteness, we will discuss the pathogen of southern corn leaf blight, *Helminthosporium maydis*. This particular fungus is propagated by multicelled asexual spores or conidia about 100 μm long and about 15 μm wide. Under suitable conditions of moisture and temperature the spore will germinate and invade the host. Characteristic of the fungal growth are aerial mycelia or conidiophores that bear the spore about 100 μm above the surface of a leaf.[1]

To reach fresh host material and begin its life cycle anew, the fungus is faced with three problems: 1) spore removal, 2) flight, and 3) landing. We are only concerned here about the flight of spores in dry air—not flight in droplets, and passive removal by wind—not active discharge mechanisms. Aerial dispersal is the integration of these three highly interdependent events: removal, flight with dilution, and catch before inoculation. The interdependency among these events is shown by the following three equations:

$$\underset{\text{spores/m}^2\text{sec}}{CATCH} = \begin{bmatrix} DEPOSITION \\ VELOCITY \\ m/sec \end{bmatrix} \cdot \begin{bmatrix} CONCENTRATION \\ \text{spores/m}^3 \end{bmatrix} \tag{1}$$

$$\underset{\text{spores/m}^3}{CONCENTRATION} = \begin{bmatrix} REMOVAL \\ \text{spores/sec} \end{bmatrix} \cdot \begin{bmatrix} DILUTION \\ \text{sec/m}^3 \end{bmatrix} \tag{2}$$

$$REMOVAL = f(instantaneous\ wind\ on\ the\ spore) \tag{3}$$

The total number of spores caught is obtained by simply integrating *CATCH* over the time or period of interest. We want to emphasize that *REMOVAL* is not a constant simply to be plugged into a diffusion formulae as can be done for material emitted from a factory chimney. Rather, *REMOVAL* depends explicitly on *instantaneous* wind speed.

Removal

For a spore to be removed, its attachment to the stalk must be broken. Mature spores of *H. maydis* are connected by a narrow (0.35 μm) isthmus of connecting material.[2] In spite of this apparently tenuous connection, these spores are not easily removed.

116

0077-8923/80/0353-0116 $01.75/0 © 1980, NYAS

FIGURE 1 shows observations of percent removal of *H. maydis* spores. The force for removal was supplied by centrifuging the spores in closed tubes: a centrifugal force caused this removal.[3] The abscissa indicates the force applied to the spore relative to its own weight, and 50% removal occurs at about 2000 on this scale, or the removal force corresponds to an acceleration of about 2000 times gravity. Most removal occurs over a fairly narrow range of forces. In fact, when the variation in spore size is accounted for, the actual removal force is remarkably near 0.02 dynes for all spores. Thus the strength of attachment of conidia is remarkably uniform.[3]

It is satisfying that a mechanical analysis using these forces yields a sensible estimate for the strength of the connecting tissue. The tensile strength is about the same as that for individual wood fibers.[2]

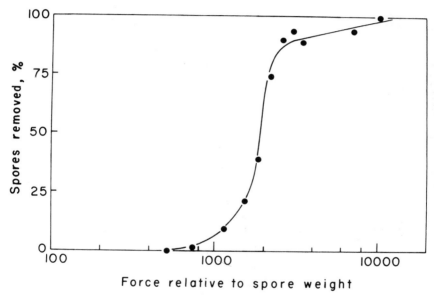

FIGURE 1. Percentage removal of *H. maydis* spores vs. centrifugal force redrawn from Aylor.[3]

If 0.02 dynes is required to remove the spore, aerodynamics should allow us to calculate how fast the wind must blow to exert a drag sufficient to remove a spore. A wind of 5 m/sec directly on the spore would exert the requisite 0.02 dynes to detach it. A wind of 5 m/sec or 11 miles per hour would, of course, be a high wind indeed to blow where the spores stand, about 100 μm above lower leaves of a corn crop.

Now let's look at how spores are removed by wind from sporophores growing from corn leaves. Shown in FIGURE 2 are observations of percentage of *H. maydis* spores removed vs. wind speed.[4] In these experiments most removal occurred near leaf edges. Two things are evident from the data. First, no spores are removed below a minimum wind speed, but once removal begins, it is essentially completed over a narrow range of wind speed just as spores were removed over a narrow range of centrifugal force. Second, the wind speed that removes 50% of the spores is about the 5 m/sec calculated from their removal in a centrifuge.

The centrifuge experiment, remember, shows that a wind of about 5 m/sec must act directly on the spore. First, this is indeed a fast wind to blow in the bulk air within a crop canopy. Second, we must account for the viscous boundary layer that normally surrounds the leaf. Nevertheless, observations in real corn-

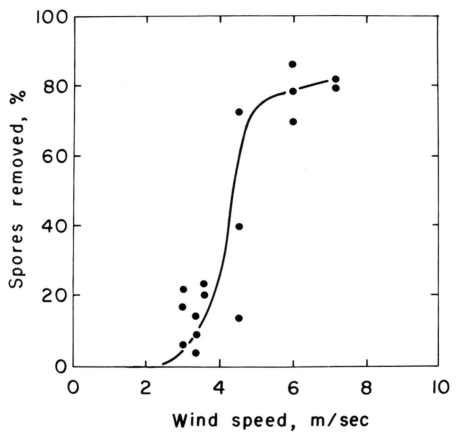

FIGURE 2. Percentage removal of *H. maydis* spores vs. wind speed redrawn from Waggoner.[4]

fields show that conidia of *H. maydis* can be removed when the average wind in the canopy is only about 1 m/sec.[5]

To resolve this paradox we must first explain that during average winds of 1 m/sec inside a crop canopy the wind occasionally reaches the critical 5 m/sec,[6] but we will not dwell on this further here.

Even with a 5 m/sec wind in the bulk air, however, resolving the paradox requires answering a second question: How can a 5 m/sec wind in the bulk air exert a force of 0.02 dynes on a spore near the leaf and within the viscous boundary layer? The growth of the boundary layer inward from the edge of a lamina like a leaf is well known. In a steady wind at the leading edge, there is no boundary layer but centimeter-by centimeter the boundary layer grows inward until, for example, the wind at the level of a spore 3 cm from the leading edge is only 1 when the wind in the bulk air is fully 5 m/sec.[7]

The viscous boundary layer also grows with time as well as growing inward along the leaf. We shall describe the growth of the boundary layer with time, beginning with the start of a gust of wind. When the air above a leaf is started suddenly, the velocity near the surface at the instant of starting is everywhere equal to the speed in the bulk air because of the small but finite inertia of the air. Immediately thereafter viscosity begins to slow the air adjacent to the surface, and the boundary layer begins to form.[7] At some relatively long time, a dynamic equilibrium exists between forces due to viscosity and inertia; the boundary layer is then fully grown, is steady, and shelters the spore. Before the boundary layer has grown, a gust of 5 m/sec can impose 5 m/sec on the spore, if for only a very brief time. Such sudden gusts of wind, as we have described, are capable of removing spores.[8] In the last section we will relate this discussion of removal by gusts to the patterns of spores caught at a distance from a source.

Flight with Dilution

Once liberated, spores are transported by turbulent wind. The signal feature of turbulent wind is the unsteady, chaotic, three-dimensional motion of individual volumes of air. It is the vertical component of turbulence that keeps heavier than air particles suspended but all three components, i.e., the vertical, the crosswind and the downwind components, dilute a cloud of spores.

The time-average concentration of spores released steadily from a point into a steady wind can be determined by the well-known Gaussian plume diffusion model, which describes the dilution of smoke plumes downwind of tall chimneys.[9] For such plumes, the concentration at a given downwind distance is generally less when the average speed and the directional fluctuations of wind are greater since the particles released sequentially are separated through a distance proportional to the speed and variance of the wind.

When clouds of spores are released infrequently by gusts, however, the spatial concentration of the cloud is specified with respect to the instantaneous downwind location of the cloud's center.[10] The dilution of the cloud depends on the time during which turbulence acts on the cloud.[11] Clouds of spores that are released by gusts with speeds exceeding some critical minimum value, as described here for H. maydis, will arrive at a nearby place downwind at about the same time whether the average wind be 0.5, 1, or 3 m/sec.[12] This produces similar dilutions and thus similar concentrations for different average winds in marked contrast to the greater dilution by fast winds of spores released steadily.

Spores clouds travelling in a crop canopy are further diluted by filtration of the air by the foliage. To determine how many spores are filtered we must examine the physics of deposition.

Catch

The number of spores caught and inoculating an area of host per unit time is given by equation **(1)**. Because particles the size of *H. maydis* spores are deposited by settling or by impaction, the deposition velocity v_D must be formulated for the alternatives of settling and impaction.

$$v_D = \begin{cases} v_s \\ f(P)U \end{cases}$$

The settling velocity v_s of a *H. maydis* spore is about 2.5 cm/sec.

The alternative of impaction prevails according to the aerodynamic field of flow around a leaf, which is determined by the size of the leaf and by the wind speed U in the bulk air, and according to the inertia of the spore given by its mass and initial velocity. These factors are summarized by a dimensionless parameter P.[13]

$$P = \frac{u_i v_s}{gL}$$

where g is the acceleration of gravity, L is a characteristic dimension of the leaf, and v_s is settling velocity. The u_i is the initial speed of the projectile before it enters the influence of the leaf and it is usually the wind speed. If P is small because a particle is small, a leaf is large, or a wind is slow, then the particle will likely remain in the air stream and be carried around the leaf. Consequently, impaction is inefficient. If P is large, on the other hand, because a particle is massive, a leaf is small, or a wind is fast, the particle will likely strike the leaf. Then impaction is efficient.

Not all spores impacting on a plant will necessarily remain there to infect the host. They can bounce off, reducing the catch below the theoretical and below the catch observed when the target is wet or sticky. Sedimentation, on the other hand, is a gentle process, and particles that settle should rarely bounce off. Consequently, sedimentation efficiencies are at present much better understood than impaction efficiencies.

Generally, the impaction parameter P will determine whether a particle is caught by impaction or settling. If P is large, impaction will predominate, and if P is small, settling will prevail by default. When ragweed pollen, which has a settling velocity v_s about half that of *H. maydis* spores, was released steadily just above a corn field, the u_i was the average wind speed in the canopy of about 1 m/sec, and observation showed that they were caught on leaves by settling, exactly as predicted by the small P for the slow u_i.[14]

In general, the impaction parameter P determines the deposition mechanism and since P depends on the particle speed u_i we expect different outcomes for spores released only in fast gusts compared with spores released continuously.

Integration of Removal, Flight and Catch

Having now discussed Removal, Dilution and Catch, let's integrate these three equations for two cases: 1) steadily released spores and 2) spores released intermittently during fast gusts. These two situations correspond to weakly and strongly held spores since weakly held spores can be removed by almost any wind but strongly held ones are only removed by fast gusts. Obviously, actively discharged spores resemble weakly held ones.

Put another way, these two kinds of spores are not selective and highly selective of the kinds of wind they ride. Strongly held spores, such as *H. maydis*, are usually removed by sudden fast gusts and ride on, and are diluted by, a different kind of wind than weakly held spores, which can be removed by slower and steadier winds. Furthermore, wind speed affects the rate of deposition of the two sorts of spores differently. Impaction on maize leaves can be important for strongly held spores borne by fast winds but weakly held spores, travelling on slower winds, settle onto leaves.[12]

FIGURE 3 shows the integration of these three equations for weakly held or actively discharged spores borne on slow winds and strongly held spores borne

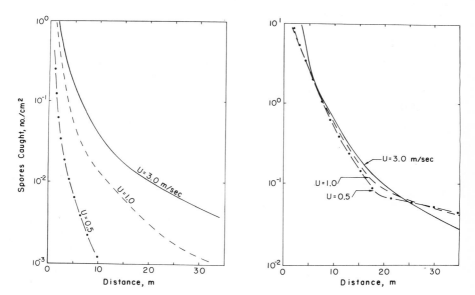

FIGURE 3. The number of spores caught per unit area of corn leaf vs. distance downwind of a source redrawn from Aylor.[12] The left panel represents steadily released spores and the right panel represents spores that are released by gusts of wind. Calculations are based on one million spores released from a source and average wind speeds U of 0.5, 1 and 3 m/sec.

on gusts.[12] Both cases represent the release of one million spores inside a canopy of maize.

The left panel represents spores removed easily and essentially at the average wind speeds of 0.5, 1 and 3 m/sec shown on the curves. At these speeds impaction efficiency on leaves 5-cm wide is small, and thus deposition is mainly by sedimentation. Therefore, in the slowest wind the spores are deposited near the source, and they are carried farther in the faster wind.

The right panel represents spores held strongly. At removal, the spores are travelling considerably faster than the average wind speed because gusts must remove them. At these speeds impaction efficiencies are large. Deposition by impaction is great in all gusts but is greatest in the fastest wind. Thus, a wind of 3 m/sec paradoxically carries the spores the shortest distance, an outcome far different than when spores are weakly held and borne on average winds. It remains to be be verified in the field that different wind speeds have different effects upon the deposition of the two kinds of spores.

SUMMARY

Pandemics of plant disease are caused by air borne fungal spores, some that are injected into the air and some that are blown into the air. A spore that is blown into the air, *Helminthosporium maydis*, is held by uniform force and most are removed from a lesion at about the same wind speed by gusts striking the spore before a viscous boundary layer forms around the leaf. Flight of spores from steady sources causes dilution roughly proportional to the average wind speed while the dilution of puffs of spores blown into the air by gusts is less affected by average wind speed. Spores settle from slow winds but strike leaves when carried by gusts. The net of becoming airborne, flying, and being caught causes a gradient of deposition away from the source that is particularly rapid for a steady source in slow wind and that is relatively unaffected by wind speed if the spores are blown into the air by gusts.

REFERENCES

1. WAGGONER, P. E., J. G. HORSFALL & R. J. LUKENS. 1972. Epimay: A simulator of southern corn leaf blight. Bulletin No. 729. Conn. Agri. Expt. Station. New Haven, Conn.
2. AIST, J. R., D. E. AYLOR & J.-Y. PARLANGE. 1976. Ultrastructure and mechanics of conidium-conidiophore attachment of *Helminthosporium maydis*. Phytopathology. **66:** 1050–1055.
3. AYLOR, D. E. 1975. Force required to detach conidia of *Helminthosporium maydis*. Plant Physiol. **55:** 99–101.
4. WAGGONER, P. E. 1973. The removal of *Helminthosporium maydis* spores by wind. Phytopathology **63:** 1252–1255.
5. AYLOR, D. E. & R. J. LUKENS. 1974. Liberation of *Helminthosporium maydis* spores by wind in the field. Phytopathology **64**(8): 1136–1138.
6. SHAW, R. H., D. P. WARD & D. E. AYLOR. 1979. Frequency of occurrence of fast gusts of wind inside a corn canopy. J. Applied Meteorol. **18**(2): 167–171.
7. SCHLICHTING, H. 1960. Boundary Layer Theory. McGraw Hill. New York.
8. AYLOR, D. E. & J.-Y. PARLANGE. 1975. Ventilation required to entrain small particles from leaves. Plant Physiol. **56:** 97–99.
9. GIFFORD, F. A., Jr. 1968. An outline of theories of diffusion in the lower layers of the atmosphere. *In* Meteorology and Atomic Energy. D. H. Slade, Ed.: 65–116. U.S. Atomic Energy Comm. Oak Ridge, Tennessee.
10. TURNER, D. B. 1970. Workbook of Atmospheric Dispersion Estimates. Environmental Protection Agency. Research Triangle Park. North Carolina.
11. CSANADY, G. T. 1973. Turbulent Diffusion in the Environment. Reidel Pub., Dordrecht, the Netherlands.
12. AYLOR, D. E. 1978. Dispersal in time and space: aerial pathogens. *In* Plant Disease: An Advanced Treatise. J. G. Horsfall and E. B. Cowling, Eds. **2:** 159–180. Academic Press. New York.
13. DAVIES, C. N. 1966. Deposition from moving aerosols. *In* Aerosol Science. C. N. Davies, Ed. 393–446. Academic Press. New York.
14. AYLOR, D. E. 1975. Deposition of particles in a plant canopy. J. Applied Meteorol. **14**(1): 52–57.

(PHILOSOPHICAL) REVIEW OF AIR CURRENTS AS A CONTINUING VECTOR

Charlotte C. Campbell*

American Society for Microbiology
Washington, D.C. 20006

INTRODUCTION

Most papers presented at this conference are directed to pathogenic microbes which, when infected individuals talk, sneeze, or cough are moved *via* air currents in droplet nuclei or in aerosols from one person to other person(s). Usually, but not necessarily, this occurs indoors or, at least, in closed environments. Humankind itself is the source of such bacteria and viruses. In contrast, this paper deals with pathogens whose source, indeed habitat, is soil or organic debris in which they exist as free living forms. To produce the upper respiratory or pulmonary infection, the characteristic primary epidosde in humans and other mammalians, infectious particles of these microbes must be inhaled; but to be inhaled they must first become airbourne, i.e., set free from the soil wafted up and dispersed by air currents. By every criterion, the diseases produced are outdoor or environmental diseases; and the infectious particles, when in the airborne state, are air pollutants. Humans and other mammalians are accidentally parasitized by these pollutants while engaging in the most elemental function for survival—breathing. Inhalation of the infectious particles (alone or in combination with the particles of soils in which they reside) is the only way in which these infections can be acquired. They cannot be transmitted from one person to other person(s); or from one mammalian to other mammalian(s). They can be acquired only by breathing air polluted with infectious particles.

Polluted air, then, *is* the continuing vector and the only source of infection. Without the air current the pathogen is usually harmless, except in rare instances when entry is made via abrasion of the skin and/or direct contact with the organism in soil, rather then via inhalation.

The pulmonary mycoses are representative of this category of infection and disease. I shall use two of the most widely known of these to illustrate points I wish to emphasize. Similar observations, however, may also apply to other diseases (some of them bacterial in origin) just beginning to command our attention, such as Legionnaires disease and the mycobacterioses, to name only two.

It is the purpose of this report to discuss briefly (1) the epidemiology and ecology of the two most widely recognized mycoses which occur in outbreaks† and increasingly in large cities[1,2] as pulmonary infections with acute onset, (2) the role of immunologic tools in defining the geographic distribution of these two mycoses, (3) the skin test vs the ecologic niche, (4) humanity's role in creating these fungal air pollutants as infective agents and as allergens, (5) the incidence and cost of fungal air pollutants in respiratory infections and allergies and (6) finally, to note preventive measures available to us now that would reduce

---

*Retirement address is 120 Pembroke Street, Boston, Mass., 02118.

†To differentiate from epidemics, representative of contagiousness and person-to-person transmissability.

0077-8923/80/0353-0123 $01.75/0 © 1980, NYAS

mycotic and other microbial infection and disease and crippling allergic and asthmatic conditions in which the air current is the continuing vector.

The Respiratory Mycoses as 20th Century Phenomena

Except as rare, debilitating and invariably fatal medical curiosities, the pulmonary mycoses were unknown until the third decade of this, the 20th century. They played no recorded role in the epidemics of person-to-person transmissable, water-, food-, or vector-borne diseases that decimated earlier populations and possibly civilizations. That they were not identified does not, of course, mean they did not occur. It is more likely, however, that such cases merely were overlooked or misdiagnosed in the morass of other infectious diseases extant before the advent of improved sanitation, cotton underwear, vaccines and antibiotics, even after acceptance of the germ theory in the late 1800s.

Disseminated, fatal coccidioidomycosis described in 1890 by Posadas[3] in Argentina was, in the 1930s, the first mycosis to emerge in the U.S. (California) as a prominent primary pulmonary infection from which most persons spontaneously "recovered".[4] Histoplasmosis, discovered in 1906 on the Isthmus of Panama[5] emerged as a clinically similar infection in the middle western United States in the mid to late 1940s.[6,7] Obviously, "recovery" meant clinical recovery and not the residues of calcified lesions, fibrosis, cavitation and other pulmonary pathology of even the pulmonarily disseminated infection.[1]

However, at that time person-to-person transmitted "tuberculosis", one of humankind's principal scourges since antiquity, still had to be conquered with the "miracle therapies" for its cure still two–five years in the future. Prior to discovery of effective antituberculosis drugs, most pulmonary disease, *ipso facto*, was diagnosed as pulmonary tuberculosis. Solitary pulmonary nodules were "tuberculomas," not coccidioidomas, histoplasmomas, or cryptococcomas, as they would later become with increasing prominence of the mycoses.[8,9] Eventually, acute onset, other similar clinical characteristics and history of exposure to sources in nature made it even more important to differentiate the primary mycosis from psittacosis, Q fever and other flu-like syndromes than from miliary tuberculosis.[10,11] With the rapid development of serologic diagnostic tests for both coccidioidomycosis[12] and histoplasmosis,[13] this could be done. Today, of course, the greater concern is over whether a solitary lesion, for example, is due to an infectious agent (its etiology is secondary) or is a neoplasm (carcinoma). The pulmonary mycosis may thus be regarded as one measure of progress of medical knowledge. In this paper I hope also to show that the probable increase in the incidence of pulmonary mycoses is not wholly unrelated to social, industrial and technological changes in contemporary life as well.[1,14,15]

There are systemic mycoses acquired by the respiratory route other than coccidioidomycosis and histoplasmosis. However, they are not characterized by outbreaks of respiratory infections with acute onset from which so much has been learned about both coccidioidomycosis and histoplasmosis, and also about the ecology and epidemiology of their causative fungi. It is also possible our diagnostic tools and skills are not yet sufficiently well advanced to differentiate such outbreaks if they do indeed occur. Consequently, we speak with much less authority concerning the entire disease spectrum of blastomycosis, cryptococcosis, paracoccidioidomycosis, sporotrichosis and aspergillosis, but especially of their primary episodes. There is merely strong evidence that the primary infection for each *is* pulmonary, suggesting that their respective etiologic agents also are to be found in nature, probably soil. Other than those shown in FIGURE 1., more specific ecological niches for the mycotic pulmonary pathogens have yet to be determined.

Epidemiological Tools/Endemic Areas

Approximately 30 to 35 years have passed since standard immunological procedures, i.e., skin and serologic tests, became available as adjuncts to differentially diagnose individual cases as well as outbreaks of coccidioidomycosis and histoplasmosis.[12,13] The skin testing of populations is most useful in defining the geographic regions in which the etiologic fungus resides in the soils and in which it is said to be endemic as evidenced by a high percentage of the indigenous populace reacting to skin tests with the fungus antigen.[12,16,17] Later studies, however, revealed that skin test reactions to histoplasmin defined not so much the geographic distribution of *H. capsulatum* as the areas in which the microfoci

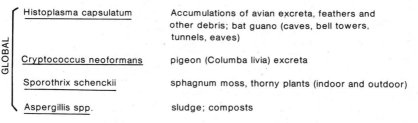

FIGURE 1. Known ecological niches of mycotic pathogens.

for this organism had been disturbed.[18,19] Serologic tests, on the other hand, are used primarily as an adjunct to diagnostically differentiate the primary flu-like illnesses due to *Coccidioides immitis* or *Histoplasma capsulatum* from each other and other clinically and radiologically similar infections.[12,13,20] In the case of coccidioidomycosis results of some serologic tests also have prognostic value.[20]

Isolation of the etiologic fungus from soils is the third way in which endemic areas have been outlined. This is a time consuming procedure ideally requiring isolated mouse facilities.[21,22,23] Nevertheless, it is the effective way to demonstrate beyond doubt that a pulmonary pathogen such as *C. immitis* or *H. capsulatum* is a resident of a particular niche in nature in a particular geographic region and does not comprise part of the overall soil ecology in that region.

The skin test as an immunological tool as well as the asparagine semisynthetic broth used to grow the etiologic fungi to prepare the antigens, coccidioidin and histoplasmin, were borrowed in their entirety from the field of tuberculosis.[12] It was, in fact, during national skin test surveys for tuberculosis that the discovery of tuberculin skin test negative healthy individuals whose chest x-rays revealed marked miliary calcifications were first observed on a wide scale basis.[16,17]

After 30 years, however, coccidiodin and histoplasmin still are the only fungal skin test antigens commercially available for epidemiologic purposes. *Paraoccid-*

ioides brasiliensis is the only other respiratory mycotic pathogen for which immunological studies still appear to be as promising and useful as in coccidioidomycosis and histoplasmosis.[24] The latter organism, of course, has been found only in Central and South America.

Endemic Areas/Ecological Niches

As shown in FIGURE 1., one type of ecological niche may harbor two very important pulmonary mycotic pathogens. This niche is soil heavily contaminated with accumulations of excreta and other debris, including feathers of various species and varieties of avians, both wild and domestic. It is thus not surprising that these two organisms are essentially global in distribution.[25] One of these agents, *Cryptococcus neoformans*, a yeast, not only is closely associated with accumulations of dried excreta of the ubiquitous pigeon (*Columba livia*) but the organism has been isolated from the pigeon's gut and from its fresh feces[26] (also feces from parakeets, budgerigars, canaries and other avians increasingly popular as pets of aging, high-rise apartment dwellers).[1] The bird itself does not acquire the disease, but appears to be merely an innocent carrier of this very serious pathogen for man.

Histoplasma capsulatum, the second pathogen associated with avian excreta and debris is dimorphic. In its yeast (tissue) phase it is unable to propagate at the 40° C internal temperature of avians. The organism has not been found in fresh feces or in the alimentary tracts of birds. However, the organism in its filamentous phase is able to at least survive within the sheaths of avian feathers. Protected by the same it is capable of competing for survival in a manure pile teeming with more rapidly growing microbes.[27] In other words, birds moult as well as defecate at roosting and nesting sites. Until the possibility that the feather is as or more important than feces in establishing microfoci of *H. capsulatum* is disproved, avian(s) must be considered carriers of this pathogen as well as for *C. neoformans*.

Although its exact mode of arrival at this microfocus is still a matter of conjecture, the fact that *H. capsulatum* has been isolated repeatedly from soils under bird roosts heavily contaminated with *accumulations* of avian excreta is not.[28] Certain herbivorous species of bats also have been implicated in the establishment of microfoci of *H. capsulatum*.[29] As flying mammalians, bats do acquire the infection; and the organism propagates in and passes through their alimentary tracts.[29a] Bats, therefore, are quite capable of establishing new microfoci of *H. capsulatum*. Since bats also frequently hibernate or roost in caves, deserted buildings (and under the eaves of inhabited ones) as well as protective tree canopies of forests or in city parks, bat guano alone and/or in combination with avian debris provides an excellent culture medium for *H. capsulatum*. However, the bat itself undeniably is capable of seeding the organism into the appropriate ecological niche.

While it seems a foregone conclusion that all the organisms shown in FIGURE 2., are also basically inhabitants of the soil, the more finite ecological niches for *Coccidioides immitis*, as well as for *Blastomyces dermatitides* and *Paracoccidioides brasiliensis* still elude us despite intensive searches for each.

It is believed by some that *C. immitis* needs no ecological niche[30] to survive other than the desert soils and climatic conditions of its well identified endemic areas in North, Central and South America, as seen in FIGURE 3. Because of the high salt content of these soils, microbial competitors of Coccidioides are

Coccidioides immitis   creosote bush?; lower Sonoran life zone?;
                                        Amerindian middens?; niche undetermined

Blastomyces dermatitidis   soil?; niche undetermined

Paracoccidioides brasiliensis   soil?; bats?; niche undetermined

FIGURE 2. Mycotic pathogens for which ecological niches are not yet determined.

relatively few.[31] From the earlier studies by Maddy[32] revealing the similarity of
the geographic distribution of coccidioidomycosis in the U.S. and the area
comprising the Lower Sonoran Life Zone in the U.S. (as shown in FIGURE 4.) no
solid evidence has come forth that the creosote bush, the only plant common to
these areas, is associated in any way with the presence of *C. immitis* in these
soils. Similarly, frequent isolation of the organism from soils in desert rat burrows
seems only to indicate that the desert rodent prefers a "cool" burrow, is as
susceptible to coccidioidomycosis as other mammalians and acquires it in the
same way.[33] When the infected rodent or other infected mammalian host dies
from coccidioidomycosis (or other causes) it is the dead end of the cycle of the
organism—until the wind again lifts the spores from the desert soils to infect
other mammalians.

Nevertheless, it is still possible that small ecological niches (microfoci) exist in
which *Coccidioides immitis* is an established resident as opposed to a mere
invader of desert soils following a high wind. Based on a 20 year study, Swatek
presents convincing evidence that Amerind middens provide a highly reliable
indicator of the ecological niche of *C. immitis* in desert soils.[34,35] The early
American Indian trails throughout the Lower Sonoran Life Zone do much to

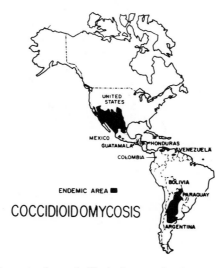

FIGURE 3. Endemic areas, shown in black, for coccidioidomycosis in North, Central and
South America.

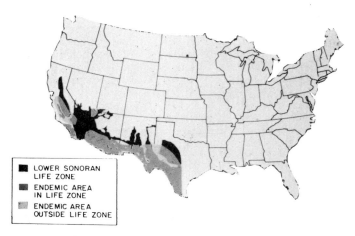

FIGURE 4. Comparison of lower Sonoran Life Zone and endemic areas of coccidioidomy-cosis in the U.S.

explain this mycotic agent's distribution. According to Swatek, movements of the early Indians may well account for the transport of Coccidioides from place to place as part of their dust laden clothing, structural and cooking material. Isolation of the fungus is especially frequent from the kitchen sites (middens).[34,35]

It is possible then, that even with *C. immitis* we are less at the mercy of the wind than it sometimes seems. *C. immitis* may yet also prove to have circumscribed niches that can be destroyed, as suggested later in this paper. Certainly treatment of a circumscribed site is more feasible than trying to sterilize soils, or introduce other microbes to compete with *C. immitis* throughout the entire endemic region.

Much has been written about the respiratory and allergenic fungi as being airborne or transmitted by air. In reality, the infectious particles of the fungus pathogens, allergens and other microbial inhabitants of the soil have no mechanisms by which to become airborne[1] and must depend on external forces to remove them from their ecological niches. The most obvious of these forces is the wind, though even rain drops can disperse spores of some nonpathogenic fungi. Without doubt, day to day winds and air currents alone are capable of releasing some fungus particles from certain kinds of soils, thereby converting them into air pollutants.[14,15,36]

For example, the filamentous form of *Coccidioides immitis* and the arid desert sands in which it thrives are each well suited for transmission by the wind. Indeed if such statistics were recorded, the number of persons acquiring coccidioidomycosis while merely passing through an endemic area by train or car on a mildly windy day would by now be an impressive figure. Unfortunately, this pulmonary mycosis as well as other mycoses is not a reportable disease. For this reason, statistics on the incidence of all pulmonary mycoses amount to little more than educated guesses at best.

There is no guessing, however, about "the large number of new cases" of primary coccidioidomycosis resulting from a spectacular windstorm that blew through Kern County, California on December 20, 1977.[30,37] Wind swept down the west face of the Sierra-Tehachapi Mountains. It scoured the topsoil to a depth of up to 15 cm., raising it in a huge dust cloud that reached an elevation of approximately 15 meters. Borne aloft near Arvin, the dust cloud was carried up the San Joaquin Valley at high altitude. As the dust settled, hazy atmospheric conditions prevailed up to 600 to 700 km. north of Bakersfield and persisted for approximately 18 hours; the dust "irritating the eyes and mucus membranes of area residents and forming a thich layer on automobiles and sidewalks." In the wake of this storm there were approximately 530 new cases of coccidioidomycosis, not only in persons exposed directly to the dust raised by the windstorm, but also among those in many areas to the north and west of the areas. All told, it was estimated that the ratio of actual to reported infections was 50:1 in this epidemic[37] although exposure to the dust borne *Coccidioides immitis* was brief because of the arrival of drenching rains (FIGURE 5).[30]

Anthropogenic Factors/Air Pollutants

It would be difficult not to remember a storm of this magnitude and intensity, but such storms are not common, even in the San Joaquin Valley in California

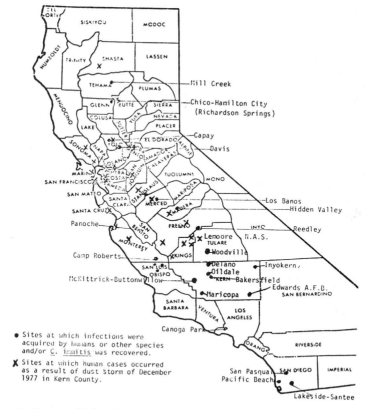

FIGURE 5. Sites at which infections were acquired by humans or other species and/or *Coccidioides immitis* was recovered (●); sites at which human cases occurred as a result of dust storm of December 1977 in Kern County, California (X). (Courtesy of Dr. D. Pappagianis, U.C., Davis.)

and other endemic areas. It is more likely, that for *C. immitis* as well as for other pathogens and fungal allergens, the activities of man, *Homo sapiens*, contribute heavily to dispersion of infectious and sensitizing particles by air currents. In fact, the continuous rotations of airplane propellers played no small role in elevating coccidioidomycosis to the leading infection among U.S. military personnel during World War II, as many training bases for the Air Force as well as the other military services were located throughout the endemic areas for *C. immitis*.[38] Though prop planes have long since been replaced by jets, coccidioidomycosis is still very much a problem in military personnel, as it is in civilian populations residing in the endemic areas.

Homo sapiens, however, began to deplete the soils with the beginning of agriculture in the unrecorded past and has continuously upheaved them ever since; not only for his crops, but also to construct more and more cities, highways and industries to expand living room to accommodate the increasing and increasingly aggregating population of our species.[1] In so doing, he was sooner or later bound to disrupt the ecological niches of fungal pathogens, as he did in Panama where the dredging up of *H. capsulatum* was indirectly recorded through the astute observation of Darling.[5] Like Coccidioides, this fungus proved to be pathogenic for man as well as sensitizing.[16] At first, the identifiable primary cases and outbreaks traceable to their sources in nature were few; but, as shown in FIGURE 6., once the proved microfoci were extended beyond the old chicken house and open top silo on the farm to include roosting sites for avians in general, the ecological niches for *H. capsulatum* were found to encompass the globe in temperate and tropical regions.[25] Birds[39] and herbivorous bats[29,29a,40] are indigenous to such areas. Undomesticated avians and bats are also partial to trees, caves and unfinished buildings as sheltered roosting and nesting sites. Thus, regardless of how it arrives in such microfoci, *H. capsulatum* flourishes in soils where there is plenty of moisture and protection from direct sunlight; soils that are much more tightly bound and fertile than the arid desert sands preferred by *C. immitis*; and, without man's help, far less easily shifted by the wind.

However, *H. capsulatum* receives plenty of help from man in its transformation from a soil microbe into an air pollutant. The identifiable outbreaks have grown increasingly larger as disturbance of its ecological niche has occurred among increasingly congregated populations.[1,2] There were more and more people to inhale the airborne infectious and sensitizing particles as man moved and progressively congregated from farm to village to city to metropolis.[1,14,15,18] The earliest recorded outbreaks involved only the farm family who were engaged in cleaning out the old chicken house or silo, simply because they were the only persons about within inhaling distance to be infected or sensitized. Once the association with avians in general had been recognized, it was also relatively easy to relate the village or small city outbreaks to a specific excavation or disruption of soil around a known bird roost. Often it is the only excavation at the time in the community; its victims are admitted as patients to that community's one or two hospitals and/or visit its smaller number of practicing physicians.[28]

However, these "props," which are so useful in locating the microfoci of small histoplasmosis outbreaks in rural areas, villages and smaller cities, may prove to be essentially useless in tracing an outbreak to its source(s) in larger metropolitan populations. In most metropolises today, the razing of old buildings, and/or excavation and/or construction activities for new buildings is literally continuous. Ill people are treated by many different physicians and admitted to the many different hospitals not only in that particular city, but also to those in its surrounding suburbs. An outbreak or an increase in the number of cases of

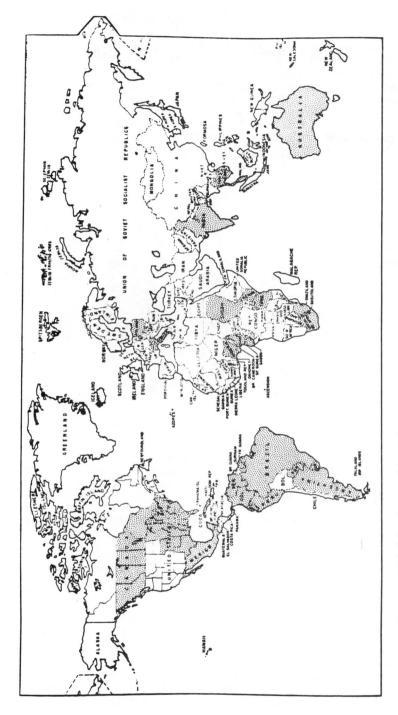

FIGURE 6. Global distribution of *Histoplasma capsulatum* is shown by the shaded areas. (Courtesy of Dr. L. Ajello, Mycology Unit. Communicable Disease Center. Atlanta, Ga.)

primary pulmonary histoplasmosis must, under the cirucumstances, be identified
by the clinical picture and confirmed or supported largely by positive serologic
findings. Since the latter rarely comprise part of an admission workup, even in
the largest and best hospitals outside the middle western, traditionally recognized endemic areas in the U.S. (FIGURE 7.), I predicted in 1974 that without the
familar "props" so useful in pinpointing the source in smaller communities, a city
outbreak might be attributed to nonspecific causes in traditionally nonendemic
areas; but if the outbreak were noted, tracking it to its source(s) might literally
prove to be impossible.[1]

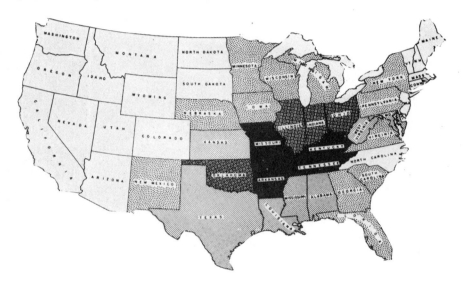

■ States with histoplasmin sensitivity levels of 50 percent or more in both rural and urban areas.

States with histoplasmin sensitivity levels of 50 percent or more in farm areas only.

States with histoplasmin sensitivity levels of 50 percent or more in one or more counties only.

Peripheral *H. capsulatum* endemic areas based on soil isolations.

FIGURE 7. Principal histoplasmosis endemic areas in the United States.

Such an outbreak did recently occur in Indianapolis, Indiana; the first to be
reported from a very large metropolis, even in the heart of the endemic area.[41,42]
In this one city, there were at least 435 diagnosed cases, 49 with disseminated
disease and 15 deaths. Serologic surveys indicated that there were an additional
20 thousand to 200 thousand infections, illustrating that the outbreak was the
largest as well as one of the most serious outbreaks of histoplasmosis yet
recorded. Although there was no spectacular windstorm to herald the outbreak's

approach, or to transport the organism, cases though concentrated in the center of the city, were scattered over a 400 square mile radius. The outbreak lasted nearly one year, from September 1978 to August 1979, suggesting a continuing disruption of the microfocus or microfoci.[43]

As also predicted[1] the latter are proving difficult to find. Two very usual sources are under investigation. Soil samples from both may be positive, or from neither, just as disruption of soils aroung both or neither might have contributed to the outbreak or had nothing to do with it. Locating the source(s) of an outbreak in a large city or metropolis is a much more complex task than locating one in a rural area, village or small town.

To illustrate, I will describe the situation around my office building in downtown Washington, D.C., which is the situation around most downtown offices in any city in the U.S. today. Within the past two and one-half years, buildings have been razed, excavations dug and large new buildings constructed on six of the possible eight corners at 19th and 20th Streets, N.W., between which the American Society for Microbiology headquarters building on I Street stands. During this time the area has been a veritable continuum of bulldozers, dump trucks (none covered) and other massive razing and earth moving equipment. A small city park occupies a seventh corner. Here people come to eat lunch, sun, relax and, of course, feed the pigeons and other birds. One possible difference from some other cities is that the soils in Washington, D.C. are known to be positive not only for *H. capsulatum*, but also for *C. neoformans*.[23,44] As noted earlier, *C. neoformans* has not been recognized in outbreaks with acute onset, but it is well recognized as a devasting CNS disease with an affinity for the meninges, especially in the compromised host; and of compromised hosts Washington, as elsewhere in the U.S., has an increasing number.

Perhaps even more important in the tracing of an outbreak of histoplasmosis in a metropolis is "the vacant lot" adjacent to the ASM headquarters building. The lot has been vacant only since April 1979! For approximately ten years prior to that time this so recently vacated lot had been the site of a dilapidated, Victorian type brick residence with all windows and doors broken out; long since abandoned except for the countless pigeons, starlings and bats, which came to roost and hibernate there day and night.

In April, without warning, the building was razed. Old bricks and salvageable building materials were hauled away. The site was leveled by bulldozers with these dusty soils heavily fertilized with avian debris and bat guano. Any pathogenic fungi present are multiplying *in situ*, awaiting disruption by the next bulldozer operator to begin the next construction.

Although there are regulations concerning the razing of buildings like this, contractors are either ignorant of, or ignore, them. The workmen throughout this entire project were as unprotected as the passersby on the adjacent sidewalk, or across the street. The workmen were obviously as ignorant of the potential hazards of their occupation as persons walking or passing by in cars several blocks away were innocent of the razing activity hidden from their view by the tall buildings in between. Moreover, consider that some of these passersby are on their way to a bus or subway in the center city, from which they will disperse to all areas of the city and its peripheral suburbs in Maryland and Virginia. If, a week or two later, these individuals develop a mild to moderate—or even quite severe—primary pulmonary illness, who among them will recall or associate this illness with something so commonplace in our contemporary lives as the razing of one more building, or the bulldozing of one more excavation site a week or two before?

The second outbreak of histoplasmosis in Mason City, Iowa, was very instructive on several counts: there could be a second outbreak from the same source; on a day with essentially no wind, air currents could move infectious particles of *H. capsulatum* from a disturbed microfocus for a distance of several blocks; and positive cultures obtained on the tops of tall buildings indicated that even in the absence of measurable wind, fungus particles were borne upward and over the taller buildings nearby by gentle convection currents.[45]

Without question the microfoci of *H. capsulatum* and the point source(s) of outbreaks in large cities will be much more difficult to locate than they are in smaller towns and rural areas, implicating a single excavation site, or other disturbed microfocus. In situations such as the vacant lot described above, there are not even birds left to suggest the recent classical microfocus of two pathogenic fungi, some of which, without treatment[46] remain positive for almost a decade.[19]

Incidence and Cost of Fungal Air Pollutants
As Infective and Sensitizing Agents

The absence of reliable statistics on the number of cases of either histoplasmosis or coccidioidomycosis (and other mycoses) makes it impossible to assess their incidence. It has been pointed out repeatedly, however, that while mortality from primary infection may be low, morbidity is extremely high and represents a major loss of productive time among residents of the endemic areas and travelers to endemic areas. It is estimated that nearly 100% of the population residing in the endemic areas for *C. immitis* will have been infected within the first or second year of residence and about a fifth of these will have had an illness severe enough to cause temporary incapacity and warrant medical care.[30]

It is of interest that both reports[30,37] describing the coccidioidomycosis outbreak resulting from the spectacular wind storm in December 1977 noted the fiscal impact. Pappagianis and Einstein[30] estimated that hospital room costs only for the 521 cases recognized through the first three months of 1978 would have amounted to $1,823,500. Since more than 500 cases per year are reported from Arizona alone, the seasonal recurrence of coccidioidomycosis in the Southwest requires a continuing and substantial medical expenditure.[30] Flynn, et al,[37] in a later report on the same outbreak, also referred to its economic impact, estimating total care costs also to be in excess of one million dollars. The figures will differ little for the histoplasmosis outbreak in Indianapolis, where there were also around 500 cases, 300 of moderate to intensive severity requiring hospitalization.[43]

When it is recalled that histoplasmosis and coccidioidomycosis are only two of the mycoses, not to mention the other diseases whose microbial agents are transported by air currents in the open environment following disruptions of the same soils, we may continue to call such infections "benign" if we wish, but they are not cheap! A study by Hammerman, Powell and Tosh[47] provides further evidence that for pulmonary mycoses alone, hospitalization costs far exceed 10 million dollars per year, without notable outbreak such as those described herein. The mycoses following dissemination have an especially poor prognosis—and a high rate of relapse in persons compromised by immuno suppressive and/or chemotherapeutic agents—and those undergoing organ transplantation or cancer chemotherapy. As noted earlier, compromised hosts represent a growing number of U.S. citizens.

However, the cost of infection—mycotic or bacterial—is only part of the cost of disease due to air as a continuing vector. We have yet to consider the allergies, the most common of the immunologic diseases. Allergies vary from sensitivities to common fungi to reactions that lead to asthma and all the management and medical problems this serious illness presents. In a report by Krause[48] it is estimated that "80 percent of children with asthma and 50 percent of adults with the disease also suffer from allergies to, among other allergens, molds (fungi). In this same category are pollens and dusts, also transported by the wind. Reexposure to these allergens after certain time intervals precipitates the more serious asthmatic attacks. In this same report, Krause provides theretofore unpublished data on the major causes for visits to U.S. physicians in 1975. Despite availability of antibiotics to treat *bacterial* infections, infections are responsible for nearly 22 percent of all visits to physicians each year. For children under 16, the percentage rises to 65. About 30 percent of the office visits, however, are to seek assisstance for asthmatic and other allergic conditions.

Not wholly unrelated to the category of allergic diseases associated with air as the vector are outbreaks of "farmers lung" among office personnel[1] striking executive directors as indiscriminately as the beginning "gofer help." Central air conditioning and heating systems may not only feed in pathogenic fungi from the environment, but because of their engineering design support the growth of thermophilic actinomycetes and other fungi whose spores are disseminated through the air ducts. The development of hypersensitivity alveolitis in office workers, home owners and apartment dwellers—all who are exposed to central air conditioning—demonstrates that this condition can be serious, crippling and even fatal if exposure is repeated or continued. Continuous nearby excavations must certainly tax the best air conditioning systems, especially those that are somewhat antiquated and/or need replacement. That these systems contribute to infections as well as allergies is well supported by recent experiences with Legionnaires disease and possibly the most ironical of all histoplasmosis outbreaks.[49] To celebrate Earth Day 1970, school children at the Willis School in Delaware, Ohio raked leaves to clean up an inner courtyard that had long been the roosting site for birds and thereby innocently fed countless infectious particles of *H. capsulatum* directly into the air intakes of the school's forced air ventilation system. The number of clinical cases was only slightly fewer than in the Indianapolis outbreak, but the number of infections was far less because of the lesser number of persons exposed.[41]

Prevention and Control

Though at first glance it might seem that we are helpless against environmental diseases and allergies that arise from polluting air with infecting and sensitizing particles of microbes, which without man's intervention are residents of the soil, this really is not the case.

The most immediate preventive step is to enforce legislation which already exists, at least in Region IV of the Environmental Protection Agency; and to extend this legislation to other regions throughout the U.S. This step is to decontaminate the very well identified microfoci of *H. capsulatum* (and *C. neoformans*) before they are disturbed by razing and/or soil moving equipment, especially in densely populated areas.[46] A pamphlet describing methods for this purpose is also available from: DHEW, Public Health Service Center for Disease Control, Bureau of State Services, Environmental Health Services Division,

Atlanta, Georgia 30333. It is of interest that the General Services Administration before renovating vacant buildings for historic preservation issues a "Hazard Alert" which informs "workers who must work around and demolish bird, especially pigeon habitations, to use extreme caution due to the potential risk of illness involved when disturbing accumulations prior to decontamination."

Unfortunately, these protective procedures seem not to have been heard of by nongovernment construction workers, certainly not in Washington, D.C. Workmen wear no respiratory masks or protective clothing. Neither buildings nor soils are wetted down to contain the dust to protect the passersby on their way to and from their own work. Contractors and job foremen profess complete ignorance of any such regulations. The Environmental Protection Agency (EPA) itself gives little emphasis to air pollutants that are microbial, pathogenic or sensitizing substances. According to the present Deputy Assistant Administrator for Health and Ecological Effects of the EPA, the first interest of this group is with drinking water contaminants in an extensive virology program. I was assured, however, that "as that group expands to give more attention to immunology and identification research, soil pathogens and bird vectors could well be included."

It is to hoped that in the future humanity will understand every thing there is to know about immunology and identification. Meanwhile, it is also hoped that those in the EPA will consider some of the tried and true environmental approaches of stemming the source in nonmedical ways, e.g., John Snow removing the handle from the pump at the Broad Street well in 1854 to quell the cholera epidemic[50] and much more recently, the massive programs to reduce cigarette smoking as a principal means of diminishing an array of pulmonary and cardiovascular diseases.[51,52] Perhaps it is now time to consider that the state of our general pulmonary and respiratory health would also be considerably improved and the vast cost of our national medical bill reduced simply by imposing and enforcing some needed constraints on those whose job in life it is to move the good earth itself. Constraints should be placed on the mass disturbance of all soils in large metropolises, but certainly on those *known* to be the ecological niches of pathogenic microbes.

Education of the general public, of scientists, physicians, veterinarians, construction workers, health workers and of city, county, state and federal legislators was recommended in an earlier report.[1] Additional research funds for the discovery of the ecological niches of other pulmonary pathogenic fungi is also recommended.[1] These recommendations, however, are merely means to treating such microfoci. In summarizing the Indianapolis report on the longest and most severe outbreak yet of histoplasmosis, Wheat et al., stated, "the short-term impact has been great. The long-term impact may be equally important. Histoplasmosis is clearly a threat to the citizens in large cities."[43]

So, too, are all the other pathogenic microbes and "nonpathogenic" allergens whose natural habitat is the soil, but which become air pollutants with man's disturbance of these soils, which in our contemporary lives is essentially continuous.

ACKNOWLEDGMENTS

I am indebted to Drs. Libero Ajello (CDC) and Demosthenes Pappagianis, University of California, Davis, for the geographic distribution maps used in the published report; to Drs. Robert. J. Weeks, and Vernon N. Houk, CDC, for slides and other materials used in the presented report; and to Mr. John Gardiner, American Society for Microbiology, for typing the manuscript.

REFERENCES

1. CAMPBELL, C. C. 1974. Respiratory mycotic infections. Preventive Medicine **3:** 517–528.
2. DRUTZ, DAVID J. 1979. Urban coccidiodomycosis and histoplasmosis. Editorial. N. Engl. J. Med. **301**(7): 381–382.
3. POSADAS, A. 1892. Un Nuevo Caso di Micosis Fungoidea con Psorospermias Circulo Med. Argentino **15:** 585–597.
4. DICKSON, E. C. & M. A. GIFFORD. 1938. *Coccidioides* infection (coccidioidomycosis) II the primary type of infection. Arch. Int. Med. **62:** 853–871.
5. DARLING, SAMUEL T. 1906. A protozoan general infection producing pseudotubercles in the lungs and focal necrosis in the liver and spleen and lymph nodes, J. Am. Med. Assoc. **46:** 1283–1285.
6. PARSONS, R. J. & C. J. D. ZARAFONETIS. 1945. Histoplasmosis in man: report of seven cases and a review of 71 cases. Arch. Intern. Med. **75:** 1–23.
7. DACK, G. M. 1948. Statement, Proceeding of the (first) seminar on histoplasmosis. National Institutes of Health, Maryland. September 13: 1.
8. PEABODY, J. P. Jr., S. KATZ & E. W. DAVIS. 1957. The so-called tuberculoma. A reappraisal. Bull. Georgetown University. Washington D.C. **10:** 141.
9. SEABURY, J. H. 1970. Discussion. Proceedings International Symposium on Mycoses. PAHO Scientific Publication No. 205:263.
10. SABIN, A. B. 1951. Nontuberculous diseases of the chest and related matters; Miliary granulomatous pneumonitis in a group of men exposed to pigeon excreta (abstract). Trans. Nat. Tuberc. Assoc. **47:** 290–293.
11. JOHNSON, J. E. & P. J. KADULL. 1966. Laboratory-Acquired Q fever: A report of fifty cases. Am. J. Med. **41:** 391–403.
12. SMITH, C. E., E. G. WHITING, E. E. BAKER. H. G. ROSENBERGER, R. R. BEARD & M. T. SAITO, 1948. The use of coccidioidin. Am. Rev. Tuberc. **57:** 330–360.
13. CAMPBELL, C. C. 1971. History of the development of serologic tests for histoplasmosis. Proc. of the Second National Conference. A. Balows, Ed.: 341–357. C C Thomas. Springfield, Ill.
14. CAMPBELL, C. C. 1967. Histoplasmosis and other respiratory mycoses in tropical climates. Industry and Tropical Health, VI. Proc. Sixth Conf. of the industrial Council for Tropical Health: 145–152. Harvard School of Public Health.
15. CAMPBELL, C. C. 1971. The Pilot Wheel, a Change in Course. Proc. first PAHO Symposium on Paracoccidioidomycosis. PAHO Scientific Publication No. 254: 306–312.
16. CHRISTIE, A. & J. C. PETERSON. 1945. Pulmonary calcification in negative reactors to tuberculin. Amer. J. Public Health **35:** 1131–1147.
17. PALMER, C. E. 1945. Nontuberculous pulmonary calcification and sensitivity to histoplasmin. Public Health Rep. **60:** 513–520.
18. CAMPBELL, C. C. 1965. The epidemiology of histoplasmosis. Ann. Int. Med. **62**(6): 1333–1336.
19. DISALVO, A. F. & W. M. JOHNSON. 1979. Histoplasmosis in South Carolina: support for the microfocus concept. Am. J. Epidemiol. **109**(4): 480–492.
20. SMITH, C. E., M. T. SAITO, R. R. BEARD, R. M. KEPP, R W. CLARK & B. U. EDDIE. 1950. Serological tests in the diagnosis and prognosis of coccidioidomycosis. Amer. J. Hyg. **52**(1): 1–21.
21. STEWART, R. A. & K. F. MEYER. 1932. Isolation of *Coccidioides immities* (Stiles) from the soil. Proc. Soc. Exp. Biol. Med. **29:** 937–938.
22. EMMONS, C. W. 1949. Isolation of *Histoplasma capsulatum* from soil. Public Health Rep. **64:** 892–896.

23. EMMONS, C. W. 1951. Isolation of *Cryptococcus neoformans* from soil. J. Bacteriol. **62:** 685–690.
24. RESTREPO, A., D. L. GREER & M. VASCONCELLOS. 1973. Paracoccidioidomycosis: A review. Commonwealth Mycological Review Institute Rev. Med. Vet. Mycol. **8**(2): 97–123.
25. AJELLO, L. 1970. The medical mycological iceberg. Proceedings International Symposium on Mycoses. PAHO Scientific Publication No. 205: 3–12.
26. STAIB, F. 1962. Vogelkot, ein Nährsubstrat für die Gattung Cryptococcus Zbl. Bakt. (Orig.) **186:** 233–247.
27. TEWARI, R. P. & C. C. CAMPBELL. 1965. Isolation of *Histoplasma capsulatum* from feathers of chickens inoculated intravenously and subcutaneously with the yeast phase of the organism, Sabouraudia, **4**(1): 17–22.
28. SAROSI, G. A., J. D. PARKER & F. E. TOSH. 1971. Histoplasmosis outbreaks: their patterns. Histoplasmosis: 123–139. Proceedings of the Second National Conference. Albert Balows, Ed. C C Thomas.
29. EMMONS, C. W. 1958. Association of bats with Histoplasmosis. Public Health Reports. **73:** 590.
29a. SHACKLETTE, M. H., F. H. DIERCKS, & N. B. GALE. 1962. *Histoplasma capsulation* recovered from bat tissue. Science **135:** 1135.
30. PAPPAGIANIS, D. & H. EINSTEIN. 1978. Tempest from Tehachapi takes toll or coccidiodes conveyed aloft and afar. Western Journal of Medicine. **129:** 527–530.
31. ELCONIN, A. F., R. O. EGEBERG & M. C. EGEBERG. 1964. Significance of soil salinity on the ecology of *Coccidioides immitis* J. Bacteriol. **87:** 500–503.
32. MADDY, K. T. 1957. Ecological factors possibly relating to the geographic distribution of *Coccidioides immitis*. Proceedings of Symposium on coccidioidomycosis. Public Health Service Publications No. 575.: 144–157.
33. EMMONS, C. W. 1943. Coccidioidomycosis in wild rodents. A method of determining the extent of endemic areas. Publ. Health Reports **58:** 1–5.
34. SWATEK, F. E. 1977. Ecology of *Coccidioides immitis* and the epidemiology of coccidioidomycosis. Second International Mycological Congress; pg 649. University of So. Florida. Tampa.
35. LACY, G. H. & F. E. SWATEK. 1974. Soil ecology of *Coccidioides immitis* at Amerindian middens in California. Applied Microb. **27**(2): 379–388.
36. CAMPBELL, C. C. 1971. The need for an improved serologic test for histoplasmosis. Proc. Second National Conf. A. Balows. Ed.: 464–467. CC Thomas. Springfield, Ill.
37. FLYNN, N. M., P. D. HOEPRICH, M. M. KAWACHI, K. K. LEE, R. M. LAWERENCE, E. GOLDSTEIN, G. W. JORDAN, R. S. KUNDARGI & G. A. WONG. 1979. An unusual outbreak of windborne coccidioidomycosis. N. Engl. J. Med. **301**(7): 358–361.
38. SMITH, C. E. 1967. Reminiscenses of "The Flying Chamydospore" and its allies. Proc. Second Symposium on Coccidioidomycosis. University Ariz. Press. L. Ajello, Ed.: XIII–XXIII.
39. SMITH, C. D. 1971. The role of birds in the ecology of *Histoplasma capsulatum*. Histoplasmosis. Proc. Second National Conf. A. Balows, Ed.: 140–148.
40. DiSALVO, A. F. 1971. The role of bats in the ecology of *Histoplasma capsulatum*. Ibid: 149–161.
41. WHEAT, L. J., T. SLAMA, H. EITZEN, R. B. KOHLER, J. BIESECKER & M. V. FRENCH. 1979. Unique features of the Indianapolis Histoplasmosis outbreak. 19th Interscience Conference on Antimicrobial Agents and Chemotherapy. Boston. Abstract 667.
42. Ibid. Abstract 666.
43. WHEAT, L. J. 1979. Personal Communication.
44. EMMONS, C. W. 1961. Isolation of *Histoplasma capsulatum* from soil in Washington, D. C. Public Health Rep. **76:** 591–596.
45. TOSH, F. E., I. L. DOTO, D. J. D'ALESSIO, A. A. MEDEIROS, S. L. HENDRICKS & T. D. Y. CHIN. 1966. The second of two epidemics of histoplasmosis resulting from work on the same starling roost. Amer. Rev. Resp. Dis. **94:** 406–413.
46. WEEKS, R. J. & F. E. TOSH. 1971. Control of epidemic foci of *Histoplasma capsulatum*. Histoplasmosis Proc. Second National Conf. A. Balows, Ed.: 184–189. CC Thomas. Springfield, Ill.

47. HAMMERMAN, K. J., K. E. POWELL & F. E. TOSH. 1974. The incidence of hospitalized cases of systemic mycotic infections. Sabouraudia **12:** 33–45.
48. KRAUSE, R. H. 1978. A matter of opportunity. A report from the director. National Institute of Allergy and Infectious Diseases, NIH.: 46–52.
49. FOSS, R. J. & S. SASLAW. 1971. Earth Day histoplasmosis: a new type of urban pollution. Arch. Intern. Med. **128:** 588–590.
50. SNOW, J. 1964. "The Broad Street Pump" in Curiosities of Medicine. Berton Roueche, Ed. Berkley. New York City.
51. Surgeon General's Report on Smoking. 1964. DHEW Publication.
52. Surgeon General's Report on Smoking and Health. 1979. DHEW Publication.

ASPERGILLUS IN PATIENT CARE AREAS

Lloyd G. Herman

Environmental Safety Branch
Division of Research Services
National Institutes of Health
Bethesda, Maryland 20205

The *Aspergilli* are among the four most common fungi of the environment.[1] They can be readily isolated from the soil, most readily from compost piles and damp basements of houses as well as the tropics, polar areas and the upper atmosphere.[2] Of the 150 described *Aspergillus* species, only about a dozen[3] are presently known to be pathogenic to man, animals and birds,[4,5] and although infections of almost every body tissue have been noted,[3] the *Aspergilli* are most frequently encountered as respiratory pathogens.[2,6] A *fumigatus* is the most commonly noted pathogenic species among cancer patients and is especially active as an allergic and invasive organism.[2,7]

Other species, e.g., *A. niger, A. terreus, A. flavus, A. nidulans, A. niveus, A. clavatus,* and *A. restrictus,*[3] have also been responsible for similar infections; some are involved in the production of aflotoxins in human and animal foods,[8] allergic broncho-pulmonary aspergillosis,[7] colonization of paranasal and sinus surfaces,[9,10] invasive diseases of lungs and other organs,[11] and are also occasionally found in systemic infections.[12]

The thermo-tolerance of some members of this group, 12°–53°C in hot or active compost piles[2,13] apparently helps them to become established in animal (37°C) and bird (40°C) host tissues. Since the spores (conidia) of *A. fumigatus* are small, only about 2–3 microns in diameter, they are readily distributed by air currents and thus not easily isolated on fallout plates. Special equipment is usually necessary to remove the viable spores from the air currents especially inside residential and public buildings e.g., hospitals and patient care units.[14] However, culturing vacuum cleaner dust will usually provide several species of viable *Aspergilli.*[15] As with every biological contamination, the numbers and species of viable spores will vary widely both seasonally[16-18] and geographically.[1,19]

A study in England[20] reported that *A. fumigatus* spores were isolated on each of 78 days at levels varying from 0.01–70 spores per cubic foot of air tested, while air samples in Nevada rarely showed spores of *A. fumigatus.*[17] Although *A. fumigatus* spores are seldom[21] transmitted from animal to man or patient to patient, still several patients in the same ward may be infected by breathing air from the same source carrying viable spores.[22,23]

Although the science of microbiology prefers to deal with readily demonstrable means of contamination, viz, "the control of contact infections and of food borne, insect borne, and water borne infections is far ahead of airborne infections,"[24] this might indicate that this conference comes at an opportune time "to cast some light on the transmission and pathogenesis of airborne disease."[25]

Sources of Aspergillus Spores

Most fungal (mold) spores can survive months to years in the dry state inside buildings[2,16] so that they can be readily isolated from undistured dust and lint

140

0077-8923/80/0353-0140 $01.75/0 © 1980, NYAS

accumulations, carpeting, mattresses, bedding, the soil and leaves of indoor plants,[26] humidifiers[27] and from virtually every soiled and continuously damp area.[2]

In the outside environment, especially in the vicinity of deciduous trees, shedding leaves from September through November, air counts can easily exceed 300 mold spores, including those of the *Aspergillus* species, per cubic foot especially on windy days.[18] Dust from construction sites, farm operations, and manufacturing processes can also provide excessive mold spore counts.[28-30] Hospital building repairs and reconstruction close to patient care areas are also prime sources of *Aspergillus* spores.[22,23] The contaminated and disturbed dust and lint settles everywhere and is readily redistributed when floors are cleaned or bedding is changed. Recent emphasis on conservation of organic matter by recommending "compost piles" in each garden in the suburban areas[2] or recycling sewage sludge by the acre may create problems close to residential areas.[13]

The ability of *Aspergilli* to grow at low levels of moisture on cellulose sound and fire proofing materials was noted in a hospital and was the suspected source of several patient infections.[23] A more direct cause of allergic broncho-pulmonary *aspergillosis* was noted in a patient who insisted on smoking moldy marijuana.[31] Other plant materials such as dry hay, straw, jute and hemp, usually also carry exceptionally high levels of viable mold spores.[30]

Monitoring and Isolation Methods

Although there is little evidence that viable and virulent spores of *A. fumigatus* are spread from person to person,[21] yet infections due to this mold have been reported post mortem[11,12] in 60% of patients dying of leukemia, up to 45% after renal transplants and in 49% of infections noted in surgical patients.[32] However, due to the small size of the spores of *Aspergillus* species, fallout plates for short periods of time are not usually satisfactory.[14,18] Nevertheless, contaminated dust and lint particles can easily be removed from dusty surfaces by a swab moistened with sterile broth and then swabbed over the surface of Czapeck or Sabourauds agar plates and incubated at room temperatures for total mold growth or at 37°–44°C for *Aspergillus* species. When *Aspergilli* are noted, more definitive studies can be made with Rodac Czapeck's or Sabouraud agar plates from surfaces close to critically ill patients; e.g., mattresses, pillows, bedding, drapes, curtains, carpets, shelves, cupboards, i.e., the environment of the patient, while more intimate checks on exposed skin, hair or clothing of the patient would indicate a probable exposure or contact.[33] Since no open surface is ever sterile, less than 5 mold colonies per plate would presuppose good sanitation, although 10 to 30 colonies might indicate poor sanitation or control, while more than 50 colonies per Rodac plate is certainly cause for caution and evidence of excessive contamination from a specific source. Weekly checks for up to two months will help to identify the areas that are properly maintained as well as those that seem to be ignored. Careful evaluation and interpretation of the results can provide much useful basic data for future studies should an increase in infections occur, especially when done by the same individual. Whatever information is acquired, it must always be remembered that total numbers are not as significant as are the species.

Air Sampling

Since spores of *A. fumigatus* are only 2–4 microns in diameter, they are readily airborne and special air sampling equipment is needed to isolate and measure the viable spores in any desired volume of air,[34] although air currents inside and outside of buildings are dynamic, rarely predictable or seldom replicable.[16] The following methods can be used to extract most of the viable spores from measured volumes of air for selected time periods and deposit them in or on suitable media, e.g., broth and Sabouraud's or Czapeck solution agar media, with added antibiotics to inhibit bacterial growth. The volumes of air sampled can vary from 1–120 cubic feet in time periods, varying from 1 minute through 120 minutes. Following the sampling, incubation of the plates should be done at 20°–28°C for total viable mold spore content and at 37°–44°C for counts of the thermo-tolerant *Aspergilli*[13] for 4–8 days.

Familiarity with routine microbiology lab procedures is helpful but any willing technician can be readily trained to handle any of the following pieces of equipment and materials and maintain low levels of contamination of the media, the equipment and the environment. The simplest controllable method for trapping, isolating and growing viable *Aspergilli* spores, from the air, in any environment, is with the membrane filter.[34] These units are available in most laboratories and with in house vacuum or with a suitable pump, a flow meter, a stop watch, plus the desired media and diluting fluid, small or large volumes of air, tropical or polar, can easily be checked for viable spores. In dusty or heavily contaminated areas, only small volumes of air, 1–10 cubic feet, should be pulled through the sterile pad at approximately 0.5 cubic feet per minute and the pad transferred directly onto the surface of the above agar plates and incubated until the colonies are easily counted, but not overgrown. Larger volumes, in cleaner areas, e.g., 30–90 cubic feet of air may also be pulled through a sterile air filter pad and also set on an agar plate or broken up in a blender and diluted with 1 ml. aliquots spread over the surface of the above agar plates. This technique, although not noted for its accuracy (50–70% recovery) will provide an indication of the levels and species of viable mold spores in the environment at any given period of time as well as the levels of the nonviable particulates, e.g., lint and dust when the larger volumes are used.

The Andersen Multi-State Sieve Sampler

This unit with a self contained vacuum pump is portable, but requires six plates of agar per sampling and may be run for a 1–30 minute sampling period, at the rate of 1 cubic foot per minute, with media and incubation (available from Andersen, 2000 Atlanta, Ga.)[35,36] With this unit one can separate air borne particles and droplet nuclei ranging in size from 1 micron or less, to over 100 microns and classify up to 2600 viable particles per cubic foot. However, exposure time should be adjusted to permit growth of about 50 colonies, on the average, per plate for ease in counting and isolation of suspect colonies. This unit is especially valuable in intensive care, isolation, critical surgery and research units, to identify numbers and species of organisms depending on the media and incubation used.

Reyniers Slit Sampler

This unit can be used with an in-house vacuum unit, a suitable pump, flowmeter and 30, 60, and 120 minute clockwork mechanisms but requires a 150 MM plastic plate with the above media. The advantage of this unit is its ability to demonstrate the actual time and level of a spore shower during its operational period, i.e., an increase in viable spores shed by people, things, activities, dusty procedures or changes in air supply or movement. However, accuracy and isolation will be a problem if the viable count exceeds 10 spores per cubic foot. On the other hand, it is a very desirable unit to demonstrate that the viable mold spore count can be controlled by air filtration, aseptic technics, protective clothing and proper maintenance,[35,37] e.g., less than 0.2 viable cells per cubic foot microbial and fungal, have been noted in a neurosurgical procedure over a period of 6 hours. (Available from the New Brunswick Instrument Co., New Brunswick, N.J.)

The Ross Sieve Sampler

This unit, adapted from the Andersen Multi-State Sampler was developed to provide maximum versatility in laboratories with trainable technicians. The sampler is easily portable, can be plugged into any 110 volt outlet, carries a self contained vacuum pump and a self-timer with a range of 1–15 minutes. The unit uses 90 mm plastic dishes, does not need sterilizing, but can be decontaminated with an alcohol swab between uses. The pump draws 0.7 cubic feet (20 liters) of air per minute or 10 cubic feet in 15 minutes.[35] The resulting colony growth is distributed over the surface of the plate which simplifies counting and isolation. The unit can be used for one minute in a heavily contaminated animal room area to imbed 100–300 viable spores from 0.7 cubic feet of air on the surface of the agar plate or for the full 15 minutes where the contamination is less than 5–10 spores per cubic foot, as in patient care, intensive care, surgical units, or other special study areas. Here, too, duplicate counts with two or more units can be set up with differential media or varying the incubator temperatures as well as using anaerobic incubation.[39] This unit, being simple to operate is an excellent teaching tool to demonstrate the various microbial life forms present in the air in patient care areas to housekeepers, nurses and doctors.

It is especially useful for checking the sterility of laminar flow hoods, filtered air supplies[38] and laboratory procedures. With an extension cord, the air outside of schools and hospitals can also be monitored on an hourly or daily basis and the efficiency of the air conditioning system evaluated. (Available from Ross Industries, Midland, Va. 22727.)

The Reuter Centrifugal Sampler

This unit is a recent European introduction and is an example of the growth and development possible in any scientific community when new ideas can be incorporated on a previously accepted instrument, viz., the "Wells Centrifugal Air Sampler."[40,41] The unit is very portable, weighs less than three pounds, is totally self contained in that it operates with four flashlight batteries and a self-timing system, to extract the mold spores from varying amounts of air onto a plastic "slide strip" filled with Czapeck agar. This media is presently only available from the company and some training is needed to handle the unit and the agar strips. The timer can be set for 30 seconds, 2, 4 and 8 minute intervals to expose 40 liters of air per minute. The strips are returned to the plastic cover and incubated at room or 37°-44°C. temperatures. The unit is especially useful for collecting samples of contaminated loose dust and lint from the patient's hair, clothing and bedding, or from the environment of intensive care, isolation and special treatment rooms. Since the operator is always behind the unit, it can be used as a probe to check the mold spores in the dust from shelf tops, corners, under beds, in incubators, laminar flow hoods inlets and exhaust air vents, or the aerosols created by laboratory equipment such as centrifuges, shakers, humidifiers, transfer hoods as well as the expulsion of viable organisms by patients during coughing and sneezing spells and especially patients with tracheostomies. Mold colonies at low levels can be readily identified but will grow over the strip on continued incubation. This is also an excellent training and psychological tool since the procedures or exposure of a patient by or to a doctor, nurse, or visitor can be readily monitored during surgery or treatment. (Available from Biotest, Moonachie, N.J. 07074.)

DISCUSSION

Although each of the above methods have limitations in the search for viable mold spores carried by air currents, yet the closer to the patient they can be found, the more likely it is that they can be considered as being responsible for an infectious process,—if and when they are also found in the tissue or infection. During a two year period of air sampling at a research hospital, a study was conducted to determined the sources and levels of *Aspergilli* within and outside various areas of the hospital. Since the *Aspergillus* species are most likely to be involved in fungal infections, especially among compromised patients,[42-44] each of the methods described above was used to isolate these potential pathogens from the air, from accumulated dust residues or from contaminated instruments and equipment. Of a total of 34 swabs taken inside the hospital, 44% were positive for *A. fumigatus*, 38% showed a mixture of other *Aspergilli* while 18% were negative. Of the 550 air samples taken with the Ross Sampler inside the hospital, 25% were positive for *A. flavus*, 12% for *A. niger*, 12% for *A. fumigatus*, 10% for *A. sydowii*, 20% grew out of various other species of *Aspergilli* and 21% were negative for *Aspergilli*.

Of the 120 air samples taken in the open air on a roof 25 feet above ground level, 30% were positive for *A. fumigatus*, 47% had other species of *Aspergilli* while 23% were negative. There was also considerable variation in the daily levels of viable mold spores outside and inside the hospital, the total mold counts varying from 0 to 300 plus per cubic foot on the outside and from 0 to 30 per cubic foot on the inside, but *Aspergilli* seldom exceeded 20% of the total count. The highest counts were noted from late September through early December, especially when fallen leaves were blown about.[18] Although the air filtering and conditioning system usually reduced the levels of mold spores in the outside air by 90% or better, additional viable mold spores could have been carried into the building by many methods, e.g., street clothes, dusty containers, animal bedding, and supplies; and especially through open doors and windows when the air pressure was negative to the outside.

Although *Aspergillus* species was first identified as a causative agent of infection in man in 1847[2] and is seldom a primary cause of death, the rate of secondary infections due to *A. fumigatus* is definitely increasing in cases of neoplastic diseases, cardiac surgery, and in kidney transplantation where the patients are on therapeutic dosages of antibiotics, cytoxic agents and/or cortico-steroids.[43] Since *A. fumigatus* can often be isolated from the air and dust particles surrounding the patient, extra precaution should be observed to prevent undue exposure of the patient to viable spores of *A. aspergilli* as well as other mold species. This is best formulated by Gaya[45]: "An understanding of the mode of spread of microbes (*and molds*) is essential for the development and mainte-nance of policies for the prevention and control of infection, and the prevention of infection is surely preferable even to its successful treatment."

ACKNOWLEDGMENT

I gratefully acknowledge the cooperation of Dr. June Kwon Jung for her encouragement and assistance in identifying the numerous cultures of *Aspergilli* isolated during the study period.

REFERENCES

1. MORROW, M. B. & G. H. MEYER. 1964. A summary of air-borne mold surveys. Ann Allergy **22**(11): 575–587.
2. SLAVIN, R. G. & P. WINZENBURGER. 1977. Epidemiologic Aspects of allergic aspergillo-sis. Ann. Allergy **38**(3): 215–218.
3. RIPPON, J. W. 1974. Medical mycology. W. B. Saunders. Philadelphia, Pa.
4. KHAN, Z. V., M. PAL, D. K. PALIWAL & V. N. DAMODARAN. 1977. Aspergillosis in imported penguins. Sabouraudia **15**: 43–45.
5. ZINKL, J. G., J. M. HYLAND & J. J. HURT. 1977. Aspergillosis in common crows in Nebraska. 1974 J. Wildlife Dis. **13**: 191–193.
6. ROSENBERG, M. & R. PATTERSON. 1977. Allergic bronchopulmonary aspergillosis. J. Chron. Dis. **30**: 193–194.
7. MALO, J. L., R. HAWKINS & J. PEPYS. 1977. Studies in chronic pulmonary aspergillosis. Thorax **32**: 254–261.
8. MOUBASHER, A. H., M. I. A. ABDEL-KADER & I. A. EL-KADY. 1978. Toxigenic fungi isolated from Roquefort cheese. Mycopathologia **66**(3): 187–190.
9. SMOLANSKY, S. J. 1978. *Aspergillus* of the paranasal sinuses. Ear, Nose & Throat J. **57**: 6–14.
10. TITCHE, L. L. 1978. Aspergillosis of the maxillary sinus. Ear, Nose & Throat J. **57**: 62–66.
11. OKUDAIRA, M., H. KURATA, F. SAKABE. 1977. Studies on the fungal flora in the lung of human necropsy cases. Mycopathologia **61**(1): 3–18.
12. MEYER, R. D., L. S. YOUNG, D. ARMSTRONG & B. YU. 1973. Aspergillosis complicating neoplastic disease. Am. J. of Med. **54**: 6–15.
13. MILLNER, P. D., P. B. MARSH, R. B. SNOWDEN & J. F. PARR. 1977. Occurrence of *Aspergillus fumigatus* during composting of sewage sludge. Appl. Envir. Microbio-logy **34**(6): 765–772.
14. SAYER, W. J., N. M. MACKNIGHT & H. W. WILSON. 1972. Hospital airborne bacteria as estimated by the Andersen Sampler versus the gravity settling culture plate. Am. J. Clin. Path. **58**: 558–566.
15. GRAVESAN, S. 1978. Identification and prevalence of culturable mesophilic micro-fungi in house dust from 100 Danish homes. Allergy **33**: 268–272.
16. LUMPKINS, E. D. SR., S. L. CORBIT & G. M. TIEDEMAN. 1973. Airborne fungi survey: 1 culture plate survey of the home environment. Ann. Allergy **31**: 361–370.

17. RICHARDS, M. 1954. Atmospheric mold spores in and out-of-doors. J. Allergy **25**: 429–439.
18. SOLOMAN, W. R. 1976. A volumetric study of Winter fungus prevalence in the air of midwestern homes. J. Allergy & Clin. Immunol. **57**(1): 46–55.
19. HARIRI, A. R., A. GHADARY, M. NADERINASAB & C. KIMBERLIN. 1978. Airborne fungal spores in Ahwaz, Iran. Ann. Allergy. **40**: 349–352.
20. NOBLE, W. C. & Y. M. CLAYTON. 1963. Fungi in the air of hospital wards. J. Gen. Microbiol. **32**: 397–402.
21. MADDY, K. T. 1967. Epidemiology and ecology of deep mycoses of man and animals. Arch. Dermat. **96**: 1–9.
22. ARNOW, P. M., R. L. ANDERSON, P. O. MAINOUS & E. J. SMITH. 1978. Pulmonary aspergillosis during hospital renovation. Am. Rev. Resp. Dis.: **118**: 49–55.
23. AISNER, J., S. C. SCHIMPFF, J. E. BENNETT, V. M. YOUNG & P. H. WIERNIK. 1976. Aspergillus infections in cancer patients. Association with fireproofing materials in a new hospital. J. Am. Med. Assoc. **235**: 411–412.
24. DOWLING, H. F. 1966. Airborne infections—Past and future. Bact. Rev. **30**: 485–487.
25. PROCTOR, D. F. 1966. Airborne disease and the upper respiratory tract. Bact. Rev. **30**: 498–511.
26. STAIB, F., B. TOMPOK, D. THIEL & A. BLISSE. 1978. *Aspergillus fumigatus* and *A. Niger* in two potted ornamental plants. Mycopathologia **66**: 27–30.
27. SOLOMON, W. R. 1974. Fungus Aerosols arising from cold mist vaporizers. J. Allergy Clin. Immunol. **54**(4): 222–228.
28. SEGRETAIN, G. 1962. Infection by fungi that ordinarily are saprophytes. Lab. Invest. **11**(11): 1046–1052.
29. SAUDHU, R. S., Z. U. KHAN & H. S. RANDHAWA. 1975. Natural occurrence of *Aspergillus fumigatus* in cane sugar mills. Sabouraudia **15**: 263–272.
30. MARSH, P. B., P. D. MILLNER & J. M. KLA. 1979. A guide to the recent literature on Aspergillosis as caused by *A. fumigatus*. U. S. D. A. Manual: ARM-NE-5.
31. LLAMAS, R., D. R. HART & N. S. SCHNEIDER. 1978. Allergic bronco-pulmonary aspergillosis associated with smoking moldy marihuana. Chest. **73**: 871–872.
32. Hospital associated infections. 1977. Infectious Diseases Research. National Institute of Allergies and Infectious Diseases.
33. FINCHER, E. L. 1965. Surface sampling, application methods, recommendations. Proceedings, Institute on Control of Infections in Hospitals. U. of Michigan, 189–199.
34. Public Health Monograph #60. 1959. Sampling microbiological aerosols.
35. ANDERSEN, A. A. 1958. New sampler for the collection, sizing and enumeration of viable airborne particles. J. Bacteriol. **76**: 471–484.
36. ROSE, H. D. 1972. Mechanical control of hospital ventilation and *Aspergillus* infections. Am. Rev. Respir. Dis. **105**: 306–307.
37. ROSE, H. D. & S. R. HIRSCH. 1979. Filtering hospital air decreases *Aspergillus* spore counts. Amer. Rev. Respir. Dis. **119**: 511–512.
38. VOXAKIS, A. C., P. P. LAMY & L. G. HERMAN. 1974. Sterility assurance through environmental monitoring. Hosp. Formul. Manage. **9**: 14–19.
39. LIDWELL, O. M. & W. C. NOBLE. 1975. Fungi and clostridia in hospital air: The effect of air conditioning. J. App. Bacteriol. **39**: 251–260.
40. WELLS, W. F. 1955. Airborne contagion and air hygiene. Harvard University Press. Cambridge, Mass.
41. STAIB, F. 1978. Raumluft untersuchung auf *Aspergillus* Arten in der wohnung eines chronisch. Lungenkranken. Bundes gesundheitsblatt. **21**(26): 471–474.
42. HUTTER, R. U. P., P. H. LIEBERMAN, & H. S. COLLINS. 1964. Aspergillosis in a cancer hospital. Cancer **17**: 747–756.
43. YOUNG, R. C., J. E. BENNETT, C. L. VOGEL, P. P. CARBONE & V. T. DEVITA. 1970. Aspergillosis: The spectrum of the disease in 98 patients. Medicine **49**(2): 147–173.
44. ROSEN, P. P. 1976. Opportunistic fungal infections in patients with neoplastic diseases. Pathobiol. Annu. **11**: 255–315.
45. GAYA, H. 1976. Infection control in intensive care. Br. J. Anaesth. **48**: 9–12.

VIRUSES AS AGENTS OF AIRBORNE CONTAGION

Vernon Knight

Department of Microbiology and Immunology
Baylor College of Medicine
Texas Medical Center
Houston, Texas 77030

The concept of airborne contagion is ancient, but serious study of airborne contagion had its beginning in the 1930s and received further impetus in World War II because of problems of respiratory illness in military populations. William Furth Wells, who was preeminent in developing knowledge of airborne infection in those years, has summarized events to about 1950 in a monograph published for the Commonwealth Fund.[1] His concepts seem valid today. The early studies on airborne transmission dealt almost exclusively with bacterial diseases while the problem of airborne viral disease had to await the development of virology as a discipline after World War II.

The greatest recent contributions to understanding of airborne infection came from the extensive studies of the U.S. Army Chemical Corps Biological Laboratories at Fort Detrick, Maryland, and from a similar institution, the Microbiological Research Establishment at Porton, England, during and after World War II. My colleagues and I began studies of airborne viral infections in 1961, and our work was greatly benefitted by collaboration with the group at Fort Detrick.

In recent years interest in the problem of airborne viral disease has waned, partly because of reduced activity at Fort Detrick and lack of interest of the civilian community in the problem. The present situation seems to be that by inference, many viral infections are disseminated by the airborne route, but proved instances of such transmission are few.

In the future, we need to follow the spread of infections from their source in the infected patient to their implantation on the mucous membranes of the susceptible host. To get a proper perspective we should study both airborne and the various forms of contact spread of infection. This is not an easy assignment, but interrupting transmission effectively will require more precise knowledge than we now possess.

The following report reviews the physical properties of aerosols that influence their distribution and the characteristics of viruses that influence their capacity to function as infections agents in aerosol.

The Role of Particle Size in Transmission

To be effective in airborne transmission, particles should be small (about 10 microns in diameter or less), because small particles will remain suspended in air for periods long enough to permit their dissemination. Ten-micron diameter particles will fall the height of a room in 17 minutes, and one-to three-micron diameter particles will remain suspended almost indefinitely, especially if they are periodically elevated by air currents.[2]

Particles 20 microns in diameter will fall the height of a room in four minutes, and particles 100 microns in diameter will fall the height of a room in 10 seconds.

147

Although particles this large are formed by coughing and sneezing and other exhalatory activities, because of rapid settling they can ordinarily transmit infection only in near proximity to a patient, making it difficult to distinguish this route of transmission from contact spread of infection.

Infection with airborne viruses requires that virus be deposited at a site or sites within the respiratory tract. The level at which deposition occurs is determined by particle size, and the pattern of deposition according to particle size is shown in FIGURE 1. Twenty-micron diameter aerosols deposit almost exclusively in the nose with a further minute fraction impacting in the pharynx and large bronchi. Larger particles deposit in the nose. As size diminishes, deposition in the lower respiratory tract increases and extends to the alveolar ducts.

Biological aerosols are hygroscopic and the effect of this property is also shown in FIGURE 1. The distribution percentages are based on theoretical and experimental studies, but there is considerable variability in these responses from person to person and at different times in the same individual.

Two important sources of physiologic variation in the fraction deposited are the rate of flow of inspiration and expiration and tidal volume.[3] Increased flow rates lead to greater nasal deposition. The effect is due to inertia and increases with particle size. With increasing tidal volume there is also an increase in the fraction deposited.[4] Of particular interest to transmission of infection by aerosol is the variation in percent deposition from person to person while breathing normally. This ranged from 22 to 62 percent in one study of 25 normal adults, a

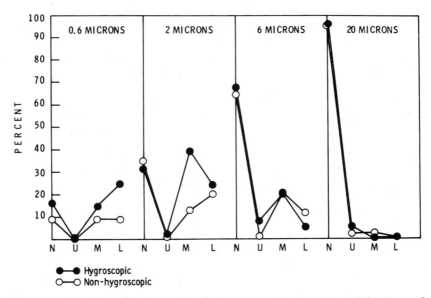

FIGURE 1. The effect of hygroscopicity and consequent increase in particle size on the site of deposition and percentage of retention of particles. (N = nose breathing {6 percent Tidal Air}. U = upper respiratory tract — pharynx to and including bronchi {10 percent TA}. M = middle respiratory tract — bronchioles {20 percent TA}. L = lower respiratory tract including alveolar ducts {63 percent TA}.)[17]

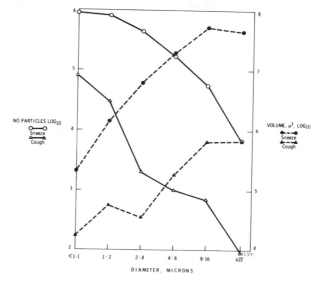

FIGURE 2. Distribution of particles by size in coughs and sneezes.[18,19]

difference that could alter appreciably the amount of virus deposited from aerosol. Anatomic differences undoubtedly influence deposition, and smokers deposit inhaled particles more proximally in the tracheobronchial tree than nonsmokers,[5] probably resulting from chronic inflammatory changes that alter the dimensions of the airways. Such effects could influence the amount and site of deposition of viruses in aerosol and affect the type of illness produced.

Sneezes and coughs produce a large and variable population of particles. The largest number are particles of one micron and less in diameter progressively diminishing in number as the particle size increases (FIGURE 2). It is a reasonable assumption that virus particles will be uniformly distributed in fluids from which aerosols are generated and therefore would correlate with volume of particles rather than numbers of particles (FIGURE 3). Nevertheless, coughs and sneezes as well as other exhalatory activities produce large numbers of small particles which can serve as vehicles of airborne transmission. Thus, large particles may contain more virus but sediment rapidly, and small particles contain less virus but disseminate widely.

Occurrence of Viruses in Natural Aerosols

Before infection can be transmitted by aerosol, virus-containing aerosols must be generated, and the virus must persist in sufficient concentration long enough to transmit infection. Couch et al.[6] found that coxasackievirus A-21 could be recovered in appreciable amounts from air of rooms occupied by volunteers acutely ill with induced infection with this agent and that the amount of virus in secretions was correlated with the amount of virus recovered from the air. Artenstein and Miller[7] recovered adenovirus type 4 from a barracks room occupied by recruits with adenovirus type 4 infection. It was not possible to measure the diameter of the virus-containing particles, but the circumstances of the study suggested that rapidly sedimenting particles were not involved in the transmission.

Isolations of virus from contaminated air are not frequently reported, and the problem seems to be related to the low titer of virus in contaminated air, and to the low efficiency of isolation methods. Only about 10 percent of airborne virus is recovered by the Litton large volume sampler, currently the best available methodology.

In another study, Couch et al.[8] demonstrated airborne transmission of coxsackievirus A-21 in volunteers. In a large barracks room divided by a 4-foot

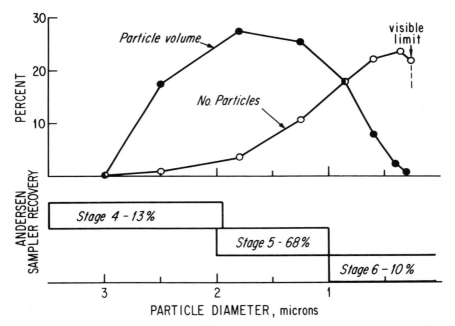

FIGURE 3. Distribution in aerosol of particles, particle volume, and virus according to particle diameter.[20]

deep double wire mesh barrier, they showed transmission of infection from volunteers on one side who had been infected with virus to uninfected suscepti-bles on the other side of the barrier. Coxsackievirus A-21 was recovered from sneezes and coughs of the infected volunteers and from the air of the barracks room on the side in which the susceptibles were quartered. Infected and uninfected susceptible volunteers were kept separate at all times.

Persistence of Viruses in Natural Aerosols

Some generalizations have emerged concerning airborne transmission of virus infections from studies by many investigators.[9] Transmission by the airborne route will usually occur indoors because of rapid dispersion of inocula out-of-doors. Indoors, inocula will probably not persist longer than one hour because of dissipation by ventilation.

The seasonal variation of some virus infections has been tentatively explained by seasonal variations of relative humidity indoors. In summer relative humidity will usually be high, 60 percent or greater, while in winter, with artificial heating, relative humidity may be 40 percent or less. Influenza, measles, mumps, rubella, chickenpox, and respiratory syncytial viral aerosols are most stable in low relative humidity, and infection with these lipid-enveloped viruses occurs most frequently during the winter season. Coxsackievirus and echovirus infections that are more stable in aerosol in high humidity are more common in summer. Foot and mouth disease caused by a picornavirus is more prevalent after periods of wet weather when transmission can occur over a distance of many miles. Paradoxically, however, rhinovirus and adenovirus infections are more common in winter. The correlation of stability in aerosol and the seasonal pattern of occurrence of several groups of virus suggests their transmission in aerosol. However, relative humidity would probably affect survival of viruses deposited on surfaces or elsewhere in the environment in much the same way as in aerosol. Other information would, therefore, be required to establish the predominant pattern of transmission.

The mode of inactivation of viruses in aerosol seems to be related to virus structure.[10] Lipid enveloped virus may be inactivated by surface effects when exposed at high relative humidities, probably due to damage to the protein coat of the virus. Lipid-free viruses appear to be damaged in aerosol by removal of structural water molecules. In some studies, viral nucleic acid retained infectivity when viral infectivity in aerosol was lost.

Not surprisingly, there are contradictions and uncertainties about the mechanisms of loss of viral infectivity in aerosols. Some factors that influence virus survival in aerosol are virus species, the nature of the suspending fluid, damage by the aerosol sampling procedures, shifts in relative humidity, temperature, and effect of additives.[11] Inositol has been shown to stabilize Rous sarcoma, Langat, influenza, and Semliki Forest virus in aerosol. It does not stabilize aerosols of poliovirus or encephalomyocarditis virus. NO_2 and SO_2 were shown to reduce viability of some viruses in aerosol. Finally, solar radiation damages viruses in aerosol.

The Infectious Dose by Aerosol

We measured the 50 percent infectious dose in man by small particle aerosol in normal volunteers for four different types of virus (TABLE 1). Based on the expected distribution of the inhaled dose of 1.5 micron diameter, the deposition at various sites in the respiratory tract was estimated. For comparison the infectious dose for virus administered in nasal drops was determined. Some inferences can be drawn from the data. These viruses by either route were highly infectious for volunteers who had no measurable antibody to the agent administered. Two of the agents, rhinovirus 15 and coxsackievirus A-21, were most infectious by nasal drops by factors of 21 and 5 respectively. Underscores in the table are doses deposited on sites in which the inhaled dose is equal to or greater than the infectious dose by the nasal route.

Since the amount of rhinovirus type 15 deposited by aerosol in the nose exceeded the dose deposited there by nasal drops, it seems reasonable to suppose that the nose is the site of initiation of infection in both situations. We are unable

Table 1

Fifty Percent Human Infectious Dose (HID$_{50}$) in Units of 50% Tissue Culture Infectious Doses (TCID$_{50}$) for 4 Respiratory Viruses by 1.5-Micron Diameter Aerosol.

% Site of Inhaled Dose	(1) Nose 37.0	(2) Pharynx, Bronchi 1.0	(3) Bronchioles 25.0	(4) Alveolar Ducts 21.0	(5) Total Ret. 84.0	(6) Exhaled 16.0	(7) Total Inhaled HID$_{50}$	(8) Nasal Drops HID$_{50}$
Rhinovirus type 15	0.24‡	0.007	0.170	0.14	0.56	0.12	0.68* (0.2–2.0)	0.032 (S.D.=0)
Coxsackievirus A type 21	10.10	0.200	7.000	5.900	23.20	4.80	28.00 (15–49)	6.00 (3–13)
Adenovirus type 4	0.18	0.005	0.125	0.11	0.42	0.08	0.50 (0.2–1.4)	35.00 (8–157)
Influenza A/2/ Bethesda/10/63	1.08	0.030	0.750	0.63	2.49	0.51	3.00 (estimate)	†

*50% human infectious doses in TCID$_{50}$, with 95% confidence limits.
†Probably 5- to 10-fold greater than HID$_{50}$ by aerosol.
‡Underlined figures represent doses approximately equal to or greater than HID$_{50}$ by nasal drops.

to determine whether or not infection was simultaneously initiated at a site or sites in the lung at the same time. The exquisite susceptibility of the nasal mucosa to this infection is remarkable. In fact, the nasal mucosa is more susceptible to infection with rhinovirus type 15 than the tissue culture used to measure the dose. Though both the nose and the lower respiratory tract are much less susceptible to infection with coxsackievirus A-21 than with rhinovirus 15, the situation otherwise resembles that with the rhinovirus.

Adenovirus type 4 is about 70-fold more infectious by small particle aerosol than by nasal drops. By electron microscopy it was shown that one 50 percent tissue culture infectious dose consisted of 13.2 virus particulates each usually

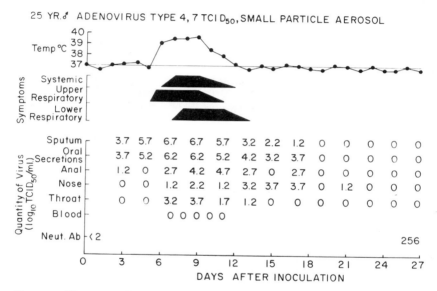

FIGURE 4. Illness in volunteer after inoculation with adenovirus type 4 by 1.5 micron diameter aerosol. Incubation period was four days with a five-day febrile illness. Predominant upper respiratory symptoms were sore throat and scanty nasal discharge. Lower respiratory symptoms were severe cough with small amount of sputum. There was hoarseness and pain over sternum with coughing. Headache was persistent, and there was pronounced malaise. (Courtesy of R. B. Couch, Baylor College of Medicine.)

consisting of a single virion.[12] Since the infectious dose of 0.5 $TCID_{50}$ contained approximately six virions, adenovirus type 4 in aerosol approaches the ultimate in infectivity. Moreover, the illness produced by these minute doses of virus was as severe as naturally occurring, acute respiratory disease (ARD) in recruits (FIGURE 4). Although the data are less complete for influenza, it appears that this virus is also highly infectious for the lower respiratory tract.

Both adenovirus type 4 and influenza virus infections appear to be transmitted by small particle aerosol, and Couch showed aerosol transmission of coxsackievirus A type 21 infection. In the case of the latter disease and rhinovirus infection, the question might be whether the aerosol caused infection in the nose or the lower respiratory tract, or both. Although some major differences in the infectious dose with these four viruses were observed, the infectious dose was low enough by each route for all the viruses that infection could reasonably be transmitted by either route.

Transmission of Infection by Contact

Transmission of infection by contact or by large particulates impacting directly on respiratory surfaces are the alternatives to small particle aerosol transmission. The conjunctival or nasal mucosa and the mouth are the potential sites for entrance of infection. Hendley et al.[13] found that rhinovirus transferred by fingers to nasal or conjunctival mucosa from contaminated surfaces regularly resulted in infection and illness. They found also that dropping virus into the mouth did not produce infection. Gwaltney et al.[14] later found that face-to-face exposure of susceptible volunteers to infected volunteers who coughed and sneezed did not result in infection (large particle exposure), nor did exposure in a room in which susceptibles were separated from infected subjects by a wire mesh barrier result in infection (small particle aerosol exposure).

Douglas and Hall and their associates (personal communication) recently showed that respiratory syncytial virus infection in infants was transferred only by contact, and not by exposure, of susceptibles in a room of infected babies when there was no contact with the child. They also found that respiratory syncytial virus introduced into the mouth did not produce infection in volunteers.

These findings point to the contact as possibly the most important means of transmission of these infections. The findings are consistent with the observations described earlier in which nasal mucosa was found to be more susceptible to infection with rhinovirus than pulmonary sites exposed by small particle aerosol.

DISCUSSION

Significant findings so far concerning transmission of virus infection by small particle aerosol are 1) the demonstration that large numbers of small particles (<10 microns MMD) are produced by sneezes and coughs and that virus can be recovered from these exhalations; 2) the recovery of virus from the air of rooms occupied by infected subjects; 3) the observation that very small doses of virus are infectious by small particle aerosol; and, finally, 4) the demonstration of airborne infection with coxsackievirus A type 21 under controlled conditions.

It is reasonable to suppose from the data that adenovirus infection in recruits is spread predominantly by small particle aerosol. Though not discussed, conjunctival inoculation by contact is certainly responsible for transmission of some adenovirus infections; and among institutionalized infants, contact may also be the major mechanism of spread. The rapidity with which influenza epidemics move through the community suggests that small particle aerosol is the predominant mode of spread of this infection. An interesting example of apparent airborne transmission of influenza was recently reported by Moser et al.[15] Following a 3-hour exposure in the cabin of a commercial aircraft grounded in an Alaskan airport with the ventilation system turned off, 72 percent of 53 passengers and crew members developed influenza caused by an influenza

A/Texas/1/77-like virus. The source of the virus was a young woman acutely ill with the disease who had boarded at the previous stop. This report emphasizes the high infectiousness of influenza by aerosol in still, dry indoor air during winter (March, 1977) and suggests a protective effect of ventilation in preventing similar outbreaks elsewhere.

The data presented also support the concept that rhinovirus infection, and possibly respiratory syncytial virus infection, may spread predominantly by contact.

If more information were available on mechanisms of airborne transmission, it should be possible to develop methods of interfering with the spread of infection. From a variety of standpoints, control of influenza would be a logical choice for early study. Influenza is responsible for much morbidity and mortality worldwide; it occurs in brief severe epidemics during which controlled studies could be made. School children are important in community spread of the disease through contact at school, and epidemics among old people in institutions are frequent and severe. Riley[16] has reviewed the problem and proposes that use of ultraviolet radiation in the upper levels of rooms might control transmission in areas where transmission of infection is likely to occur. Schools and institutions for old people would be logical places to study the problem. Controlled ventilation, air filtration, and no doubt other measures would also be subjects for study.

REFERENCES

1. WELLS, W. F. 1955. Airborne Contagion and Air Hygiene. Published for the Commonwealth Fund by Harvard University Press. Cambridge.
2. KNIGHT, V. 1973. Airborne transmission and pulmonary deposition of respiratory viruses. In Viral and Mycoplasmal Infections of the Respiratory Tract. V. Knight, Ed.: 1–9. Lea & Febiger. Philadelphia.
3. HEYDER, J. & G. RUDOLF. 1977. Deposition of aerosol particles in the human nose. In Inhaled Particles IV, part 1. W. H. Walton, Ed.: 107–126. Proceedings of an International Symposium organized by The British Occupational Hygiene Society. Pergamon Press. New York.
4. GIACOMELLI-MALTONI, G., C. MELANDRI, V. PRODI, & G. TARRONI. 1972. Deposition efficiency of monodisperse particles in human respiratory tract. Amer. Ind. Hyg. Assoc. J. **33:** 603–610.
5. PALMES, E. D., & M. LIPPMANN. 1977. Influence of respiratory air space dimensions on aerosol deposition. In Inhaled Particles IV, Part 1. W. H. Walton, Ed.: 127–135. Proceedings of an International Symposium organized by the British Occupational Hygiene Society. Pergamon Press. New York.
6. COUCH, R. B., T. R. CATE, R. G. DOUGLAS, JR., P. J. GERONE, & V. KNIGHT. 1966. Effect of route of inoculation on experimental respiratory viral disease in volunteers and evidence for airborne transmission. Bact. Rev. **30:** 517–531.
7. ARTENSTEIN, M. S., & W. S. MILLER. 1966. Air sampling for respiratory disease agents in army recruits. Bact. Rev. **30:** 571–575.
8. COUCH, R. B., DOUGLAS, R. G., JR., LINDGREN, K. M., P. J. GERONE. & V. KNIGHT. 1970. Airborne transmission of respiratory infection with coxsackievirus A type 21. Amer. J. Epidem. **91** (1):78–86.
9. DE JONG, J. C., T. TROUWBORST, & K. C. WINKLER. 1973. Mechanisms of incativation of viruses and macromoles in air. 31. The mechanism of virus decay in aerosols. In Airborne Transmission and Airborne Infection. J. F. Ph. Hers & K. C. Winkler, Eds.: 124–130. Concepts and methods presented at International Symposium on Aerobiology held at the Technical University at Enschede, The Netherlands. Oosthoek Publishing Co. Utrecht, the Netherlands.
10. TROUWBORST, T., & J. C. DE JONG. 1973. Surface inactivation, an important mechanism

of aerosol inactivation for viruses, inactivated at high relative humidity. *In* Airborne Transmission & Airborne Infection. J. F. Ph. Hers & K. C. Winkler, Eds.: 137–140. Concepts and methods presented at International Symposium on Aerobiology held at the Technical University at Enschede, the Netherlands. Oosthoek Publishing Co. Utrecht, the Netherlands.

11. AKERS, T. G. 1973. Some aspects of the airborne inactivation of viruses. *In* Airborne Transmission and Airborne Infection. J. F. Ph. Hers & K. C. Winkler, Eds.: 73. Concepts and methods presented at International Symposium on Aerobiology held at the Technical University at Enchede, the Netherlands. Oosthoek Publishing Co. Utrecht, the Netherlands.

12. HAMORY, B. H., R. B. COUCH, R. G. DOUGLAS, JR., S. H. BLACK, & V. KNIGHT. 1972. Characterization of the infectious unit for man of two respiratory viruses. Proc. Soc. Exp. Biol. Med. **139**(3): 890–893.

13. HENDLEY, J. O., R. P. WENZEL, & J. M. GWALTNEY, JR. 1973. Transmission of rhinovirus colds by self-inoculation. New Engl. J. Med. **288**: 1361–1354.

14. GWALTNEY, J. M., JR., P. B. MOSKALSKI, & J. O. HENDLEY. 1978. Hand-to-hand transmission of rhinovirus colds. Ann. Int. Med. **88**: 463–467.

15. MOSER, M. R., T. R. BENDER, H. S. MARGOLIS, G. R. NOBLE, A. P. KENDAL, & D. G. RITTER. 1979. An outbreak of influenza aboard a commercial airliner. Amer. J. Epidem. **110**(1): 1–6.

16. RILEY, R. L. 1977. Ultraviolet air disinfection for protection against influenza. Johns Hopkins Med. J. **140**: 25–27.

17. LANDAHL, H. D. 1972. The effect of gravity, hygroscopicity and particle size on the amount and site of deposition of inhaled particles, with particular reference to hazard due to airborne viruses. *In* Assessment of Airborne Particles. T. T. Mercer, P. E. Morrow, and W. Stober, Eds.: 421–428. Charles C Thomas. Springfield, Ill.

18. DUGUID, J. P. 1946. The size and duration of air-carriage of respiratory droplets and droplet-nuclei. J. Hyg. (Camb.) **44**: 471–479.

19. GERONE, P. J., *et al.* 1966. Assessment of experimental and natural viral aerosols. Bact. Rev. **30**: 576.

20. COUCH, R. B., *et al.* 1965. Preparation and properties of a small-particle aerosol of coxsackie A-21. Proc. Soc. Exp. Biol. Med. **118**: 818.

AN ASSESSMENT OF THE AIRBORNE ROUTE
IN HEPATITIS B TRANSMISSION

Norman J. Petersen

Hepatitis Laboratories Division, Bureau of Epidemiology
Center for Disease Control, U.S. Public Health Service
Phoenix, Arizona 85014

INTRODUCTION

During the past decade, rapid advances in viral serodiagnostics and accompanying seroepidemiologic studies of hepatitis B in a variety of human populations have significantly increased our understanding of this disease. We now know that hepatitis B can be transmitted by means other than the traditional percutaneous mechanisms of direct transfusion or needle inoculation of infective blood or blood products. Based on this newly developed information Maynard has suggested the following principal modes of hepatitis B virus transmission:[1] (a) direct percutaneous inoculation by needle of contaminated serum or plasma or transfusion of infective blood or blood products, (b) nonneedle percutaneous transfer of infective serum or plasma, (c) introduction of infective serum or plasma onto mucosal surfaces, (d) introduction of infective secretions other than serum or plasma onto mucosal surfaces, and (e) indirect transfer of infective serum or plasma via vectors or inanimate environmental surfaces.

It is clear that if the hepatitis B virus (HBV) can penetrate mucosal surfaces to reach the circulatory system and ultimately the liver, that airborne transmission of hepatitis B is theoretically possible. Whether, in fact, the airborne route is involved in any meaningful number of naturally occurring hepatitis B infections is not clear at this time. Airborne transmission of hepatitis B under controlled experimental conditions in which the possibility of direct contact via droplets and indirect contact via contaminated fomites is eliminated has not been reported. In one study conducted before the development of serologic tests for hepatitis B, serum presumed to contain HBV was inoculated directly into the noses of volunteer subjects. In these challenges reported by MacCallum and Bauer[2] jaundice was observed in one of 10 subjects and bilirubin elevations were detected in three subjects. More recently, confirmed transmission of hepatitis B via the oral mucosa has been documented in susceptible human volunteers by Krugman[3] and in susceptible nonhuman primates at our laboratory[1]. The inadvertent introduction of hepatitis B surface antigen (HBsAg) positive blood into the eye of a hospital employee has resulted in infection further suggesting transmission via mucosal surfaces.[4] However, Bancroft and associates were unable to infect susceptible gibbons with an aerosol spray of saliva that was shown to be infectious when administered subcutaneously.[5]

Epidemiologic evidence for airborne transmission of hepatitis B appears to be inconclusive. Reports of two incidents in hemodialysis centers and of one incident in the home of a hemodialysis patient suggest that airborne transmission may have played a role in the occurrence of hepatitis B infections among

---

*World Health Organization Collaborating Center for Reference and Research on Viral Hepatitis.

0077-8923/80/0353-0157 $01.75/0 © 1980, NYAS

individuals present when sizeable quantities of HBsAg positive blood were released into the immediate environment during bleeding accidents.[6-7] However, contact with surfaces contaminated with the infective blood cannot be ruled out in these instances since it has been shown that HBsAg can frequently be detected on environmental surfaces associated with a hemodialysis patient even in the absence of major blood spills.[9,10] Other epidemiologic investigations of outbreaks of hepatitis B in hemodialysis centers and clinical laboratories, high risk areas where aerosolization of blood is possible, have not ruled out airborne transmission.[11-14] However, major risk factors have been identified and the data argue against airborne transmission as a significant mechanism of spread.

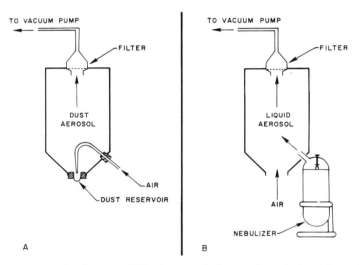

FIGURE 1. During development of filter-rinse technique, a dynamic aerosol test chamber determined efficiency and sensitivity.

Laboratory Tests

In the absence of conclusive experimental and epidemiologic evidence of airborne transmission of hepatitis B, we elected to approach the question by sampling for airborne HBsAg in several high risk environments. We had demonstrated the stability of HBsAg on environmental surfaces[15] and concluded that the presence of this antigenic marker in samples from the environment could serve as presumptive evidence of the presence of HBV. McGarrity used this approach to sample air in a hemodialysis center with a high-volume air sampler operated at a flow rate of 1100 lpm.[16] HBsAg was detected in four of 15 samples collected while HBsAg positive patients were being dialyzed and in none of 10 samples obtained when negative patients were treated. However, it could not be ascertained that the positive samples did not result from droplet contamination rather than from airborne particles since the sampler was located within the range of spatter from the patient care procedures and the sampler intake could not be oriented to prevent the sampling of droplets. Additionally, swab samples of the floor at the sampler locations also showed the presence of HBsAg suggesting that spatter had occurred.

We felt that a desirable sampling technique would be one that: (a) could be conveniently used under field conditions, (b) could sample at a rate that would not markedly distrub normal air movement patterns, (c) could sample in the breathing zone and be oriented to avoid direct contamination with droplets, and (d) could detect low levels of HBsAg quantitatively. Unfortunately, we were unable to be more specific concerning the sensitivity requirement in the last criterion because nothing is known about the size of the HBV dose required for airborne infection and there is no correlation between the titer of HBsAg and the infectivity titer of infectious blood.[17] A filter-rinse technique was devised that met most of the stated requirements.[18] With this technique air was drawn through a membrane filter in an aerosol field monitor (Millipore MHWG 037HO, pore size 0.45 μm) at a flow rate ranging from 12-25 lpm using a vacuum pump and flexible vacuum tubing. After sampling, the monitor was returned to the laboratory, the filter removed and rinsed in 1 ml of 1.0% bovine serum albumin in normal saline (BSAS) with the use of ultrasonic energy. The rinse fluid was tested for HBsAg by radioimmunoassay using Ausria II kits (Abbott Laboratories) and for occult blood with Hemastix (Ames Co.), a test capable of reacting with as little as 0.3 mg hemoglobin/100 ml.

During the development of the technique a dynamic aerosol test chamber was used to determine efficiency and sensitivity (FIGURE 1). Both liquid and dust aerosols containing HBsAg were used and assay results, expressed in counts per minute (CPM), were converted to HBsAg dilution equivalents using the proportional range of the RIA dilution response curve.[19] FIGURE 2 shows a typical conversion curve in which fresh aerosol fluid and aerosol fluid remaining in the nebulizer after a series of experiments were used as standards to calibrate an assay kit. Aerosol chamber tests showed the procedure to have an efficiency of 22% with a coefficient of variation of 11% and a capability of detecting as little as 5×10^{-5} ml of aerosolized HBsAg positive serum in a single air sample.

Field Tests—Hemodialysis Centers and Laboratory

Since its development the filter-rinse air sampling technique has been used in several different environments where the likelihood of detecting airborne HBsAg positive blood or other body fluids seemed high. In one case,[18] a 20-bed hemodialysis center in a large metropolitan area was selected because the patient population served by this center exhibited an HBsAg seropositivity prevalence in excess of 50%, and the occurrence of hepatitis B in both patients and staff was a continuing problem. Mechanical ventilation in the patient area of the center was essentially nonexistent. Kiil dialyzers were used by most patients and were disassembled and cleaned in a poorly ventilated area adjoining the patient area. Hematology and blood chemistries were also performed in a small laboratory adjoining the patient area. These conditions appeared to favor the generation of persistent aerosols. Sampling sites were selected to achieve the highest probability of obtaining an HBsAg positive air sample. Samples from the patient area were collected throughout the dialysis session at the bedside of patients seropositive for HBsAg. This included the time when patients were connected to and disconnected from the dialyzer as well as the clean-up period when bed linens were stripped. The dialyzer processing area was sampled while dialyzers were being disassembled, cleaned, and reassembled. Samples from the laboratory area were collected while blood samples were being processed and tested. In all cases the sampler face was oriented to prevent droplets or particles from settling or impacting on the filter.

The results of air sampling in this center are presented in TABLE 1. HBsAg was not detected in any of the 60 samples collected, and all samples were negative for the presence of blood. Based on the mean volume of air per sample and the calculated sensitivity of the technique, it was estimated that the mean concentra-

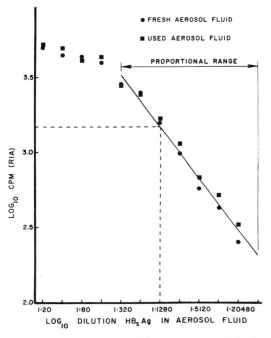

FIGURE 2. Typical conversion curve in which fresh aerosol fluid and aerosol fluid remaining in nebulizer after a series of experiments were used as standards to calibrate an assay kit.

tion in this dialysis center did not exceed 6×10^{-8} ml of HBsAg positive serum per liter of air.

In a second dialysis center a small, crowded isolation room containing four recirculating single pass dialysis systems (open bath cannisters) used only for dialyzing HBsAg positive patients was selected for air sampling. Inadequate ventilation and housekeeping combined to produce conditions conducive to the generation and maintenance of aerosols. Samples were collected at two sites in the room during three shifts of four patients each. Each sampler operated at a flow rate of 15 lpm for a mean sampling period of 35 minutes. Forty-six samples

TABLE 1

RESULTS OF AIR SAMPLING FOR HEPATITIS B SURFACE ANTIGEN
IN A HEMODIALYSIS CENTER

Area Sampled	Number of Samples	Mean Volume of Air Per Sample in Liters	Number of Samples Positive for HBsAg
Patient	37	877	0
Dialyzer processing	18	679	0
Laboratory	5	962	0

each with a mean volume of 525 liters were collected. Each filter was assayed for both blood and HBsAg in a manner described previously.

The sampling period covered the spectrum of usual activities associated with the dialysis procedure and an unusual event that appeared to present a situation in which an HBsAg positive aerosol might be generated. In this case a massive blood leak occurred in a coil dialyzer, and the dialysate immediately became heavily contaminated with HBsAg positive blood. The coil was clamped off and removed from the cannister, but the dialysate continued to recirculate for several minutes before it was drained. Neither blood nor HBsAg was detected in the air sample collected within two meters of the recirculating cannister. Similarly, the remaining 45 air samples collected during more routine procedures were negative for both blood and HBsAg.

For comparison purposes 48 swab samples of environmental surfaces also were collected in this room and the results are presented in TABLE 2. It was evident that within the dialysis setting contaminated surfaces appear to present a much more likely source of contact than does contaminated air.

A British Working Party approached the problem of environmental contamination with infected blood during hemodialysis in a comprehensive quantitative study conducted in four centers.[20] Blood contaminated with tracer organisms was used in a variety of simulated hemodialysis procedures, both routine and catastrophic in nature. The most striking negative finding was the uniform failure to detect airborne spread of blood when dramatic emergencies causing gross surface contamination were simulated. The Working Party suggested that blood does not readily form an aerosol because of its viscosity. However, they did find that the insertion and removal of certain needles from tubing containing blood did produce measurable numbers of small airborne particles. The quantity of aerosol was apparently related to the bore and length of the needle as well as the technique of the operator.

In an effort to confirm these observations we investigated this procedure to

TABLE 2

RESULTS OF SURFACE AND AIR SAMPLING FOR HEPATITIS B SURFACE ANTIGEN
IN A HEMODIALYSIS CENTER

Sample	Number of Samples	Number of Samples Positive for HBsAg	Percent Positive
Air	46*	0	0
Surface	48	7	14.6

*Mean volume of air per sample = 525 liters.

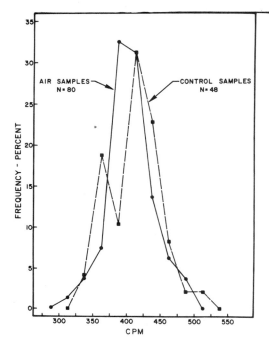

FIGURE 3. Data were analyzed by comparing the frequency distribution of sample CPM results with control CPM results.

determine whether HBsAg could be detected in the immediate vicinity of needle insertion and withdrawal. In the laboratory we were able to confirm that low levels of tracer bacteria were aerosolized during the needling of a latex injection sleeve on a blood line filled with blood spiked with *Bacillus subtilis* var. *niger* spores. Accordingly, arrangements were made with a dialysis center to collect air samples during various needling procedures on HBsAg positive patients.

The sampling program called for three samples from each of five positive patient stations on five different days: (a) during the injection of local anesthetic and the insertion of the arterial and venous needles (approximately 2–4 minutes), (b) during the collection of a blood specimen from a latex sleeve injection site on the venous blood line (approximately 30–60 seconds), and (c) during the withdrawal of the venous and arterial needles at the termination of dialysis (approximately 1–2 minutes). Each sample was collected by holding the filter face of the sampler 5 cm above the injection site while a remote vacuum pump drew air through the filter at a rate of 20 liters/minute. All samples were collected according to schedule providing a total of 25 needle insertions samples, 25 blood specimen collection samples and 25 needle withdrawal samples. Five additional samples were collected on one day when a potentially hazardous procedure was observed. This procedure occurred during termination of dialysis while the extracorporeal blood was being returned to the patient. The venous pressure monitor line was disconnected from the monitor and the end was allowed to hang in a waste container. Air pressure used to force the blood back to the drip chamber escaped through the pressure line with the result that foam and bursting bubbles of residual blood formed at the end of the line within the waste container. Samples of air in the waste container were collected during five such procedures.

All 80 air sample filters were returned to the laboratory and rinsed within four hours of collection. The BSAS sample eluates along with 48 BSAS negative controls were assayed by RIA. The data were analyzed by comparing the frequency distribution of sample CPM results with control CPM results (FIGURE 3). It was evident that the distributions were similar with comparable centering tendency and no evidence of sample CPM skewing toward higher counts. In TABLE 3 the mean CPM value for each type of sample is listed. No statistically significant differences between means were found.

Based on our mean sample volume we concluded that if aerosols were formed the concentration of blood must be less than 1×10^{-6} ml/liter of air at a point 5 cm from the source of the aerosol. During the sampling procedure we frequently observed spatter involving visible drops of blood. No visible blood was observed on any of the 80 sample filters and tests for occult blood (Hemastix) on the eluates were all negative. Spattered blood was observed on one filter holder.

Field Tests—Dental Operatory

Dental operatories constitute another environmental setting where hepatitis B transmission occurs as indicated by studies that show dentists are at risk in terms of both clinical hepatitis[21] and serologic markers for hepatitis B.[22,23] HBsAg has been found in saliva, even in the absence of blood[24,25] and experimental transmission of hepatitis B to two gibbons and a chimpanzee using percutaneous injections of bloodfree saliva has been documented.[5,26] Although direct contact of hands with infectious fluids probably constitutes the major route of transmission, it has been speculated that airborne HBV from aerosols generated during various dental procedures may also be involved in transmission of hepatitis.[27,28]

To determine whether measurable aerosols of HBsAg are generated during various dental procedures performed on HBsAg positive patients, air samples were collected during the treatment of 24 patients in the dental operatory of an institution whose residents exhibited a high prevalence of HBsAg seropositivity.[29] Sera from 21 of the 24 test patients were positive for HBsAg and gingival swabs from 20 of the 21 positive patients were positive for HBsAg. TABLE 4 lists the procedures performed on the 21 seropositive patients.

Samples were collected at a site located behind the patient's head on the

TABLE 3

RESULTS OF HBsAg TESTS PERFORMED ON AIR SAMPLES COLLECTED DURING FOUR HEMODIALYSIS PROCEDURES INVOLVING BLOOD

Procedure	Number of Samples	Mean RIA Values CPM
Needle insertion	25	404
Specimen collection	25	405
Needle withdrawal	25	408
Venting of venous pressure line	5	412
Control	48	406

TABLE 4

DENTAL PROCEDURES PERFORMED ON 21 SEROPOSITIVE PATIENTS DURING
SAMPLING OF AIR

Procedure	Patients Undergoing Procedures (%)
Hand scaling	71
Polishing (prophy cup)	67
Extraction	19
Drilling (high-speed, water-cooled)	14

headrest of the dental chair and at a site within the dentist's breathing zone. Sample filters were located to prevent materials ejected from the mouth from either impacting or falling directly on the filter face. This was done to assure that only airborne particles would be sampled. Each sampler was operated at a flow rate of 15 lpm for the duration of each patient's treatment. TABLE 5 presents a summary of the results obtained from air sampling. It was found that measurable levels of HBsAg, known to be present in the blood and saliva of the positive patients, were not detected in the volumes of air sampled. All samples were also negative for occult blood.

Based on the sensitivity of the air sampling technique and the occult blood test along with the mean volume of air per sample in this study, it was estimated that the mean concentration at the two sampling sites was less than 1×10^{-6} ml of HBsAg positive fluid or blood per liter of air. Because of the orientation of the filter of the sampler in these tests, the results apply only to airborne material as distinguished from droplets or particulates that may pass through the air and reach a sampling device or susceptible host as a result of imparted velocity or gravity. Droplets of saliva may contain HBsAg as was shown in one study in which HBsAg was detected in 17 of 40 (43%) samples from sneezes collected at a distance of 30 cm from the faces of antigenemic patients[24] and droplets of blood can be visually detected in the spatter generated during certain dental procedures.

SUMMARY

The experimental and epidemiologic evidence for airborne transmission of hepatitis B is inconclusive and our efforts to detect airborne HBsAg or blood in

TABLE 5

RESULTS OF SAMPLING OF AIR FOR HBsAg IN A DENTAL OPERATORY

Patients Undergoing Treatment	Number of Samples	Mean Volume of Air Per Sample in Liters	No. of Samples Positive for HBsAg	No. of Samples Positive for Occult Blood
21 patients (HBsAg positive)	40	104	0	0
3 patients (HBsAg negative)	6	116	0	0

environments where hepatitis B transmission occurs have been uniformly unsuccessful. In the specific areas investigated: dialysis centers, laboratories, and dental operatories, other major routes of transmission that can explain the spread of hepatitis B invariably are present. Therefore, while airborne transmission is theoretically possible and probably has occurred, at this time its contribution to the overall hepatitis B problem cannot be quantitated. We feel comfortable in concluding that airborne HBV does not play a major role in hepatitis B transmission and that true airborne infections are probably rare. Because of the fine line that separates airborne transmission from contact transmission via droplets, we feel it important to emphasize the need to take those precautions that protect against the latter. These include the use of gloves where surfaces become contaminated and masks and glasses to protect the eyes, nose and mouth where the possibility of spatter exists.

REFERENCES

1. MAYNARD, J. E. 1978. Modes of hepatitis B virus transmission. *In* Hepatitis Viruses (Proceedings of the 1976 International Symposium on Hepatitis Viruses, Tokyo, 18–20 November 1976). Japan Medical Research Foundation, Eds.: 125–137. University of Tokyo Press.
2. MACCALLUM, F. O. & D. J. Bauer. 1944. Homologous serum jaundice, transmission experiments with human volunteers. Lancet **11:** 622–627.
3. KRUGMAN, S., J. P. GILES & J. HAMMOND. 1967. Infectious hepatitis: Evidence for two distinctive clinical, epidemiological, and immunological types of infection. J. Am. Med. Assoc. **200:** 365–373.
4. KEW, M. C. 1973. Possible transmission of serum hepatitis via the conjunctiva. Infect. Immun. **7:** 823–824.
5. BANCROFT, W. H., R. SNITBHAN, R. McN. SCOTT, *et al.* 1977. Transmission of hepatitis B virus to gibbons by exposure to human saliva containing hepatitis B surface antigen. J. Infect. Dis. **135:** 79–85.
6. ALMEIDA, J. D., G. D. CHISHOLM, A. E. KULATILAKE, *et al.* 1971. Possible airborne spread of serum hepatitis virus within a hemodialysis unit. Lancet **2:** 849–850.
7. KAPPENBERGER, L., A. COLUMBI & G. LOCHER. 1973. Bleeding accident in dialysis patients leading to hepatitis outbreak. Helv. Med. Acta. **37:** 227–234.
8. GARIBALDI, R. A., F. E. HATCH, A. L. BISNO, *et al.* 1972. Nonparenteral serum hepatitis. Report of an outbreak. J. Am. Med. Assoc. **220:** 963–966.
9. FAVERO, M. S., J. E. MAYNARD, N. J. PETERSEN, *et al.* 1973. Hepatitis-B antigen on environmental surfaces. Lancet **2:** 1455–1456.
10. DANKERT, J., J. UITENTUIS, B. HOUWEN, *et al.* 1976. Hepatitis B surface antigen in environmental samples from hemodialysis units. J. Infect. Dis. **134** (2): 123–127.
11. PATTISON, C. P., J. E. MAYNARD, K. R. BERQUIST, *et al.* 1973. Serologic and epidemiologic studies of hepatitis B in hemodialysis units. Lancet **2:** 172–174.
12. SNYDMAN, D. R., J. A. BRYAN, E. J. MACON, *et al.* 1976. Hemodialysis-associated hepatitis: Report of an epidemic with further evidence on mechanisms of transmission. Amer. J. Epidemiol. **104** (5): 563–570.
13. PATTISON, C. P., K. M. BOYER, J. E. MAYNARD, *et al.* 1974. Epidemic hepatitis in a clinical laboratory. J. Am. Med. Assoc. **230:** 854–857.
14. LEVY, B. S., J. C. HARRIS, J. L. SMITH, *et al.* 1977. Hepatitis B in ward and clinical laboratory employees of a general hospital. Amer. J. Epidemiol. **106** (4): 330–335.
15. FAVERO, M. S., W. W. BOND, N. J. PETERSEN, *et al.* 1974. Detection methods for study of the stability of hepatitis B antigen on surfaces. J. Infect. Dis. **129:** 210–212.
16. McGARRITY, G. J., A. S. DION & J. SHEFFIELD. 1976. Environmental detection of mycoplasmas and viruses. Presented at 19th Biological Safety Conference, October 18–20, Frederick, Md.

Annals New York Academy of Sciences

17. BARKER, L. F. & others. 1975. Hepatitis B virus infection in chimpanzees: titration of subtypes. J. Infect. Dis. **132** (4): 451–458.
18. PETERSEN, N. J., W. W. BOND, J. H. MARSHALL, et al. 1976. An air sampling technique for hepatitis B surface antigen. Hlth. Lab. Sci. **13**: 233–237.
19. BOND, W. W., N. J. PETERSEN & M. S. FAVERO. 1977. Viral Hepatitis B: Aspects of environmental control. Hlth. Lab. Sci. **14** (4): 235–252.
20. Medical Research Council Subcommittee on hepatitis prevention in renal and associated units. 1975. Experimental studies on environmental contamination with infected blood during hemodialysis. J. Hyg. **74**: 133–148.
21. FELDMAN, R. E. & E. R. SCHIFF. 1975. Hepatitis in dental professionals. J. Am. Dental Assoc. **232** (12): 1228–1230.
22. MOSLEY, J. W. & others. 1975. Hepatitis B virus infection in dentists. N. Engl. J. Med. **293** (15): 729–734.
23. SMITH, J. L., J. E. MAYNARD, K. R. BERQUIST, et al. 1976. Comparative risk of hepatitis B among physicians and dentists. J. Infect. Dis. **133** (6): 705–706.
24. VILLAREJOS, V. M. et al. 1974. Role of saliva, urine and feces in the transmission of type B hepatitis. N. Engl. J. Med. **291** (26): 1375–1378.
25. PETERSEN, N. J., D. H. BARRETT, W. W. BOND, et al. 1976. Hepatitis B surface antigen in saliva, impetiginous lesions, and environment in two remote Alaskan villages. Appl. Environ. Microbiol. **32** (4): 572–574.
26. ALTER, H. J. & others. 1977. Transmission of hepatitis B to chimpanzees by hepatitis B surface antigen-positive saliva and semen. Infect. Immun. **16** (3): 928–933.
27. CRAWFORD, J. J. 1977. Sterilization, disinfection and asepsis in dentistry. In Disinfection, Sterilization and Preservation. S.S. Block, Ed.: 685. Lea & Febiger. Philadelphia.
28. Council on Dental Materials and Devices and Council on Dental Therapeutics. 1978. Infection control in the dental office. J. Amer. Dental Assoc. **97** (4): 673–677.
29. PETERSEN, N. J., W. W. BOND & M. S. FAVERO. 1979. Air sampling for hepatitis B surface antigen in a dental operatory. J. Amer. Dental Assoc. **99**: 465–467.

AEROSOL SPREAD OF PLANT VIRUSES: POTENTIAL ROLE IN DISEASE OUTBREAKS

Ernest E. Banttari

Department of Plant Pathology
University of Minnesota
St. Paul, Minnesota 55108

James R. Venette

Department of Plant Pathology
North Dakota State University
Fargo, North Dakota 58102

INTRODUCTION

There is voluminous literature concerning aerial dissemination of biotic disease agents of animals, man and plants.[1,6,12,14,15,25,27,29] Local and long distance aerial transport of propagules of some plant pathogenic fungi and, more recently, aerosol dissemination of certain plant pathogenic bacteria have been convincingly demonstrated.[11,20,27] However, the possibility that certain mechanically transmitted plant viruses could be disseminated as aerosols has received little attention. The paucity of information concerning plant virus aerosols may be for at least two reasons. First, the transmissibility of these viruses by many kinds of mechanical contact or wounding appears to adequately explain, in most situations, the spread of these viruses in nature. Secondly, the devices for detecting plant virus aerosols were not available or were untested for this purpose. The hypothesis that aerosol dissemination might be an additional means of spread of certain mechanically transmitted viruses may be difficult to prove. Nevertheless, the findings that plant viruses could occur as aerosols may, in itself, be of considerable interest. There is at least one report that alludes to an aerially transported virus pathogenic to plants in the greenhouse.[24] The suction devices used to filter the virus from air in those experiments apparently were effective in collecting an airborne virus. However, there appear to be no further references to this example. In discussing the potential aerial dissemination of plant pathogenic viruses, only those that are mechanically transmissible will be considered. Plant viruses that have aerially disseminated insect or mite vectors will not be included in this discussion.

A plant virus with the greatest potential for aerosol dissemination would be one that develops a high titered systemic infection in host plants. It would be stable *in vitro* and highly infectious. Certain plant viruses have these characteristics. For example, tobacco mosaic virus (TMV) may replicate as many as 6×10^7 particles/cell in trichomes of *Nicotiana tabacum*.[18] As much as 2 gr of virus/litre of leaf sap of tobacco has been extracted.[9] Trichomes of TMV-infected plants contain large crystalline inclusions easily visible in a light microscope and the inclusions consist almost solely of virus particles.[7,9] Trichomes on leaf surfaces of some plants can be easily injured. If such trichomes are disrupted, the inclusions probably will disperse, releasing large quantities of virus. If wounding occurs as

167

0077-8923/80/0353-0167 $01.75/0 © 1980, NYAS

the result of harsh weather including hail, driving rain and wind, it is possible that virus aerosols could be formed. These aerosols could consist of virus particles, parts of virus inclusions as well as virus particles attached to fragmented cellular structures. Water droplets (rain) striking plant surfaces will cause formation of splash from which surface particles can become airborne.[12] It has been shown that 1 μm pure water droplets evaporate completely in 0.5 second in air not saturated with water vapor and that 90 μm droplets evaporate in about one second in air at 50% relative humidity.[15] Virus particles could also be dispersed in a film of water over the surface of injured foliage and become dried. Secondary aerosol formation could occur from dried plant surfaces when virions or clumps of virions are dislodged by wind, by foliage rubbing and by machinery moving through the field.

The distance of dispersal of plant virus aerosols could be considerable, although wind velocity, particulate sizes and density largely determine how far aerosols can be moved. Aerosol particles 0.5 μm can be carried 624.7 km falling 3m in a 4.8 KPH wind while 20 μm particles move only 0.3 km under the same conditions.[4] TMV is highly resistant to desiccation and would remain infectious even after lengthy periods in vitro.[19,23]

The factors affecting deposition of virus aerosols on plant surfaces are not known. However, wind tunnel studies on deposition of $PbCl_2$ and uranine dye aerosols on sunflower, Helianthus annuus L., and tulip poplar, Liriodendron tulipifera L. indicate that the pubescent foliage of sunflower more efficiently trapped these materials than did glabrous foliage of tulip poplar.[28]

Finally, the method(s) by which virions initiate infection of host plants has not been completely elucidated. The most commonly supported hypothesis is that mechanically transmissible viruses enter host tissues through wounds.[8,16,22,26,30] Virus deposited from aerosols could initiate infections of plants through wounds. In large fields of closely spaced plants, abrasion could cause sufficient wounding to permit occasional entry of virus into host tissues. Further spread of viruses in the field from these primary foci could readily occur by several methods.[5,10]

Experimental Generation and Detection of Plant Virus Aerosols in the Laboratory

Before any experiments could be made to detect virus aerosols from plants, it was necessary to identify an aerosol sampler that was capable of collecting plant virus aerosols. Therefore, methods for generation of plant virus aerosols as well as their detection had to be developed simultaneously since there were no reported experiences with either. These experiments were made at Environmental Research Co., St. Paul, MN. Two types of aerosol generators were used to produce aerosols from purified preparations of tobacco mosaic virus (TMV) and potato virus X (PVX). An Environmental Research Company Model 8330 Spinning Disc Aerosol Generator that produces aerosols in the 1.0–10.0 μm range and an Environmental Research Company Model 7330 Fluid Atomization Aerosol Generator that produces aerosols in the 0.03–3.0 μm range were used. The aerosols generated from 75 ml of 0.11 mg/ml of purified PVX or from 75 ml of purified TMV (0.05 mg/ml) were discharged into a stainless steel wind tunnel (running at 21.2–28.3 m^3/minute) over a 30 minute period. Local lesion indicator plants (Gomphrena globosa for PVX or Nicotiana glutinosa for TMV) that had been lightly dusted with silicon carbide abrasive (600 Carborundum) were placed in a rack that held the leaves in position perpendicular to the flow of air in the wind tunnel. After a 30 minute exposure to the discharges, the plants were removed and the leaves were rubbed with pipet cleaner applicators dipped in buffer. In three repetitions of this experiment, means of 12 PVX and 8 TMV local lesions/leaf occurred on G. globosa and N. glutinosa, respectively. An Andersen 2000 six-stage aerosol sampler (Andersen 2000, Inc., P.O. Box 20769, Atlanta, Ga. 30320) using metal stages for nonviable particulates was also used to sample for airborne virus in the wind tunnel. The collections were assayed by inoculating indicator plants. Approximately 100 μl of 0.01 M phosphate buffer pH 7.0 was placed on each plate, the surface was swabbed with a pipet cleaner applicator and the moistened applicator was rubbed onto silicon carbide-dusted leaves of indicator plants. Although the flow and impacting characteristics of either TMV or PVX in an Andersen six-stage nonviable sampler have not been thoroughly investigated, the viruses could be detected on all stages of these aerosol samplers (TABLE 1). These experiments demonstrated that the Andersen six-stage nonviable aerosol sampler could be used to collect aerosols of either PVX or TMV.

To test the possibility that aerosols could be formed from plants subjected to

TABLE 1

INFECTION OF INDICATOR PLANTS WITH TOBACCO MOSAIC VIRUS (TMV) AND
POTATO VIRUS X (PVX) COLLECTED FROM AEROSOLS BY AN
ANDERSEN 6-STAGE SAMPLER* IN A WIND TUNNEL

TMV Local Lesions		PVX Local Lesions	
Stage	Nicotiana glutinosa	Stage	Gomphrena globosa
1	3	1	33
2	3	2	54
3	24	3	20
4	15	4	30
5	8	5	27
6	1	6	28

*Andersen Sampler Collections: 1 = 7+ μm, 2 = 4.7-7 μm, 3 = 3-4.7 μm, 4 = 2.1-3.3 μm, 5 = 1.1-2.1 μm, 6 = 0.65-1.1 μm. Viruses were removed from plates in each stage of the sampler and leaves of each indicator host were inoculated.

artificial conditions that simulated wind, hail, abrasion and driving rain in the field, experiments were made to approximate these conditions. A plywood chamber 1.3m × 1.3m × 2.2m was constructed. In separate experiments potato plants systemically infected with PVX and tomato plants systemically infected with TMV were placed in the chamber. An Andersen six-stage nonviable aerosol sampler placed in the center of the chamber was used to collect aerosols. In each experiment air sampled prior to placing plants in the chamber served as a control. In one treatment compressed air at approximately 4-6 kg/cm^2 was directed on the plants for two minutes; in other treatments water at 4-6 kg/cm^2 was sprayed on either uninjured or injured plants. After a two minute settling period, the sampler was run for 30 minutes after which the plates were assayed on indicator plants for each virus (TABLE 2). Tobacco mosaic virus aerosols developed readily by any of treatments. Little PVX was collected after any of the treatments. Since the wind tunnel experiments demonstrated that PVX could be collected in an Andersen six-stage aerosol sampler, these results suggested that little or no PVX was generated by the treatments applied to the potato plants.

TABLE 2

LOCAL LESIONS ON INDICATOR PLANTS WHEN INOCULATED WITH TOBACCO MOSAIC
VIRUS (TMV) AND POTATO VIRUS X (PVX) AEROSOLS GENERATED FROM INFECTED
PLANTS AND COLLECTED IN AN ANDERSEN 6-STAGE SAMPLER*

Virus/ Source	Treatment	Indicator Host	Stage†	Local Lesions
TMV Tomato	Air blast	Nicotiana glutinosa	1 2 3 4 5 6	2 3 4 8 16 7
TMV Tomato	Water spray (plants injured)	Nicotiana glutinosa	1 2 3 4 5 6	1 4 7 7 14 2
PVX Potato	Water spray (plants not injured)	Gomphrena globosa	1 2 3 4 5 6	0 1 0 1 0 0
PVX Potato	Water spray (plants injured)	Gomphrena globosa	1 2 3 4 5 6	0 0 0 1 1 4

*Andersen Sampler Collections from 0.85 m³ of air after plants were treated.
†Virus removed from the plates of each stage of the sampler and applied to leaves of
Nicotiana glutinosa (TMV) and Gomphrena globosa (PVX). $1 = 7+$ μm, $2 = 4.7-7.0$ μm, $3 =$
$3.3-4.7$ μm, $4 = 2.1-3.3$ μm, $5 = 1.2-2.1$ μm, $6 = 0.65-1.1$ μm.

Detection of Naturally Occurring Plant Virus Aerosols in the Field

Ultimately, it was important to determine if naturally-formed plant virus
aerosols occur in the field; how abundantly and under what conditions they are
formed; how far they move from their origins; and finally, if they produce
infections in plants. To test for naturally occurring TMV aerosols in 1977 and
1978, a 0.25 hectare plot of tobacco, Nicotiana tabacum was established (at the
rate of approximately 12,300 transplants/hectare). When the plants were approximately 25 cm tall, they were inoculated with a common strain of TMV. When the
plants were approximately 0.5 meter tall, a Sierra Model 235 High Volume
Aerosol Sampler (Sierra Instruments, P.O. Box 909, Village Square, Carmel
Valley, CA. 93924) was placed in the center of the plot. This device samples
approximately 48-60 m³ of air/hour. A mesh stainless steel screened box was
placed over the intake to prevent entrance of insects. A record of weather
conditions within 0.5 km of this plot was available from a weather station of the
University of Minnesota. The procedure for assays of collected fractions was
similar to the procedure used with the Andersen samplers, using N. glutinosa as

the local lesion indicator host. A Type A fiberglass back-up filter was inserted into the collector after the fifth stage to trap particulates that might not become impacted on the plates and might otherwise pass through the sampler. To assay for virus in this filter, it was ground in 25 ml of 0.02 M phosphate buffer pH 7.2 in a Waring Blendor, the slurry was squeezed through cheesecloth and the filtrate was centrifuged 79,000 g for 2 hr. The pellets were resuspended (0.25 ml of buffer each), composited and the suspension was applied to silicon carbide-dusted *N. glutinosa*. During two seasons, 1977 and 1978, collections were made during 30 sampling periods ranging from 2 to 24 hr and TMV was collected on at least some plates in 14 of these assays (TABLE 3). A summation of weather conditions during which virus was collected indicate that TMV was most frequently collected when there was at least 25 km/hr wind with or without precipitation or overhead irrigation during the assay period. Plant height appeared to have some bearing on occurrence of virus aerosols since no virus was collected until the plants were approximately 1.5 m tall.

To test for natural occurrence of PVX aerosols, a 40 hectare field of Russet Burbank potatoes infected with PVX was assayed. The Sierra High Volume Aerosol sampler was placed approximately 100m into the field. Collections were assayed as for TMV except that *Gomphrena globosa* was used as the local lesion indicator. No backup fiberglass filter was used in these assays. Twenty assay periods of approximately 24 hr each were made. A variety of weather conditions occurred during these assays although no close weather station was available for a record. No PVX was detected in any of these assays.

DISCUSSION

The evidence is that plant virus aerosols can be produced in the laboratory and that at least TMV aerosols can develop naturally in the field.[2,3] Over a two-year period, TMV was collected in the Sierra High Volume Aerosol Sampler in 14 of 30 sampling periods. No quantitative studies have been done with this collector; therefore its effectiveness in sampling for plant virus aerosols is unknown. These experiments did not show what minimum number of airborne

TABLE 3

DETECTION OF NATURALLY OCCURRING TOBACCO MOSAIC VIRUS AEROSOLS FROM A FIELD OF TOBACCO IN 1977-78 AS INDICATED BY LOCAL LESIONS ON *Nicotiana glutinosa**

Sierra Cascade Aerosol Sampler Stage or Filter	Local Lesions on *N. glutinosa*†
1	1.26
2	0.69
3	0.80
4	0.85
5	0.79
Backup Filter	0.04
Check	>10.00

*14 Aerosol collections ranged from 2–24 hr in 0.25 hectares of TMV infected tobacco at St. Paul during 1977–78.

†Average number of local lesions on 42 leaves of *N. glutinosa* in 14 air samples for stages 1–5; average number of local lesions on 100 leaves in 10 air samples for the backup filter.

particles resulted in positive biological assays. Attempts to find virus in these samples using the electron microscope were made, but excessive dust or dirt that was also impacted in the sampler plates obscured the grids. Dispersal of mechanically transmitted viruses on surface contaminated pollen has been shown[13] and could account for some virus collected in the field. Because of the relatively large size of pollen, it would probably be deposited on the upper stages of the Sierra Hi-Volume Sampler and would not account for all the fractions that were collected.

Weather conditions that occurred during sampling periods when TMV was collected indicated that wind (above 25 km/hr) with or without precipitation or overhead irrigation favors TMV aerosol formation.

Dispersal distance from points of origin of TMV aerosols is not known. Because of the apparent size range of airborne virus particulates (< 0.61 to more than 10 μm), it is likely that some fractions of such aerosols would remain suspended almost indefinitely and may be moved long distances from their source.

Although TMV aerosols collected in the field caused local lesions when rubbed on leaves of the indicator plant, N. glutinosa, the natural infectivity of these aerosols to plants in the field has not been demonstrated. However, when potentially infective aerosols are deposited on closely spaced plants in which there is substantial foliage contact, it is likely that during windy weather sufficient wounding could occur to permit virus entry and occasional infection. Wounding also could be caused by hail or movement of agricultural implements through the field. Even if only occasional infections were established in fields that originally were free from virus diseases, the trace infections attributed to aerosols would be epidemiologically highly significant.

Although TMV, because of the characteristics already mentioned, has the greatest potential for dispersal as aerosols, other mechanically transmissible viruses might also occur as naturally formed aerosols. Tomato bushy stunt virus, barley stripe mosaic virus and brome mosaic virus, among others, could possibly form aerosols. None have been investigated for this potential. Since only the Sierra Cascade 235 Aerosol Collector has been effective in the field, the utilization of other aerosol samplers or development of more efficient aerosol collection devices might permit the detection of yet other plant virus aerosols. Several additional kinds of aerosol collectors have been designed and some types will fractionate particulates according to size.[17,21]

The dissemination of viruses as aerosols may or may not have significance to the epidemiology of virus diseases of plants. Nevertheless, the detection of airborne TMV supports the hypothesis that there can be aerial dispersal of particles of certain plant viruses and serves as a foundation for future studies.

REFERENCES

1. ANDERSEN, A. A. 1958. New sampler for the collection, sizing and enumeration of viable airborne particles. J. Bacteriol. 75: 471–484.
2. BANTTARI, E. E. 1978. Formation, dispersal, and detection of plant virus aerosols. Fourth International Cong. for Virology: 153. Centre for Agric. Pub. and Doc. Wageningen, the Netherlands. (Abstr.)
3. BANTTARI, E. E. & J. R. VENETTE. 1975. Potato virus X and tobacco mosaic virus aerosols. Proc. of the American Phytopathol. Soc. 2: 51. (Abstr.)

4. BROOKS, F. A. 1947. The drifting of poisonous dusts applied by airplanes and land rigs. Agric. Eng. **28**: 233–239.
5. COCKERMAN, G. 1958. Observations on the spread of virus X. *In* Proc. Third Conf. on Potato Virus Dis.: 144–148. Wageningen, the Netherlands.
6. DIMMICK, R. L. & A. B. AKERS. 1969. An Introduction to Experimental Aerobiology. Wiley-Interscience. New York.
7. ESAU, K. 1967. Anatomy of plant virus infections. Annu. Rev. Phytopathol. **5**: 45–76.
8. GEROLA, F. M., M. BASSI, M. A. FAVALI & E. BETTO. 1969. An electron microscopy study of the penetration of tobacco mosaic virus into leaves following experimental inoculation. Virology **38**: 380–386.
9. GIBBS, A. & B. HARRISON. 1976. Plant Virology: The Principles. John Wiley and Sons. New York.
10. GOODING, G. V. 1969. Epidemiology of tobacco mosaic virus on flue-cured tobacco in North Carolina. North Carolina Tech. Bull. No. 195:1–24.
11. GRAHAM, D. C. & M. D. HARRISON. 1975. Potential spread of *Erwinia* sp. in aerosols. Phytopathology **65**: 739–741.
12. GREGORY, P. H. 1973. The Microbiology of the Atmosphere. 2nd Edit. John Wiley and Sons. New York.
13. HAMILTON, R. I., E. LEUNG & C. NICHOLS. 1977. Surface contamination of pollen by viruses. Phytopathology **67**: 395–399.
14. HATCH, T. F. and P. GROSS. 1964. Pulmonary Deposition and Retention of Inhaled Aerosols. Academic Press. New York.
15. HENDERSON, D. W. 1952. An apparatus for the study of airborne infection. J. Hyg. **50**: 53–68.
16. KADO, C. I. 1972. Mechanical and biological inoculation principles. *In* Principles and Techniques in Plant Virology: 3–24. Van Nostrand Reinhold. New York.
17. MARPLE, V. A. & B. Y. H. LIU. 1974. Characteristics of laminar jet impactor. Environmental Sci. and Tech. **8**: 649.
18. NIXON, H. L. 1956. An estimate of the number of tobacco mosaic virus particles in a single hair cell. Virology **2**: 126–128.
19. ORLOB, G. B. & P. R. LORENZ. 1968. Survival of toabcco mosaic virus in space. Phytopathology **58**: 955–956.
20. PEROMBELON, M. C. U., R. A. FOX and R. LOWE. 1979. Dispersion of *Erwinia caratovora* in aerosols produced by the pulverization of potato haulm prior to harvest. Phytopath. Z. **94**: 249–260.
21. Samplings Microbiological Aerosols. 1964. Public Health Monograph No. 60. U.S. Dept. of Health, Education and Welfare.
22. SCHNEIDER, I. R. 1965. Introduction, translocation and distribution of viruses in plants. Adv. Virus Res. **11**: 163–221.
23. SMITH, K. M. 1957. Tobacco mosaic virus. *In* A Textbook of Plant Virus Diseases: 505–524. Little, Brown & Co. Boston.
24. SMITH, K. M. 1937. An airborne plant virus. Nature **139**: 370.
25. STAKMAN, E. C. & C. M. CHRISTENSEN. 1946. Aerobiology in relation to plant disease. Bot. Rev. **12**: 205–253.
26. THOMAS, P. E. & R. W. FULTON. 1968. Correlation of ectodesmata number with nonspecific resistance to initial virus infection. Virology **34**: 459–469.
27. VENETTE, J. R. & B. W. KENNEDY. 1975. Naturally produced aerosols of *Pseudomonas glycinea*. Phytopathology **65**: 737–738.
28. WEDDING, J. B., R. W. CARLSON, J. J. STUKEL & F. A. BAZZAZ. 1976. Aerosol deposition on plant leaves. Proceedings of the First International Symposium on Acid Precipitation and the Forest Ecosystem: 897–903. USDA Forest Service Technology Report NE-23.
29. WELLOCK, C. E. 1960. Epidemiology of Q fever in the urban east bay area. Calif. Health **18**: 72–76.
30. YARWOOD, C. E. & R. W. FULTON. 1967. Mechanical transmission of plant viruses. *In* Methods in Virology I: 237–266. Academic Press. New York.

OVERVIEW OF AIRBORNE CONTAGION IN ANIMALS*

Lawrence A. Falk, Jr. and Ronald D. Hunt

New England Regional Primate Research Center
Harvard Medical School
Southborough, Massachusetts, 01772

INTRODUCTION

Airborne spread of viral infections is a predominant mode for transmission of various diseases in man. Although a number of viral infections can be transmitted by airborne route, the common cold and influenza are probably the two viral diseases transmitted most frequently by the airborne route. Airborne transmission of viral diseases is of particular importance in veterinary medicine because of the economic impact outbreaks of severe infections can have on the food production industry.

This overview seeks to highlight factors favoring and promoting survival of viruses in air and to summarize three viral diseases to illustrate the magnitude of losses resulting from major viral disease epidemics in the poultry and livestock industry.

Suspension of Particles in Air

Normally air is not a suitable or favorable environment for viruses and the presence of viruses in air is a result generally of contamination from infected materials. Infectious virus in air is associated with two types of particles: droplet nuclei and dust particles. These two particle types have uniquely different properties and behavior.[1]

Droplet Nuclei

These particles are generated from evaporated droplets expelled from the respiratory system as a result of sneezing, coughing and talking. Because of their small size, they remain suspended indefinitely because of minor air currents: average settling velocity is 0.04 feet per minute. Generally droplet nuclei contain only one infectious particle which may be deposited in the lungs of susceptible contacts. Droplet nuclei are associated with propagated epidemics in which infection is transmitted from person to person.

Dust Particles

These larger particles are shed from skin or clothing and because of their larger size they settle rapidly: 1.5 feet per minute. Dust particles generally contain more than one infectious particle that may be deposited on external body

*Preparation of this review was supported in part by Grant No. RR-00168-18, Animal Resources Branch, National Institutes of Health and Grant No. RO1 CA22725-01, National Cancer Institute.

surfaces and in the respiratory tract. Localized epidemics are associated with infections transmitted via dust particles.

Factors Affecting the Survival of Virus in Air

Harper[2] studied the survival of poliovirus (small, RNA-containing virus) and vaccinia virus (large, DNA-containing virus belonging to the pox-virus group) at various relatively humidity (RH) values. Poliovirus, whether suspended in crude tissue culture medium, water, phosphate buffer or gelatin showed 66%–120% survival after one minute at RH values of 50% and 80%; in the same suspending fluids at 20% RH, survival values of <1%–20% were obtained. Prolonged aerosolization of poliovirus for 23 hours showed that at 20% and 50% RH only trace infectivity was detected whereas infectivity values of 23%–89% were obtained at 80% RH.

TABLE 1

SOME ANIMAL VIRUSES WHICH MAY BE TRANSMITTED BY THE AIRBORNE ROUTE

Avian encephalomyelitis	Hog cholera
Avian leukosis	Infectious bovine rhinotracheitis
Aleutian disease of mink	Infectious bronchitis of fowls
Canine distemper	Infectious laryngotracheitis of fowls
Canine herpesvirus	Infectious porcine encephalomyelitis
Eastern equine encephalomyelitis	Marek's disease
Equine infectious arteritis	Newcastle disease
Equine influenza	Porcine enterovirus
Equine rhinopneumonitis	Poxviruses
Feline rhinotracheitis	Rabies
Feline pneumonitis	Swine influenza
Foot-and-mouth disease	Transmissible gastroenteritis of swine
Fowl plaque	Wester equine encephalomyelitis

Directly opposing results were obtained when similar evaluations were performed with vaccinia virus. Survival values of 52%–112% were obtained after one minute aerosolization at 20%, 50%, or 80% RH. After aerosolization for 23 hours, infectivity at 50% or 80% RH ranged from <1%–12% but 15%–37% infectivity was retained at 20% RH.

These marked differences observed between poliovirus and vaccinia virus serve to emphasize the importance the virus type plays in the maintenance and survival of viral infectivity in the airborn state.

Similarly, Rechsteiner[3] examined what influence RH had on the survival of respiratory syncytial virus: high infectivity (81%) was maintained after one minute aerosolization at high RH and low at low RH.

In studies Hyslop[4] performed with poliovirus, foot-and-mouth disease virus and rinderpest virus, there was a progressive decreased resistance to desiccation at RH values of 15% or 75%. Furthermore, it was suggested from these data that the survival, particularly of poliovirus and foot-and-mouth disease virus, was sufficient to allow transport over distances of several miles at normal wind velocities.

Although RH is generally regarded as the most important environmental factor affecting infectivity of viruses as well as other pathogenic microorganisms, other factors, i.e., irradiation and visible light of short wave length are also important.[5-6] It is difficult to measure and to assess precisely how environmental factors affect the infectivity of viruses in the airborn state because it is difficult to duplicate under laboratory conditions the complex interactions of environmental factors.

Transmission of Viral Diseases of Veterinary Importance

Documentation has been gathered supporting airborn transmission of viral diseases and in TABLE 1 is a partial listing of viruses which can be transmitted by this mode.[7]

Newcastle disease and Marek's disease of chickens and foot-and-mouth disease of cattle aptly illustrate the severe economic losses which can result from epidemics of viral diseases in the poultry and livestock industry. Large outbreaks of Marek's disease amongst chickens appear to be an event of the past.

Newcastle Disease Virus

Newcastle disease virus is an RNA-containing virus belonging to the paramyxovirus group. Newcastle disease virus produces pneumoencephalitis in young chickens and an influenza like disease in older chickens. Infection in man is generally an occupational disease in laboratory personnel and poultry workers handling infected birds; disease in man is characterized by conjunctival inflammation.[1] The last major outbreak in the United States occurred in California in 1972 resulting in the slaughter of 13 million chickens with a cost of $55 million to the poultry industry. Isolated and confined outbreaks occurred in California and Florida in 1979; in both outbreaks, the index cases were imported birds (personal communication, U.S. Department of Agriculture).

Marek's Disease Virus of Chickens

Marek's disease is a lymphoproliferative disease of chickens affecting nerves and producing visceral tumors. A herpesvirus, Marek's disease virus (MDV) was isolated in cell culture after cultivation of tumor tissues in vitro.[8-9] Although all attempts to recover infectious virus or to demonstrate herpesvirus particles or antigens in tumor tissues were negative, later studies showed that virus replicated in epithelial cells of the feather follicles. This site of active viral replication favored and promoted dispersal of infectious virus into the surrounding environment and presumably accounted for the high infectivity of MDV amongst flocks of chickens.

A virus of turkeys, herpesvirus of turkeys, was isolated in 1970[10] and it was demonstrated to be antigenically related to MD. The herpesvirus of turkeys has been used successfully as a vaccine against MDV. Therefore in a few short years after the discovery of the herpesvirus of turkeys, it was possible to eliminate Marek's disease from most poultry farms. Previously, the widespread incidence of MDV amongst poultry farms imparted severe economic losses to the poultry industry. The story with Marek's disease shows how effective control measures can be achieved for complete eradication of a recurring disease.

Foot-and-Mouth Disease

Foot-and-mouth disease (FMD) virus is a highly infectious virus infecting cloven hoofed animals. FMD virus is an RNA-containing virus, 23 nm in diameter and labile at acid ph (ph 3.0). The virus is very hearty as it survives freezing and is unaffected by drying at ordinary temperatures. There are at least 53 subtypes divided into seven antigenic types. Generally infection with one type fails to prevent infection with other types.[1]

Naturally FMD virus infects cattle, sheep, goats and swine but wild ruminants, i.e., deer, goats and antelopes may also be infected. Natural infection may occur in man resulting in a mild disease characterized by acute fever and vesicles on hands, feet and oral mucosa.

Susceptible animals most likely become infected by the oropharyngeal route and shortly thereafter viremia develops and virus can be recovered from blood during the febrile stage of disease. Virus becomes concentrated in the fluid of epithelial vesicles developing on the tongue. Mortality is low, <5%, although mortality rates of >60% have been reported with some virus strains.[1,11]

There have been nine major recorded outbreaks of FMD in the United States and the last episode occured in 1929.[12-14] The cost to eliminate all outbreaks in the United States amounted to greater than $9 million. The United States assisted Mexico in eliminating FMD after the disease occurred within Mexico in 1946: the total cost for eliminating the disease was in excess of $134.5 million. Similarly the United States also assisted Canada in eliminating FMD in 1952 after an outbreak occurred in 1951. The North American continent has remained free of FMD since 1952 because of an aggressive survelliance policy particularly at importation stations.

A major outbreak of FMD occurred in England in 1967-68 which became the subject of several extensive investigations.[15-21] The outbreak began after a consignment of infected meat was imported from Argentina in October, 1967. The course of the outbreak ran approximately 120 days and 2,339 farms were affected, resulting in the slaughter of 443,000 animals.[18]

Hurst examined meterological records covering periods of previous FMD outbreaks in England and the data suggested that some of the outbreaks occurred during a key period which would favor a windborne transport of infection from the continent.[18] Hugh-Jones and Wright studied the spread of disease from the initial focus and also found evidence pointing to a windborne spread of infection. Snow and rain were also factors contributing to the spread of FMD: specific periods when greatest outbreaks occurred coincided with periods with average daily rain falls of two-three hours' duration. Precipitation in effect will bring droplet nuclei or infectious dust particles out of suspension and deposit them on grazing and fodder crops and will also produce a ground level aerosol capable of blowing into buildings housing livestock. These studies also revealed that although weather accounted for much of the behavior of the epidemic, after the peak of the epidemic, spread of infection thereafter appeared to be less controlled by weather and continued to decrease in intensity even under what appeared to be suitable weather conditions for a high rate of spread. This decreased intensity could be accounted for by: 1) decreased availability of susceptible animals as result of slaughter, 2) during the epidemic peak, more animals were grazing in open fields. This correlated well with wind speed during the early part of the epidemic. 3) Delay in slaughtering infected animals: in the early part of the epidemic more herds were being slaughtered the day after confirmation of infection than in the decline period of the epidemic when herds were slaughtered on the day of confirmation of disease.

Recognition that wind is responsible for most of the spread of FMD makes it difficult to devise means of limiting spread of infection during epidemics. However, knowledge of wind directions and speed during epidemics can be used to identify areas in which fresh outbreaks are likely to occur.

REFERENCES

1. JAWETZ, E., J. L. MELNICK & E. A. ADELBERG. 1976. Review of Medical Microbiology: 91,418 Lange Medical Publications. Los Altos, Calif.
2. HARPER, G. J. 1965. Proc. 5th International Symposium on Aerobiology: 335,341. Naval Biological Laboratory. Oakland, Calif.
3. RECHSTEINER, J. 1970. 3rd International Symposium on Aerobiology: 267.
4. HYSLOP, N. St. G. 1978. International Symposium on microbial ecology: 197–205.
5. HYSLOP, N. St. G. 1971. Amer. Vet. Med. Assoc. 159: 1500–1507.
6. HYSLOP, N. St. G. 1972. Trop. Anim. Health Prod. 4: 28–40.
7. DIMMICK, R. L. & ANN B. AKERS, Eds. 1969. An Introduction to Experimental Aerobiology: 465 Wiley-Interscience. New York.
8. CHURCHILL, A. E. & P. M. BIGGS. 1967. Nature 215: 528–530.
9. NAZERIAN, K., J. J. SOLOMON, R. L. WITTER & B. R. BURMESTER. 1968. Proc. Soc. Exp. Biol. Med. 127: 173–176.
10. WITTER, R. L., K. NAZERIAN, H. G. PURCHASE, G. H. BURGOYNE. 1970. Am. J. Vet. Res. 31: 525–538.
11. SMITH, H. A., T. C. JONES & R. D. HUNT. 1972. Veterinary Pathology: 395–397. Lea & Febiger. Philadelphia.
12. U.S. Department of Agriculture Pamphlet 600. 1963. Foot and mouth disease, a foreign threat to U.S. livestock.
13. Agriculture Research Service/U.S. Department of Agriculture. 1969. Foot-and-Mouth Disease: a menace to North American livestock.
14. SCHWABE, C. W. 1969. In Veterinary Medicine and Human Health: 463–465 The Williams & Wilkins Company. Baltimore.
15. DAVIES, W. K. D., G. B. LEWIS & H. A. RANDALL. 1968. Nature 219: 121–125.
16. DONALDSON, A. I., K. A. HERNIMAN, J. PARKER & R. F. SELLERS. 1970. J. Hyg. Camb. 68: 557–564.
17. HENDERSON, R. J. 1969. J. Hyg. Camb. 67: 21–33.
18. HUGH-JONES, M. E. & P. B. WRIGHT. 1970. J. Hyg. 68: 253–271. Cambridge.
19. HURST, G. W. 1968. The Veterinary Record, June 1st, 1968.
20. SELLERS, R. F. & J. PARKER. 1969. J. Hyg. 67: 671–677. Cambridge.
21. SMITH, L. P. & M. E. HUGH-JONES. 1969. Nature 223: 712–715.

SPREAD OF PLANT VIRUSES AND SPIROPLASMAS THROUGH AIRBORNE VECTORS

Karl Maramorosch

Waksman Institute of Microbiology
Rutgers, The State University
P. O. Box 759
Piscataway, New Jersey 08854

INTRODUCTION

Plant pathogens belong to fungi, bacteria, mycoplasmas (spiroplasmas), viruses and viroids. Most fungi and bacteria can enter plant cells and infect plants without the intermediary of vectors. No vectors are known for viroids.[8] Most viruses and mycoplasmas require the intermediary of vectors to infect plants. The term "vector" is used here in its broad sense, describing a carrier of a pathogen. In this context vectors comprise insects (TABLE I) and other arthropods, such as eryophyid mites.[11] Several "soilborne" viruses are transmitted by nematode vectors[31] and by lower fungi.[32] A number of plant viruses are transmitted via airborne pollen that can be considered as a vector in the broad sense of the word.[16] The airborne vectors of viruses play an important role in the epidemiology of plant diseases. The interactions between pathogens and vectors, as well as the dispersal of the vectors determine the mode and the area of contagion. We shall discuss here the spread through airborne vectors of plant pathogenic viruses and mycoplasmas.

Aphid Vectors

The largest single group of vectors of plant viruses is comprised by aphids. The large number and diversity of aphid-borne viruses indicated the nearly perfect adaptation of aphids for virus transmission.[29] Aphids feed on plants without causing much damage and they penetrate superficial tissues as well as phloem tissues. Among aphid-borne viruses are single-stranded RNA and double-stranded DNA viruses. Aphid-transmitted viruses belong to two distinct groups as far as virus-vector interaction is concerned. One group is retained in the vectors for prolonged periods and such persistent viruses can be carried for considerable distances by airborne aphid vectors. The second is nonpersistent and transmission is limited to short distances. The above generalization grossly oversimplifies the actual interrelationships. Rhabdoviruses have been shown to multiply in aphid vectors, and their vectors are thus alternate hosts of plant viruses.

The terminology of vector-virus interrelationships has undergone considerable changes in recent years. Based on the length of virus retention, Watson and Roberts[35] classified aphid-borne viruses as nonpersistent, semipersistent and persistent. Newer classification systems, dealing with stylet-borne and circulative virus vector interactions,[14] and the ingestion-egestion hypothesis[10] better describe the actual interrelationships. However, for the purpose of airborne contagion the system proposed by Watson and Roberts still seems adequate. The

0077-8923/80/0353-0179 $01.75/0 © 1980, NYAS

migration of aphid vectors depends on the available food plants, aphid species, time of year, and weather conditions, specifically winds. Low-level jet winds have been studied in the southern Plain States and Northern Central States of the United States in relation to the spread of barley yellow dwarf virus by aphids.[34] Nonpersistent viruses can be carried for short distances downwind.[1] Winged and nonwinged aphids (alatae and apterae) can be carried by wind. Comparatively little is known of the actual long-range dispersal of aphid-borne viruses and it seems logical to assume that persistent viruses can be carried for considerable distances by their aphid vectors.

Mite Vectors

Eriophyid mites, primarily *Aceria tulipae* has attracted much attention since it has been demonstrated as the vector of wheat streak mosaic virus.[27] Nearly a dozen other plant viruses are now known to be carried by mites belonging to the Eriophyidae.[28] The very small mites, approximately 0.2 mm in length, are dispersed by wind during warm weather, and the virus persists in its vector for

TABLE 1

INSECT VECTORS OF PLANT PATHOGENS

Vector group	Disease agent
1. Aphids	Viruses
2. Leafhoppers and planthoppers	Viruses, MLO, bacteria
3. Whiteflies	Viruses
4. Beetles	Viruses, fungi, bacteria
5. Thrips	Viruses
6. Mealybugs	Viruses
7. Psyllids	MLO, viruses
8. Membracids	Viruses

long periods, up to 9 days, and is retained through the molts. However, mites are susceptible to dryness and seldom, if ever, carry viruses over large distances.

Leafhopper and Planthopper Vectors

Most leafhopper- and planthopper-transmitted viruses are circulative in their vectors. Many have been shown to be propagative and some are carried to the progeny of vectors transovarially.[18,22,26] Leafhopper vectors may move between plants in a field, or may disperse from breeding areas to crops. Besides, leafhoppers may move over large distances—up to several hundred miles, depending on the life history of the insect, the host range, host preference and the physical factors of the environment.[4] Light intensity and temperature also influence leafhopper movement.[7,15] Of special interest is the long distance dispersal via airborne leafhopper vectors. In the Western United States beet leafhoppers (*Circulifer tenellus-Neoaliturus tenellus* (Baker) were found to migrate normally 30 to 60 miles, but instances of migrations up to 400 miles are documented.[7] This airborne dispersal is caused by prevailing winds. Since the curly top virus of beets is retained in its leafhopper vectors, the virus is carried, and later transmitted to plants growing at distant locations. Several years ago, the curly top virus of sugar beets, as well as its leafhopper vector, appeared as far east from the Rocky Mountains as the state of Illinois.

In Rhodesia, three species of the leafhopper Cicadulina, that act as vectors of maize streak virus, are composed of two morphs.[25] One morph is a short-distance flier, the other a long-distance flier and the flying ability is inherited. The shortflying leafhoppers move from 2 to 12 meters, while the long distance fliers carry the virus to plants in a radius of 1.8 kilometers.

The largest airborne distance reported for leafhopper vectors concerns the spiroplasma agent of aster yellows and its vector *Macrosteles fascifrons*. The disease agent was considered a virus until 1967, when Doi et al.[9] described mycoplasma-like bodies in aster plants in Japan, and Ishiie et al.[13] found that these microorganisms temporarily disappeared when diseased plants were treated with tetracycline antibiotics. This was confirmed for American aster yellows by Maramorosch et al. in 1968,[23] Since then, more than 100 different plant diseases have been shown to be caused by, or associated with, mycoplasma-like organisms (MLOs).[38] Chiykowski and Chapman[6] showed the *M. fascifrons* migrates northward from the Mississippi delta several hundred miles each spring and that adults, carrying the aster yellows spiroplasma[20] arrive as far north as Wisconsin, and even the prairie provinces of Canada.[36] Chiykowski[5,7] found that the migrant population of *M. fascifrons* contained a larger percentage of spiroplasma-carrying individuals than did populations that acquired the spiroplasmas later in the season. Therefore areas affected by airborne leafhopper vectors are subject to aster yellows infection earlier than those involving local populations. Consequently, the airborne vectors of aster yellows spiroplasma were more important in the epidemiology of the disease than were the populations that acquired the spiroplasma locally.[24]

The same vector, *M. fascifrons*, also carries the oat blue dwarf virus,[2] and a high percentage of migratory leafhoppers, blown as far north as Manitoba, were found to carry this virus.[37]

Spiroplasmas and MLOs, that have not yet been properly classified, are carried biologically and specifically by leafhoppers and psyllids. One MLO disease will be mentioned here, because it illustrates the impact an airborne vector can have on the economy, and even geopolitical developments of an area. The disease caused by this MLO is called lethal yellowing of coconut palms. It has been known in the Caribbean Islands since the beginning of the 19th century.[17] The same disease under different names occurs in Ghana, Togo, Nigeria and the Cameroons in West Africa, and apparently also in Tanzania in East Africa.[19,30] Recent reports indicate that the disease may have been present for many years in Malaysia and Indonesia.[12] The suspected vector, *Haplaxius* sp. is being studied in Florida and in Jamaica and confirmation of the role of this leafhopper as a vector of the lethal yellowing MLO can be expected shortly.[33] In Jamaica the disease has been confined for many years to the east end of the island, where it was called the East End Bud Rot.[17] After 1963 the disease suddenly appeared in the western part of the island where it now kills millions of coconut palms each year.[30] The same disease appeared for the first time in Key West in the 1950s[17] but disappeared for a while, only to return to southern Florida a few years later and to destroy not only coconut palms, but several other palm species.[19] Why did the disease or its suspected leafhopper vector remain confined to certain islands or parts of an island for long periods without moving to adjoining areas? If the vector were carried in a similar manner as the vector of the aster yellows spiroplasma, it would be expected to move for hundreds of miles with air currents. It probably does move that way, but the prevailing winds in Jamaica and some Caribbean Islands are from west to east. Only during hurricanes, and even then but rarely, does the direction of the wind shift.

Lethal yellowing has wiped out coconut palms on Cuba at the turn of the century and this epiphytotic changed the agriculture and the economy of the island. When attempts to replant coconut palms had failed, sugarcane plantations were started, changing drastically the agriculture and economy of the island. Instead of numerous owners of small coconut groves, a few large landowners began to dominate the island's agricultural production, mainly sugarcane. After 50 years the extreme wealth of the sugar barons and the dire poverty of the rural population provided a fertile ground for Castro's rise to power. The tremendous impact of the coconut lethal yellowing disease on Cuba and, more recently, on other Caribbean islands in terms of economy and politics is comparable to the impact of major airborne contagions of man in the middle ages.

Virus Transmission Through Pollen

Less than 10% of all plant viruses are able to infect pollen of plants. Pollen may be carried by insects, such as bees, during pollination. It can also be airborne in plants that are air pollinated. If pollen carries a virus, contagion can be considered as airborne. An example of such transmission is the pollen-borne barley stripe mosaic virus, where from 10% to 35% of the barley plants become infected. Some plant viruses prove lethal to the gametes they infect. Tobacco ring spot virus causes sterility of tobacco, and lettuce mosaic virus causes sterility in lettuce. Barley stripe mosaic, even though it infects barley plants via airborne pollen, can induce sterility of gametes. Infected ovules seem to be affected to a lesser degree and some virus transmission does occur when viable pollen fertilizes the infected ovules.[3]

CONCLUSIONS

Airborne virus contagion per se is seldom considered by plant disease epidemiologists, but airborne transmission of vectors of viruses plays an important role in plant disease epidemiology. The virus, the host, the vector and the environment influence disease epidemiology. Airborne vectors are influenced by the size of the population, number of generations per year, longevity, diapause, patterns of dispersal, feeding behavior, food plants, and by the reaction to the pathogen.[7] Environmental factors include temperature, air currents, humidity, predators, and pollutants in the atmosphere. Many of these factors are well understood, but their combined action creates highly complex problems.

The complexity of the airborne dispersal of vectors adds to the difficulties in controlling airborne contagion of plants. Complete elimination of vectors needed to prevent disease appearance is not feasible. This cannot be accomplished by insecticides or other approaches considered for the prevention of plant virus and mycoplasma diseases. Selection and breeding are the methods of choice, and efforts to develop resistant varieties provide the best solution. In addition, new approaches, in which the airborne insect vectors are diverted from host plants by repellents, or by thin layers of oil, have proven successful in selected crops. In addition to breeding for resistance to disease agents, resistance to specific vectors can be incorporated in breeding programs.[21] A combination of integrated control and proper breeding and selection might reduce considerably, but not eradicate, airborne vectors of plant viruses and mycoplasmas.

SUMMARY

Natural transmission of plant pathogenic viruses and of spiroplasmas requires specific vectors, some of which are airborne. The principal vectors of viruses belong to the following groups: aphids, leafhoppers, planthoppers, whiteflies, beetles, thrips, mealybugs, psyllids, mites, membracids, nematodes, and fungi. Spiroplasmas are transmitted by leafhoppers. Several as yet poorly defined mycoplasma-like agents are transmitted by leafhoppers, planthoppers and psyllids. Leafhopper vectors of the aster yellows spiroplasma can be carried by air currents over distances exceeding 1,400 kilometers, surviving without food, at low temperature, and retaining their infectivity. This illustrates one of the difficulties in preventing the natural, "airborne" spread of leafhopper-borne plant disease agents. Stylet-borne, nonpersistent viruses are less likely to be carried over great distances by airborne vectors. Airborne virus contagion via airborne pollen is known to occur in several instances. In its broad meaning, pollen can be considered a vector in such transmission. Eriophyid mites can be airborne but their sensitivity to low humidity limits the distance of actual contagion. Control measures such as breeding for resistance to disease agents, resistance to vectors, and integrated vector control can diminish, but not completely eliminate vector-borne plant contagion.

REFERENCES

1. ADLERZ, W. C. 1974. Wind effects on spread of watermelon mosaic virus 1 from sources to watermelon. J. Econ. Entomol. **67:** 361–364.
2. BANTTARI, E. E. & R. J. ZEYEN. 1979. Interactions of Mycoplasma-like organisms and viruses in dually infected leafhoppers, planthoppers and plants. *In* Leafhopper Vectors and Plant Disease Agents. K. Maramorosch & K. F. Harris, Eds. 327–347. Academic Press. New York, N.Y.
3. BENNETT, C. W. 1969. Seed transmission of plant viruses. Adv. Virus Res. **14:** 221–261.
4. CARTER, W. 1961. Ecological aspects of plant virus transmissions. Ann. Rev. Entomol. **6:** 347–370.
5. CHIYKOWSKI, L. N. 1958. Studies on migration and control of the six spotted leafhopper, Macrosteles fascifrons (Stål) in relation to transmission of aster yellow virus. Ph.D. Thesis. U. Wisconsin, Madison.
6. CHIYKOWSKI, L. N. & R. K. CHAPMAN. 1965. Migration of the six-spotted leafhopper *Macrosteles fascifrons* (Stål). Part 2. Migration of the sixspotted leafhopper in central North America. Univ. Wisconsin Research Bull. **261:** 21–45.
7. CHIYKOWSKI, L. N. 1980. Epidemiology of diseases caused by leafhopper-borne pathogens. *In* Vectors of Plant Pathogens. K. F. Harris & K. Maramorosch, Eds. Academic Press. In press.
8. DIENER, T. O. 1979. Viroids and Viroid Diseases. Wiley-Interscience. New York, N.Y.
9. DOI, Y., M. TERENAKA, K. YORA & H. ASUYAMA. 1967. Mycoplasma or PLT-goup-like microorganisms found in the phloem elements of plants infected with mulberry dwarf, potato witches' broom, aster yellows or paulownia witches' broom (in Japanese). Ann. Pytopathol. Soc. Japan **33:** 259–266.
10. HARRIS, K. F. 1977. Leafhoppers and aphids as biological vectors: vector-virus relation-

ships. *In* Leafhopper Vectors and Plant Disease Agents. K. Maramorosch & K. F. Harris, Eds.:217–308. Academic Press.

11. HARRIS, K. F. & K. MARAMOROSCH. Eds. 1980. Vectors of Plant Pathogens. Academic Press.

12. HUNT, P. 1979. A coconut disease of uncertain etiology in Indonesia. Abstracts 4th Meeting Intern. Council Lethal Yellowing, Fort Lauderdale, Fla.

13. ISHIIE, T., Y. DOI, K. YORA & H. ASUYAMA. 1967. Suppressive effects of antibiotics of tetracycline group on symptom development in mulberry dwarf disease (in Japanese). Ann. Phytopathol. Soc. Japan **33**: 367–375.

14. KENNEDY, J. S., M. F. DAY & V. F. ESTOP. 1962. A conspectus of aphids as vectors of plant viruses. Commonwealth Inst. Entomol. London.

15. KUWAHARA, M. 1974. Studies on the daily activity of the rhombic-marked leafhopper, *Hishimonus sellatus Uhler.* Jap. J. Appl. Entomol. Zool. **18**: 89–83.

16. MANDAHAR, C. L. 1978. Introduction to Plant Viruses. S. Ghand & Co. New Delhi.

17. MARAMOROSCH, K. 1964. A Survey of Coconut Diseases of Unknown Etiology. Food & Agriculture Organization of the United Nations. Rome.

18. MARAMOROSCH, K., Ed. 1969. Viruses, Vectors, and Vegetation. Wiley-Interscience.

19. MARAMOROSCH, K. 1978. Amarelecimento letal do coqueiro: distribuicao impacto implicacoes mindiais. Fitopatol. Brasileira **3**: 135–148.

20. MARAMOROSCH, K. 1979. Aster yellows spiroplasma ATCC 29747. ASM Abstracts Annual Meeting 1979:85.

21. MARAMOROSCH, K. 1980. Insects and plant pathogens. *In* Breeding Plants for Insect Control. F. Maxwell & P. Jennings, Eds. Wiley.

22. MARAMOROSCH, K. & K. F. HARRIS, Eds. 1979. Leafhopper Vectors and Plant Disease Agents. Academic Press.

23. MARAMOROSCH, K., E. SHIKATA, & R. R. GRANADOS. 1968. Structures resembling mycoplasma in diseased plants and in insects. Trans. N.Y. Acad. Sci. **30**: 841–855.

24. MEADE, A. B. & A. G. PETERSON. 1964. Origin of populations of the six-spotted leafhopper, *Macrosteles fascifrons* in Anoka County, Minnesota. J. Econ. Entomol. **57**: 885–888.

25. ROSE, D. J. W. 1978. Epidemiology of maize streak disease. Ann. Rev. Entomol. **23**: 259–282.

26. SINHA, R. 1980. Plant pathogens: Vertical transmission. *In* Comparative Aspects of Animal and Plant Pathogen Vectors. J. J. McKelvey, B. F. Eldridge & K. Maramorosch, Eds. Praeger.

27. SLYKHUIS, J. T. 1953. Wheat streak mosaic in Alberta and factors related to the spread of wheat streak-mosaic. Can. J. Agr. Sci. 195–197.

28. SLYKHUIS, J. T. 1969. Mites as vectors of plant viruses. *In* Viruses, Vectors and Vegatation. K. Maramorosch, Ed.:121–141. Wiley-Interscience.

29. SHEPHARD. R. J. 1977. Intrinsic properties and taxonomy of aphid-borne viruses. *In* Aphids as Virus Vectors. K. F. Harris & K. Maramorosch, Eds.:121–136. Academic Press.

30. SHERMAN, K. & K. MARAMOROSCH. 1977. Present status of the lethal yellowing disease of the coconut palm. J. Plantation Crops **5**: 67–130.

31. TAYLOR, C. E. 1980. Nematodes. *In* Vectors of Plant Pathogens. K. F. Harris & K. Maramorosch, Eds.:375–416. Academic Press.

32. TEAKLE, D. S. 1980. Fungi. *In* Vectors of Plant Pathogens. K. F. Harris & K. Maramorosch, Eds.:417–438. Academic Press.

33. TSAI, J. H. 1979. Progress in search of lethal yellowing vector(s). Abstracts 4th Meeting Intern. Council Lethal Yellowing Fort Lauderdale, Fla.

34. WALLIN, J. R. & D. V. LOONAN. 1971. Low-level jet winds, aphid vectors, local weather, and barley yellow dwarf virus outbreaks. Phytopathology **61**: 1068–1070.

35. WATSON, M. A. & F. M. ROBERTS. 1939. A comparative study of the transmission of Hyoscyamus virus 3, potato virus Y, and cucumber virus 1 by the vectors *Myzus persicae* (Sulz.), *M. circumflexus* (Buckton) and *Macrosiphum gei* (Koch). Proc. Roy. Soc. London, Ser. B. **127**: 543–576.

36. WESTDAL, P. H., C. F. BARRETT & H. P. RICHARDSON. 1961. The six-spotted leafhopper, *Macrosteles fascifrons* (Stål) and aster yellows in Manitoba, Canada J. Plant Sci. **41:** 320–331.
37. WESTDAL. P. H. 1968. Host range studies of oat blue dwarf virus. Can. J. Bot. **46:** 1431–1435.
38. WHITCOMB, R. F. & J. G. TULLY, Eds. 1979. The Mycoplasmas III: Plant and Insect Mycoplasmas. Academic Press.

LONG-RANGE TRANSMISSION OF BACTERIA

Åke Bovallius, Roger Roffey and Eva Henningson

National Defence Research Institute
S-901 82 Umeå, Sweden

INTRODUCTION

Information on the occurrence and the mechanism of long-range transport of airborne bacteria is scarce, although Pasteur and Miquel could show that airborne bacteria were found in practically all environments.[1,2] Since then there have been several symposia, monographs and reviews dealing with microorganisms in the atmosphere but only a few of these have discussed aspects of long-distance transport and in these cases fungal spores dominates.[3-8] This may partly be due to the fact that long-range airborne transmission of bacteria is not regarded as a dominant health or economic problem. Instead the interest has been focused on short-range airborne transmission of medical or hygienic importance, usually indoors, as well as more basic studies on the behavior of bacterial aerosols.

Studies of long-range transmission of bacteria are difficult to accomplish partly because of the methodological difficulties encountered. The extramural airborne bacterial flora is often very difficult to identify due to the fact that identification systems mainly takes medically important bacteria into account. The few qualitative studies made show a complex flora with a large number of different species both when traditional classification methods[9-13] and numerical taxonomy[14] were used. Comparisons of airborne bacterial studies are also difficult to make depending on different sampling situations and different sampling methods both regarding apparatus[5,15,16] and methods of analysis.[4,5,17,18] In practice cultural growth and viable counts are the only common ways for enumeration and detection of bacteria while in fungal studies both cultural and microscopic methods can be used.

Long-range transmission in this article means passive airborne outdoor transport of viable bacteria or particles containing bacteria. Thus, transport with living vectors, organisms like birds and insects as well as with different means of conveyance like airplanes and ships will not be discussed. Digressions to other microorganisms, especially fungal spores, are made in a few cases when correct parallels can be drawn. One question is how to define the distance for long-range transport of bacteria, is it 10 m or 100 km? This will apparently depend on the prerequisite of bacteria to remain in the airborne state and remain alive.

Conditions for Long-Range Transmission

Bacteria may be aerosolized in many ways. Coughing, dental drilling, air humidifiers, and microbiological laboratory work are examples of small scale local take-off processes. In these cases there is practically no outdoor aerosol dispersal of any significance although the initial concentration can be considerable.[3,6] In somewhat larger scale active take-off can be found in connection with different industrial or agricultural activities like sewage treatment, waste water irrigation and animal rendering.[19-25]

186

0077-8923/80/0353-0186 $01.75/0 © 1980, NYAS

For large scale passive take-off of airborne bacteria little hard evidence is available,[7] but water, soil, dust and decaying material are commonly said to be the main sources. Studies have been made on fungal spore liberation from the ground at different wind speeds. In these cases the wind was the dominating take-off factor. A similar behavior is possible for bacteria. Other possible take-off mechanisms are rain splash, sea-spray in connection with high winds and waves. Rain splash take-off has been shown for such species as *Pseudomonas*, *Xanthomonas* and *Streptomyces*.[7]

When a microorganism becomes airborne the immediate fate of the particle largely depends on the local meteorological conditions. A cloud of particles follows the movements of the wind. Depending on the turbulence of the air, the cloud will become more or less dispersed. The turbulence is dependent on the ground topography, the temperature in the air mass and the wind speed. The height of the turbulent zone varies but is often 100–1000 m in height and separated from higher regions in the atmosphere by an inversion layer that prevents further vertical diffusion. If bacteria or particles containing bacteria passes the inversion layer they reach a region with low turbulence and often high wind velocities. From that zone the bacteria can reenter the turbulent region by wash-out or by a change in the atmospheric layering.

In still air or during laminar flow conditions, small particles like bacteria sediments with a steady-state settling speed and follows Stokes' law, which has been shown to be valid for *Streptomyces spp* and for many fungal species.[7] Bacteria, usually with a mean diameter of 1–5 μm, have a very low terminal sedimentation velocity (e.g., 2 μm = $1.3 \cdot 10^{-2}$ cm/s) and can travel long distances without settling to the ground during laminar flow conditions. As an example a 1 μm particle could be transported 170 km and a 5 μm particle 7 km during a one meter sedimentation if the wind speed is 5 m/s. In general it can be stated that in the case of single bacteria, or small aggregates with diameters below 10 μm, the influence of sedimentation is limited and not a significant factor in preventing a long-distance transport. Despite the negligible sedimentation rate airborne bacteria or bacterial debris sooner or later reach the ground. This has been shown to be due to a combination of several mechanisms, e.g., diffusion, electrical charges, impaction and slow sedimentation.[7] Few studies on the overall quantitative deposition of bacterial species in natural environments have however been carried out.[26]

In connection with biological insecticide field testing (performed by the Swedish National Institute of Plant Protection) *Bacillus thuringiensis* was used.[26] Some aerosol and surface samples were taken at different distances from the source. From the obtained values a comparison was made between the spore concentration just above the ground and the amounts of spores deposited per time unit at the same place. Each pair of values was divided to get a deposition value with the same denomination as the before mentioned sedimentation rate (TABLE 1). The found deposition rates are noticeable higher than the theoretical sedimentation velocity for a 2 μm particle (0.01 cm/s). Outdoor experiments with fungal spores show a ground deposition for *Lycopodium clavatum* (32 μm in diameter) of 1.75 cm/s and for *Ganoderma applanatum* (8 μm in diameter) of 0.18 cm/s.[7]

An important factor for long-range transmission of airborne bacteria is the survival in the aerosolized state. Most studies concerning bacterial survival have been done in laboratory environments by using closed chambers or outdoor using the "microthread technique," usually with one specific bacteria and varying one parameter at a time.[27] A large number of factors influence the viability: type of

TABLE 1

DEPOSITION VALUES (MEAN VALUES AND STANDARD DEVIATIONS) OF B. *THURINGIENSIS*
SPORES ON DIFFERENT SURFACE MATERIALS

Type of Surface	Deposition Value (cm/s)
Dry iron plates	0.051 ± 0.040 (n = 29)
Water	0.071 ± 0.053 (n = 26)
Grass and agar surfaces	0.16 ± 0.08 (n = 14)

microorganisms, earlier growth conditions, type of dispersal, ultraviolet-light, temperature, relative humidity, chemical vapors in the atmosphere and physical protection by other microorganisms, dust or growth media.[6] In general it can be stated from this that bacterial spores have extremely long decimal reduction times (DRT) the time for a 90% reduction in viability. Many bacteria, e.g., *Flavobacterium sp, Sarcina sp, Serratia sp,* and *Erwinia sp* found in outdoor environments have DRTs in the range of hours while pathogenic bacteria often have DRTs in the order of seconds to minutes.[6,28]

Naturally occurring airborne bacteria have been shown to have significantly lower death rates in comparison with laboratory strains when exposed on surfaces in the open air, which can be seen in FIGURE 1. It is generally believed that the natural airborne bacterial flora at ground level consists of mostly resistent forms originating from the soil.[7]

Theoretical Models of Dispersal

The downwind concentration of particles from small sources may be estimated by using mathematical models which either empirically or theoretically take into consideration meteorological parameters like diffusion, wind speed, and turbulence.[29,30] Most such models, however, do not include microbiologically important factors but a few that add deposition and viability have been described.[31-33] The described models become, to some extent, less reliable as the downwind distance from the source increases since the models do not take into account the rapid variations in the atmospheric conditions with time and space. In literature these models are said to be approximatively valid up to a distance of 1–10 km from the source.[31,32] The importance of microbiological parameters in a model of this type, a gaussian plume-model, is exemplified in FIGURE 2.

The concentration of airborne bacteria has been calculated for an initial source strength of 8.10^3 bacteria/m^3, which is a concentration that can be expected to be found at for instance a sewage treatment plant. The effects of deposition (0.16 cm/s) and death rate (DRT 1 minute or 0.5 hour) are also shown in the figure. These calculations show that under the existing meteorological conditions, in this case neutral thermal stratification, the dispersed bacteria, with a particle size of 2 μm, will not theoretically be transported for longer distances downwind than about 3 km. The main factor that influences the dispersal picture is the meteorological situation. Very short DRTs around one minute will shorten the distance of transport significantly while the value of dry deposition does not influence the distance of transport to any great extent.

Concerning estimations of long-distance downwind concentrations from large scale sources different types of air pollution models may be used.[34,35] In the box-model[34] the transport is assumed to take place between the ground level and an inversion layer where complete mixing vertically is assumed. Also in these types of models viability values and deposition values can be added. In addition, during long-range transmissions the deposition by precipitation processes can be of great importance (FIGURE 3).

Using the box-model, assuming a homogeneous concentration of just over 1000 bacteria/m³ in a large volume of air, inert small particles can be expected to be found at very long distances, more than 1000 km from the source. In this case dry deposition starts to become a factor of importance. As the time of transportation may be in the range of days, precipitation by rain or snow is a factor to take into consideration. Survival is however the most important factor and even rather

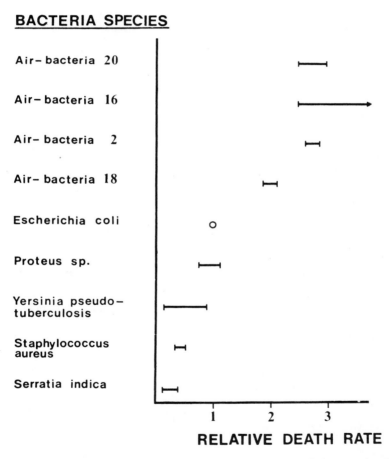

FIGURE 1. Relative death rates for bacteria, laboratory strains and strains isolated from the air, in comparison with the death rate of *E. coli.* The relative death rates are expressed as the decimal reduction time for the studied bacteria to the decimal reduction time of *E. coli.* (DRT bact/DRT *E. coli.*)

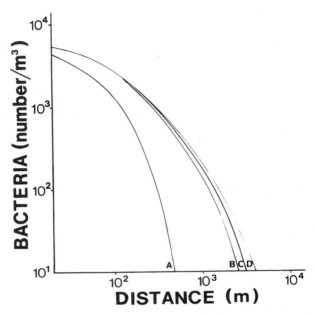

FIGURE 2. Variation in concentration of airborne particles with distance, decimal reduction time (DRT) and dry deposition (V_d) as calculated by using a plume model for dispersal from a small continuous source during neutral thermal stratification. Windspeed 5 m/s, bacteria size 2 μm and particle density 1 g/cm^3.

A $v_d = 0.16$ cm/s $DRT = 1$ min
B $v_d = 0.16$ cm/s and $DRT = 0.5$ h
C $v_d = 0.16$ cm/s and $DRT = \infty$
D $v_d = 0$ and $DRT = \infty$

resistant bacteria with long decimal reduction times will decrease considerably in viable numbers. If the dispersed bacteria passes the inversion layer the above described models are no longer valid. In this case, due to the jet airstreams and the low turbulence, the aerosol density does not decrease so rapidly and the condition for long-range transport will be favorable. Wash out is the dominating factor in bringing back the aerosol to ground level.

Dispersal from Small Sources

Some industrial and agricultural activities generate aerosols. Examples of these kinds of activities are waste water treatment plants and waste water irrigation where a large number of microorganisms become airborne. As some of these may be pathogenic or spoilage-prone, it is in the interest of health to study both the aerosol generation from such activities and also the aerosol dispersal. The concentration just above or beside the aerosolizing site may be in the range of 10^4–10^5 bacteria/m^3.[21,24,36,37] During the first seconds in the aerosolized state a very rapid decrease in viable bacteria occurs due to desiccation and fallout of large droplets. After this a slower decrease in the number of viable bacteria follows due to the meteorological conditions and the death rate of the organisms.

Some examples of downwind dispersal distances for bacteria from sewage treatment plants and waste water irrigation are collected in TABLE 2.

From the table it can be seen that a measurable increase in the total count or coliform counts in comparison with the background level very seldom could be found at distances exceeding one kilometer. These distances are in the same magnitude of order as could be expected from the mathematical models described earlier and a direct comparison,[37,38] shows a good correlation in the case of the total number of bacteria. Among bacteria that have been isolated from downwind aerosols are *Escherichia, Aerobacter, Klebsiella, Salmonella, Streptococcus, Proteus* and *Pseudomonas*.[21,22,29]

In many articles there has been speculation on theoretical grounds about the health hazard for workers near a waste water treatment plant, but little conclusive evidence have been uncovered. In one investigation a 50% higher incidence of influenza and a 20% increase in common colds, but no increase in pneumonia, have been found among workers in waste water treatment plants in contrast to workers in water works.[44] Comparison of kibbutzes in Israel that used or did not use waste water spray irrigation showed an increase in enteric diseases in the former case. The increase of shigellosis, salmonellosis, typhoid fever and infectious hepatitis was two to four times higher in communities practising waste

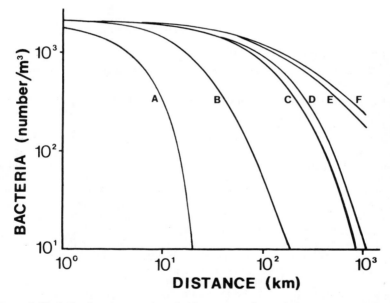

FIGURE 3. Variation in concentration of airborne particles with distance, decimal reduction time (*DRT*), dry deposition v_d and wash out as calculated by using a box model.[29] Windspeed 7 m/s; the height of the inversion layer 10^3 m and width of the source 20 km. Particle size 2 μm and particle density 1 g/cm^3.

A $v_d = 0.16$ cm/s and $DRT = 0.5$ h
B $v_d = 0.16$ cm/s and $DRT = 3$ h
C $v_d = 0.16$ cm/s and $DRT = 24$ h
D $v_d = 0.16$ cm/s, wash out 1 mm/h and $DRT = \infty$
E $v_d = 0.16$ cm/s and $DRT = \infty$
F $v_d = 0$ and $DRT = \infty$

TABLE 2

EXAMPLES OF DISTANCES WHERE DISPERSAL FROM SEWAGE TREATMENT PLANTS AND WASTE WATER IRRIGATION HAS BEEN OBSERVED

Bacteria Measured	Longest Recorded Distance Downwind (m)	Source of Dispersal	Reference
Total number	90	Sewage treatment plant	23
	270		23
	80		38
	100		20
	100		36
	200		24
	400	Spray irrigation	39
	198		37
	400		40
	650		41
Coliforms	90	Sewage treatment plant	42
	1290		23
	20		38
	700		20
	150		19
	200		24
	350	Spray irrigation	43
	152		37
Klebsiella aerogenes	90	Sewage treatment plant	42
Salmonella	60	Spray irrigation	43

water irrigation.[43] Thus in general the health and food spoilage hazard due to airborne microorganisms from waste water treatment plants must be regarded as very low and limited to the very near surroundings of the plants.[22]

Evidence for long-range transmission of pathogenic bacteria from infected humans or animals or their surroundings are very few and the discussed distances are in the range of a few kilometers. Coxiella burnetii, Chlamydia psicatti and Bacillus anthracis spores are examples of organisms that have been discussed.[3,25] Dispersal of fungi causing diseases like coccidiomycosis and histoplasmosis are better studied and so are animal viruses causing foot and mouth disease and Newcastle disease.[3] Most plant pathogens that have been shown to be transmitted by air are fungi[8] but a few bacteria have also been described. Among these, black arm of cotton, caused by Xantomonas malvacearum in the Sudan is said to be dispersed over many kilometers.[3] The spread of Erwinia amylovara that causes fireblight on apple and pear trees have been studied since the last century and it has often been noted that fireblight seems to spread in the direction of prevailing winds.[45,46] However for real long-distance transportation birds or insects are suggested as carriers.[45]

Dispersal from Large Sources

Transmission Below the Inversion Layer

For the transmission of microorganisms at distances longer than those discussed earlier the size of the source needs to be large if the initial aerosol concentration is in the range of what could be expected in natural environments. Examples of such sources can be densely populated areas, wind erosion of soil and sea-spray where the turbulent airflow cause microorganisms to become airborne. Dispersal of bacteria from these sources can be expected but there are few systematic investigations concerning this. It is claimed that bacteria originating from the sea can be separated from terrestrial bacteria by using fresh or salt water in the cultural medium.[47] Using this method, terrestrial bacteria have been found to decrease with increasing distances out to sea but as far out as 160 km they could still be detected.[65] Of the bacteria found during a similar study out at sea about 40% were cocci, 25% gram negative rods and 35% gram positive spore forming rods. In reverse during sea-breeze, "sea-bacteria" were found 32 km and 54 km inland.[47] By using the same culturing methods it was found that on average the number of fungi decreased with increasing distance from land up to 800 km and that terrestrial bacteria could also be found at this distance.[10] Sampling from airplanes in a land air mass as it traversed an ocean up to 640 km from the coast showed a consistent pattern of decrease in the number of land originating bacteria with increasing distance from the coast. At 152 m above the sea level the number of bacteria decreased from 600 bacteria/m^3 at the coast to 40 bacteria/m^3 640 km from the coast.[48]

Observations in Sweden show that the percentage of spore-forming bacteria is larger (57%) in air masses that have travelled across the sea than in air masses originating over land (7%).[15] This could also be an indication that a natural selection in favor of sporeformers occurs when the air mass travels over long distances. As a general rule the number of bacteria as well as fungal spores decreases over the ocean with increasing distance from land, but of course the numbers found at individual sampling stations and between stations varies widely.

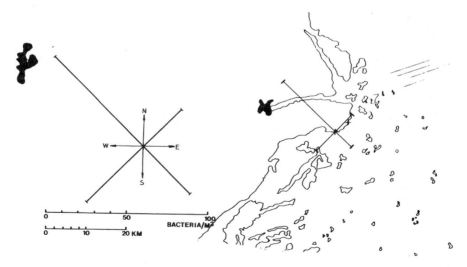

FIGURE 4. Mean number of bacteria in four wind directions during a three-year period. The samples were collected fortnightly at two stations in the center of Sweden. Towns are represented by the shaded areas.

Bacterial concentrations of 1000 to 10000 bacteria/m³ have been found in and above cities.[7,18,49] These values are significantly higher than those normally recorded over agricultural land and over the open sea.[10,12,18,50] At an inland and coastal station in Sweden mean values of collected bacteria have been calculated as a function of four wind directions (FIGURE 4). Increased mean concentrations of bacteria were found when the wind came from the city areas, which may indicate a registration of bacteria transported from the cities.

Transmission Above the Inversion Layer

Perhaps the most favorable circumstances for long transmission will be when the bacteria are transferred up to the low turbulent and often fast moving air masses above the ground friction layer. In and above this level bacteria have been sampled by a number of investigators which implies that frequent long-distance transport does also occur in this part of the atmosphere. In air sampling studies at high altitudes up to 3 km the concentration has been reported to vary a lot between different sampling events; values from 1–25 bacteria/m³ [51] to 3000 bacteria/m³ [17] have been recorded. Over the North Pole at 902 meters neither bacteria nor fungi were caught but at greater heights up to 6770 meters a few bacteria and fungi were found, thus indicating long-distance transports.[52] Identi-

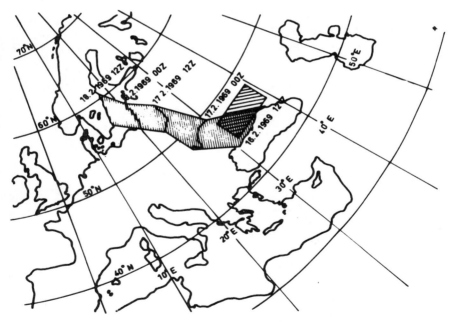

FIGURE 5. Result of trajectory calculations, indicating the air transport route from the Black Sea surroundings to the Swedish east coast in connection with a long-range transmission event. The rectangle with dashed lines represents the area where sandstorms had been reported during this period.

TABLE 3

COMPARISON OF SOME CHARACTERISTICS FOR THE MEAN AIRBORNE BACTERIAL FLORA
AND THE BACTERIAL FLORA FOUND IN CONNECTION WITH A
LONG-RANGE AIR TRANSMISSION STUDY

	Mean Airborne Bacterial Flora	"Red Snow" Airborne Bacterial Flora
Total number (bacteria/m³)	39–74	144–245
% outgrowth in two days	10–20	85–90
% less than 6.0 µm in size	41–44	80–85
% spore formers	20–30	85–90
% outgrowth at 37°C	30–50	70–80

fication of bacteria found at these heights shows that *Bacillus* spp and *Micrococcus* spp predominate[9,11] but also *Achromobacter sp* and *Micrococcus sp* have been found. At still higher heights sampling from balloons have shown 0.14 bacteria/m³ (all of the genus *Bacillus*) at 3.6–6.9 km[53] and 10^{-2}–10^{-3} bacteria/m³ at 9–27 km.[54] These latter results can be questioned as the balloon was not sterile. By using a rocket microorganisms were detected as far up as 48–77 km.[55] The bacteria were of the genera *Mycobacterium* and *Micrococcus*. Five of the six species had chromogenic pigments that is claimed to be more resistant to ultra-violet rays.[55] However in this investigation no *Bacillus* spores were detected. The described investigations at higher altitudes thus suggest that long-distance trans-mission occurs, but they support no evidence of the sources locality or the eventual degree of fallout. Examples of this type of microbial transport are rare and in the case of bacteria practically nonexistent. However, one example will be discussed in detail.[56,57]

In connection with an air sampling study it was possible to prove that airborne bacterial spores collected in the center of Sweden originated from the Black Sea area, a distance of 1800 km.[57] On one occasion significantly higher amounts than usually obtained were simultaneously found at two sampling stations 40 km apart. At both stations brown-red colored snow was falling during the air sampling. Bacterial sampling was also performed from the snow profile. The bacteria collected from both air and snow samples were similar but distinguished from the common airborne flora by a number of properties (TABLE 3). In the snow profile the amount of bacteria above, in and below the colored layer were estimated to 1, 70–120 and < 1 bacteria/ml, respectively.

For further examination 36 colonies randomly selected from the air and from the snow samples were typed. The bacteria were all of the genus *Bacillus*. Roughly 35% were *Bacillus megaterium*, 15% *Bacillus pumilus*, 10% *Bacillus mycoides*, 30% *Bacillus firmus/lentus* type and 10% of the *Bacillus subtilis/liche-niformis* type.

The air transport route was calculated by using a computer-based horizontal geostrophic trajectory program. The altitude 1500 m was chosen because of the prevailing meteorological situation and that this level was above the ground friction layer. Trajectory calculations from the same days with similar results have been shown by other authors.[58,59] During the period an area of low pressure covered central Europe and a strong high pressure the eastern part of European Russia. In an area between these, two steep pressure gradients gave rise to strong northwesterly winds (21–36 m/s). The trajectories were calculated backwards

TABLE 4

IDENTIFICATION OF 36 RANDOMLY SELECTED COLONIES FROM AIR AND SNOW SAMPLES
COLLECTED AT AN INLAND AND COASTAL STATION IN CONNECTION WITH A
LONG-RANGE AIR TRANSMISSION STUDY

Type of Bacteria	Source	
	Snow	Air
Bacillus megaterium	8	6
Bacillus pumilus	1	3
Bacillus mycoides	1	2
Bacillus firmus/lentus type	4	4
Bacillus subtilis/licheniformis type	4	3

from the Swedish Baltic coast where red snowfall had been observed and coincided both in time and place with a sandstorm in the area north of the Black Sea. The turbulent air movements during such weather conditions is able to transport eroded material up to high altitudes.[58] Due to the positions of the mentioned high- and low-pressure areas winds were able to transport suspended material between these along a concentrated "corridor" towards Scandinavia without any large degree of dispersion. The ground north of the Black Sea area was snow covered so it is not probable that further additions of airborne material occurred. Computations show that the material was transported about 1800 km in 36 hours. During that time the bacterial flora was exposed to lethal ultraviolet light from the sun that must have affected the nonsporulating more ultraviolet-sensitive organisms. The temperature during the airborne transport on the other hand—5 ± 2°C is regarded as relatively favorable for the airborne bacteria. Thus the absence of nonspore-formers in the air samples and in the red snow layer probably is due to them being killed off during the transport.

To further prove the long range transport of the *Bacillus* species some tracers from the brown-red snow could serve as evidence. The composition of the soil particles were analyzed. The mineral part consisted of mica-like material and complex clay material including a high content of iron, the same composition as loess.[60] The dust also contained organic matter (9–12%) including pollengrains.[59] The composition of the pollen species as well as the ratio of pollen from trees, bushes and herbs indicates that the source was of southern origin.[58,59] In the case of fungal spores the same type of high altitude transport has been studied in detail using airplane sampling between England and Denmark. The concentration of *Cladosporium* decreased rapidly on leaving the coast but unexpectedly it increased again at 400–500 km out over the North Sea. Further, 100–200 km and at 500–600 km maxima of spores usually liberated at night were found. From these results it was suggested that the airplane passed first the daytime cloud at the English coast, then the cloud of the previous night, then the daytime cloud from the day before and finally the nighttime cloud the night before that.[61]

In general many examples of long-distance fungal spore transport have been indicated in different parts of the world. From a Scandinavian point of view rust spores (*Puccinia sp.*) are said to be transported from Russia and the Balkans to different parts of Scandinavia,[62] from Britain to the Faroes and from England to Denmark.[63] Transport of milldew (*Erysiphe graminis*) from England to Germany and Denmark was shown by trajectory studies.[64]

Conclusion

Theoretically by using meteorological models of dispersal where relevant physical and biological factors are inserted it can be shown that long-range transmission of bacteria may occur. To enable long-distance transport of naturally generated bacterial aerosols it is required that the size of the source is large, the bacteria be either resistant or protected against the atmospheric environment, the particle size not too large (e.g. <10 μm) and the meteorological conditions favorable (e.g. high wind speed and suitable stratification). In the literature there are only a few examples of long-range transmission of bacteria and these have often only been indirectly proved. However, the existence of airborne bacteria in various concentrations in different geographical localities and at high altitudes, has been shown and studies of spores and particles have proved that long-distance transport is possible. In view of that long-range transmission of bacteria is highly probable. Although it may be a fairly common phenomenon it has not been subject to systematic investigations, which could be of medical, ecological as well as of evolutionary interest.

Acknowledgment

We express our gratitude to Edvard Karlsson, National Defence Research Institute, Umeå, for his valuable help with the mathematical models of dispersal.

References

1. Pasteur, L. 1861. Mémoire sur les corpuscles organisés qui existent dans l'atmosphère. Examen de la doctrine des générations spontanées. Ann Sci. Nat. (Zool.) 4e sér., **16**: 5–98.
2. Miquel, P. 1883. Les organismes vivants de l'atmosphère. Gauthier-Villars, Paris.
3. Hers, J. F. & K. C. Winkler, Eds. 1973. Airborne transmission and airborne infection. Concepts and methods presented at the 6th International Symposium on Aerobiology held at the Technical University at Enschede, the Netherlands. Oosthoek Publishing Company. Utrecht, the Netherlands.
4. Gregory, P. H. & J. L. Monteith, Eds. 1967. Airborne microbes. Seventeenth Symposium of the Society for General Microbiology held at the Imperial college. London. Cambridge University Press. London.
5. Wolf, H. W., P. Skaliy, L. B. Hall, M. M. Harris, H. M. Decker, L. M. Buchanan & C. M. Dahlgren. 1964. Sampling Microbiological Aerosols. U.S. Public Health Service. Public Health Monograph 60.
6. Dimmick, R. L. & A. B. Akers, Eds. 1969. An Introduction to Experimental Aerobiology. Wiley-Interscience, Wiley & Sons. New York.
7. Gregory, P. H. 1973. The Microbiology of the Atmosphere, 2nd. Edt. Leonard Hill Books. Aylesbury, Bucks. Great Britain.
8. Edmonds, R. L. 1979. Aerobiology, The Ecological System Approach. Dowden, Hutchinson & Ross. Stroudsburg, Pennsylvania.
9. Fulton, J. D. 1966. Microorganisms of the upper atmosphere. III. Relationship between altitude and micropopulation. Appl. Microbiol. **14**(2): 237–240.
10. Rittenberg, S. C. 1939. Investigations on the microbiology of marine air. J. Mar. Res. **2**: 208–217.
11. Proctor, B. E. 1935. The microbiology of the upper air. II. J. Bacteriol. **30**: 363–375.

12. KELLY, C. D. & S. M. PADY. 1953. Microbiological studies of air over some nonarctic regions of Canada. Can. J. Bot. **31:** 90–106.
13. MANCINELLI, R. L. & W. A. SHULLS. 1978. Airborne bacteria in an urban environment. Appl. Environ. Microbiol. **35(6):** 1095–1101.
14. ÅNÄS, P. & Å. BOVALLIUS. 1978. Investigation of natural airborne bacteria by numerical taxonomy. Proc. 1st Int. Conf. Aerobiology, 13–16 August, Munich.
15. ROFFEY, R., Å. BOVALLIUS, P. ÅNÄS & E. KÖNBERG. 1977. Semicontinuous registration of airborne bacteria at an inland and a coastal station in Sweden. Grana **16:** 171–177.
16. BOVALLIUS, Å., B. BUCHT, T. CASPERSSON, J. LUNDIN & M. RITZEN. 1968. Methods for enumeration of airborne microorganisms (In Swedish), Försvarsmedicin **4:** 85–96.
17. ANDERSON, D. T., R. B. MITCHELL, H. W. DORRIS & D. E. TIMMONS. 1950. Studies on microorganisms of the upper atmosphere. IV. The selection of culture media for investigation of airborne microorganisms. U.S. Air Force School of Aviation Medicine. Project 21-02-118. Report No. 4. Randolph Field, Tex.
18. BOVALLIUS, Å., B. BUCHT, R. ROFFEY & P. ÅNÄS. 1978. Three-year investigation of the natural airborne bacterial flora at four localities in Sweden. Appl. Environ. Microbiol. **35(5):** 847–852.
19. NAPOLITANO, P. J. & D. R. ROWE. 1966. Microbial content of air near sewage treatment plants. Water Sewage Works. Dec. 480–483.
20. GOFF, G. D., J. C. SPENDLOVE, A. P. ADAMS & P. S. NICHOLES. 1973. Emission of microbial aerosols from sewage treatment plants that use trickling filters. Health Serv. Rep. **88:** 640–652.
21. HICKEY, J. L. S. & P. C. REIST. 1975. Health significance of airborne microorganisms from waste water treatment processes. Part II. Health significance and alternatives for action. J. Water Pollut. Control. Fed. **47:** 2758–2773.
22. DART, R. K. & R. J. STRETTON. 1977. Air pollution and microorganisms. In Microbiological aspects of pollution control. 29–51. Elsevier. New York.
23. ADAMS, A. P. & J. C. SPENDLOVE. 1970. Coliform aerosols emitted by sewage treatment plants. Science **169:** 1218–1220.
24. ANDERSSON, R., B. BERGSTRÖM & B. BUCHT. 1973. Airdispersal of bacteria from a sewage treatment plant (In Swedish). Vatten **2:** 117–123.
25. SPENDLOVE, J. C. 1957. Production of bacterial aerosols in a rendering plant process. Public Health Rep. (U.S.) **72:** 176–180.
26. BOVALLIUS, Å & P. ÅNÄS. 1978. Bacterial spores in the air and on the ground in connection with biological insect control. 107–110. Proc. 1st Int. Conf. Aerobiology, 13–16 August, Munich.
27. MAY, K. R. & H. A. DRUETT. 1968. A microthread technique for studying the viability of microbes in a simulated airborne state. J. Gen. Microbiol. **51:** 353–366.
28. ANDERSON, J. D. & C. S. COX. 1967. Microbial survival **17:** 203–226. Symp. Soc. Gen. Microbiol. Cambridge University Press. London.
29. HÖGSTRÖM, U. 1964. An experimental study on atmospheric diffusion. Tellus XVI (2):205–251.
30. PASQUILL, F. 1974. Atmospheric Diffusion. The Dispersion of Windborne Material from Industrial and Other Sources. 2nd Edt. J. Wiley & Sons. New York.
31. ÅNÄS, P. & C. HOLMBERG. 1978. A stocastic model to evaluate the dispersal of aerosols in the air (In Swedish). National Defence Research Institute, Sweden. FOA rapport C 40090-B1.
32. PETERSON, E. W. & B. LIGHTHART. 1977. Estimation of downwind viable airborne microbes from a wet cooling tower, including settling. Microb. Ecol. **4:** 67–79.
33. LIGHTHART, B. & A. S. FRISCH. 1976. Estimation of viable airborne microbes downwind from a point source. Appl. Environ. Microbiol. **31(5):** 700–704.
34. SCRIVEN, R. A. & B. E. A. FISHER. 1975. The long range transport of airborne material and its removal by deposition and washout–I. General Considerations. Atmos. Environ. **9:** 49–58.
35. DRAXLER, R. R. & W. P. ELLIOTT. 1977. Long range travel of airborne material subjected to dry deposition. Atmos. Environ. **11:** 35–40.

36. WANNER, H.U. 1975. Mikrobielle Verunreinigung der Luft durch Belebtschlammbecken. Zbl. Bakt. Hyg. I Abt. Orig. B. **161:** 46–53.
37. SORBER, C. A., H. T. BAUSUM, S. A. SCHAUB & M. J. SMALL. 1976. A study of bacterial aerosols at a waste water irrigation site. J. Water Pollut. Control Fed. **48:** 2367–2379.
38. RAYGOR, C. & K. P. MACKAY. 1975. Bacterial air pollution from an activated sludge tank. Water, Air Soil Pollut. **5:** 47–52.
39. PARKER, D. T., J. C. SPENDLOVE, J. A. BONDURANT & J. H. SMITH. 1977. Microbial aerosols from food processing waste spray fields. J. Water Pollut. Control Fed. **49**(12): 2359–2365.
40. VON REPLOH, H. & M. HANDLOSER. 1957. Untersuchungen über die keimvershleppung bei der Abwasserverregnung. Arch. Hyg. Berlin **141:** 632.
41. SHTARKAS, E. M. & D. G. KRASIL'SHCHIKOV. 1970. Abst. Hyg. San. **35:** 330.
42. ALBRECHT, C. R. 1958. M. S. Thesis. Univ. of Florida, Gainesville.
43. KATZENELSON, E. & B. TELTCH. 1976. Dispersion of enteric bacteria by spray irrigation. J. Water Pollut. Control Fed. **48:** 710–716.
44. LEDBETTER, J. O. & C. W. RANDALL. 1965. Ind. Med. Surg. **34:** 130–133.
45. VAN DER ZWET, T. 1970. New outbreaks and current distribution of fireblight of pear and apple in northern Europe. FAO Pl. Prot. Bull. **18:** 83–88.
46. STEVENS, F. L., W. A. RUTH & C. S. SPOONER. 1918. Pearblight wind borne. Science XLVIII (1244):449–450.
47. ZOBELL, C. E. & H. M. MATHEWS. 1936. A qualitative study of the bacterial flora of sea and land breezes. Proc. Nat. Acad. Sci. U.S.A. **22:** 567–572.
48. FULTON, J. D. 1966. Microorganisms of the upper atmosphere. IV. Microorganisms of a land air mass as it traverses an ocean. Appl. Microbiol. **14**(2): 241–244.
49. WRIGHT, T. J., V. W. GREENE & H. J. PAULUS. 1969. Viable microorganisms in an urban atmosphere. J. Air. Pollut. Control. Assoc. **19:** 337–341.
50. PADY, S. M. & C. D. KELLY. 1954. Aerobiological studies of fungi and bacteria over the Atlantic Ocean. Can. J. Bot. **32:** 202–212.
51. TRÄDGÅRD H. C. 1977. Sampling of aerobiological material from a small aircraft. Grana **16:** 139–143.
52. POLUNIN, N. & C. D. KELLY. 1952. Arctic aerobiology: fungi and bacteria caught in the air during flights over the geographical North Pole. Nature **170:** 314–316. London.
53. MEIER, F. C. 1936. Effects of conditions in the stratosphere on spores of fungi. Nat. Geo. Soc. Stratosphere Series, No. **2:** 152–153.
54. GREENE, V. W., P. D. PEDERSON, D. A. LUNDGREN & C. A. HAGBERG. 1964. Microbiological exploration of stratosphere; results of six experimental flights. Proc. Atmospheric Biology Conf. April. Tsuchiya, H. M. & A. H. Brown, Eds. 199–211. University of Minnesota. Minneapolis.
55. IMSHENETSKY, A. A., S. V. LYSENKO & G. A. KAZAKOV. 1978. Upper boundary of the biosphere. Appl. Environ. Microbiol. **35**(1): 1–5.
56. BUCHT, B., B. RYDGREN & T. WALLIN. 1971. Detection of airborne bacteria emanating from a distant source (In Swedish). National Defence Research Institute, Sweden. FOA-rapport A 1530–34.
57. BOVALLIUS, Å., B. BUCHT, R. ROFFEY & P. ÅNÄS. 1978. Long-range air transmission of bacteria. Appl. Environ. Microbiol. **35:** 1231–1232.
58. LUNDQVIST, J. & K. BENGTSSON. 1970. The red snow—a meteorological and pollen analytical study of long transported material from snowfalls in Sweden. Geologiska Föreningens i Stockholm Förhandlingar **92:** 288–301.
59. AARTOLAHTI, T. & A. KULMALA. 1969. Dust-stained snow of the winter 1968–1969 in Finland (In Finnish). Terra **81**(3): 98–104.
60. LINDQVIST, B. & C. CARLSSON. Personal communications. Department of mineralogy and geology. The University of Uppsala. Sweden.
61. HIRST, J. M. & G. W. HURST. 1967. Long-distance spore transport. In Airborne Microbes. Symp. Soc. gen. Microbiol. 17. Gregory, P. H. & J. L. Monteith, Eds.:307–344. Cambridge University Press. London.
62. ZADOKS, J. C. 1967. International dispersal of fungi. Neth. J. Pl. Path. **73**(1): 61–80.

63. HERMANSEN, J. E. & A. WIBERG. 1972. On the appearance of *Erysiphe graminis* f. sp. *hordei* and *Puccinia hordei* in the Faeroes and the possible primary inoculum. Friesia **10**(1): 30–34.
64. HERMANSEN, J. E. & E. STIX. 1974. Evidence of wind dispersal of powdery mildew conidia across the North Sea. Kgl. Vet. Landb. Årsskr.: 87–100.
65. ZOBELL, C. E. 1942. Microorganisms in marine air. *In* Aerobiology S. Moulton, Ed. Amer. Assoc. Adv. Sci. Pub. No. 17, 55–68.

SURF-TO-WIND TRANSFER OF VIRUSES

Edward R. Baylor

Marine Sciences Research Center

Martha B. Baylor

Department of Cellular and Developmental Biology
State University of New York at Stony Brook
Long Island, New York 11794

The purpose of the work reported here is to show that virus particles in sea water adsorb to bubbles, which, on bursting at the sea surface, eject concentrated virus particles into the air in the form of jet droplets. These droplets, lofted by the wind, can be carried great distances as shown by Schaeffer,[1] finding marine algae and diatoms 100 miles down wind from the sea coast in the rhyme frost on top of Mt. Washington, New Hampshire, during a northeast snow storm. Similarly, Maynard[2] captured marine diatoms and algae in aerosols 40 miles inland from the nearest surf. Moreover, the data of Gruft et al.[3] suggest that the causative organism for the Battey Infection, a near relative of the tubercule bacillus, is lofted from the surf and distributed to humans by an onshore breeze for over 100 miles inland. Finally, closer to home, *Legionella*, the causative organism for Legionnaire's Disease, has been found in the aerosols created by air conditioning cooling towers.[4]

The importance to public health of the work reported here is that we have now added viruses to a growing list of microorganisms that may not remain in the ocean or other receiving waters to which they were consigned but instead may be lofted into the wind by white caps at sea, breakers in the surf or the wake of a ship. The wholly unanticipated aspect of our work[5,6] and of Blanchard's[7] is that both viruses and bacteria are actually concentrated by the process of aerosol formation. MacIntyre[8] has shown that virtually the entire skin of the bubble and the materials adsorbed to it are relegated to the uppermost drop of the jet that forms when bubbles burst.

The formation of aerosol drops by bursting bubbles has been described by Woodcock et al.[9] and by MacIntyre[8] using high speed motion picture photography. FIGURE 1 is a series of selected motion picture frames showing a rising bubble just after it has contacted the liquid surface. The burst sequence begins with a tiny hole opening where the buble is tangent to the liquid-air interface. Surface tension of the bubble skin rapidly opens the hole. The bubble skin accelerates toward the bottom of the bubble cavity where it arrives with a suddenness and force that propels the skin upwards in a tiny jet of fluid. The jet is an unstable configuration which breaks up into five or more separate tiny drops which rise 5 to 15 cm into the air depending on the initial acceleration of the jet.

Because the skin of the bubble forms the jet and because most of the bubble skin is in the uppermost drop of the set of jet drops, then the material adsorbed to the bubble skin is thereby greatly enhanced in concentration. For example,

*This work was supported in part by NOAA (MESA, New York Bight Project Grant 31-5088) and the New York Sea Grant Institution.

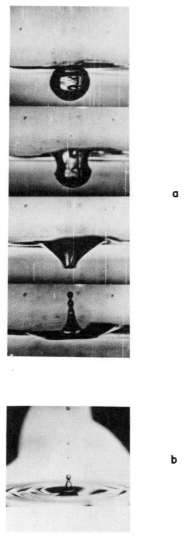

FIGURE 1 Blanchards Jet Formation. **a.** Selected high speed motion picture photographs illustrating some of the stages in the bursting of a bubble and the formation of the jet and the jet drops upon the collapse of a 1.7 mm diameter bubble. The time interval between the top and bottom frames is about 2.3 msec. The angle of view is horizontal through a glass wall. The surface irregularities are due to a meniscus. **b.** Oblique view of the jet from a 1 mm diameter bubble. Figure courtesy of D. C. Blanchard, Atmospheric Sciences Research Center, State University of New York, Albany, New York.

Blanchard[7] using a suspension of the gram negative bacterium, *Serratia marcescens*, obtained concentration enhancements of one thousand-fold. The data we report here show concentration factors of less than one thousand-fold but our experiments were less rigorous than Blanchard's because we collected the two or three top drops of the jet set. The lower less concentrated drops dilute the concentration of the top drop if all are collected together.

The experiments we describe here were designed to ask three questions: First, we asked whether bacterial viruses, like many other microbes, are concentrated in aerosol drops. Second, we asked whether the high shearing forces encountered in jet drop formation rupture or inactivate the virus particles and third, we asked whether the surf could generate a virus containing aerosol if viruses were present in the surf.

To ask whether viruses are concentrated in aerosol drops we produced aerosol drops small enough to examine conveniently with the electron microscope. To the bulk fluid was added a mixture of the coliphage T2 or T4 and a resistant strain of *E. coli*. These coliphages were used because of their distinct shape and because the condition of their external morphology gives a clear indication of their viability.

The best preparations were those which contained a small amount of lysate so the cell debris marked the periphery of the drop as it dried *in situ* on the electron microscope screen. FIGURE 2 is the electron micrograph of a captured aerosol drop containing both bacteria and bacterial viruses which are the tadpole shaped objects. This slide was prepared and photographed for another study by my colleague Virginia Peters.[10] The data from this and other photographs show that the coliphages, T2 and T4 are 50 times more concentrated in the aerosol drop than they were in the bulk fluid from which they were ejected on the jets of bursting bubbles. Similarly, in this study, the bacterium (*Escherichia coli*) showed a 30-fold increase in concentration.

In none of the hundreds of drops we photographed did we find evidence of the shearing forces of the jet rending the virus particle head from tail or even pulling off the tail fibers.

Let me recapitulate here to point out that with these experiments we have answered the first two of the questions we initially posed: namely, whether bacterial viruses are incorporated in aerosol drops and whether they suffer damage from the shearing forces of the jet formation. It is important to note in connection with the degree of concentration enhancement in our experiments that both phage and bacterial counts made by electron microscope are probably low because of material washed away during staining and rinsing. The concommitant bioassays were unsatisfactory. Aerosol drops produced in rapid succession were caught on moist tryptone agar for 10 to 40 seconds. Soft agar (0.7%) containing sensitive host cells was immediately added to the surface of the petri dish and spread by shaking. The phages diffused into the tryptone agar before they could be spread. In later experiments, the aerosol drops were captured in hanging drop of buffer suspended over the rising jets so as to catch the top drop. Concentrations exceeding 50-fold were achieved in this manner.

Having satisfied ourselves that the bacterial viruses, T2 and T4 were ejected from liquids to the atmosphere on jets of bursting bubbles, we proceeded to the next question and asked whether viruses injected into the surf would appear in the aerosol blowing toward the beach from the surf. A part of this work was done with Duncan Blanchard and has been reported elsewhere.[5] The first thing we learned in these experiments was that field work is bafflingly dissimilar to laboratory work. For example we rapidly learned that if you plan to throw viruses into the surf and collect them downwind on the beach, you had better learn something about the currents along the shore. A study by Inman et al.[11] of the Scripps Institution of Oceanography shows that the currents along the shore are difficult to predict. Such currents can carry the dye marker and virus completely out of range of the experiment if their action and locations are not understood. Some of the currents move out perpendicularly from the shore line. These are rip currents and the water feeding such currents moves toward them from both directions along the shore. Under ideal conditions you can inject the viruses and a dye marker (fluorescein) into the surf so the along shore currents

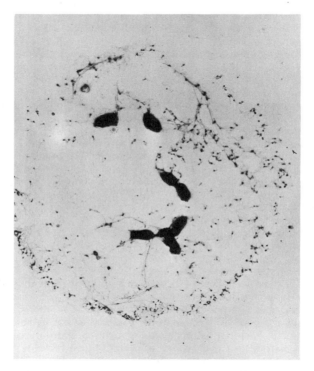

FIGURE 2. Single aerosol drop showing bacterial cells and bacterial viruses. Saturated aqueous uranyl acetate stain ×3600.

carry the virus and dye slowly past the sampling arrangements on the beach. Hence, prior to each experiment the speed and direction of along shore currents were established by watching the movements of small amounts of dye placed in the surf near the shore. Once the speed and direction of the along shore currents were established, we injected the virus and dye so the aerosol fallout plume would move past the sampling array on the beach. It is important to stress here that the speed of the alongshore currents as well as the turbulent mixing in the surf varied greatly from one day to the next. As a result, the residence time of the dye-virus patch in front of the sampling array varied by a factor of 5 in our experiments. As a further result, the concentration of phage in the dye-virus patch of seawater varied 2 to 3 orders of magnitude from day to day.

The matrix of sampling stations on the beach was designed to yield the following data: (1) the number of aerosol drops per unit area, (2) the number of viruses per drop, (3) aerosol drop size and (4) the number of T2 particles relative to the number of T4 particles for analysis by Poisson statistics. Aerosol samples were collected by allowing the droplets to fall on settling plates that were arranged in a matrix of three or more columns parallel to the wind direction and three or more rows parallel to the water's edge. Each row or column was approximately 10 meters from its nearest neighbor and the bottom row was 2 meters above the swash line. The settling plates were placed in the bottom of shallow buckets to protect them from the blowing sand. Each bucket contained three different kinds of settling plates: (1) a clean disposable plastic petri dish for size measurement of fallen drops, (2) an agar plate seeded with appropriate host cells for counting the number of virus-bearing drops per unit area, and (3) a liquid surface for estimating the total number of virus particles contained in the drops falling on each unit area. The plates were uncovered when the injected dye and virus in the surf approached a position downwind of the sampling array. The plates were re-covered when the dye patch in the surf had moved away from a position down wind of the sampling array. Speed of the alongshore currents in our experiments ranged from 0.2 to 1.0 meters per second which carried the dye and virus patch in the surf past the sampling array within 3 to 10 minutes.

At each injection of dye and virus one of us walked into the surf carrying the two flasks which were emptied into a wave trough 1.5 meters deep. We used 200 grams of fluorescein and 2×10^{15} phages. Turbulent mixing in the surf reduced the phage concentration to about 10^6 per milliliter in 30 minutes.

The number of phage bearing aerosol drops per unit area frequently exceeded 16 per square centimeter on plates within two meters of the water's edge but decreased rapidly as function of the logarithm of the distance from the water's edge as seen in FIGURE 3. The sharply decreasing rates of fallout shown by the data of FIGURE 3 are due to the dilution of virus containing aerosol with uncontaminated aerosol by the turbulent vertical mixing of the sea breeze as it moves across the surf zone. Neither solar ultraviolet inactivation nor drying can account for the rapid decrement because the travel time from the surf to the collecting matrix did not exceed six seconds.

The number of viruses per drop can be found in two ways: The simple way is to divide the number of phages per square centimeter of impact area by the volume of drops falling per square centimeter on the liquid settling plates. This method gave satisfactory results only when iced tryptone broth was used for the liquid impact surface. The second method requires simultaneous injection of T2 and T4 phages into the surf. The relative numbers of phages found in the aerosol drops allowed us to determine the average number of phages per drop by Poisson statistics. The use of Poisson statistics when employing two types of distinguishable particles is a very powerful technique. The two particle types segregate independently and randomly in the aerosol drops ejected from the surf so that some drops contain only one kind of either particle and some drops contain both particles. Such a population of drops is amenable to Poisson statistical analysis. Poisson statistics constitute an elegant way of getting something for nothing provided only that you know how often you have nothing. We assume that pure plagues of T2 are zero counts of T4. Similarly, pure plaques of T4 are zero counts of T2 and those plaques having T2 plus T4 contain at least one or more than one

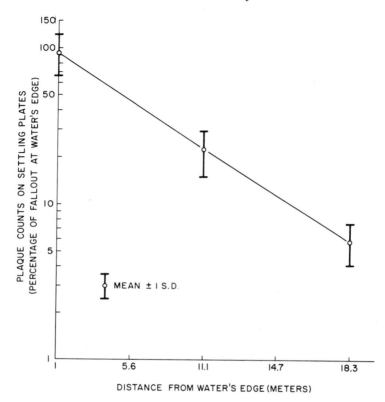

FIGURE 3. The number of plaque counts per petri dish settling plate on the beach plotted against the distance from the water's edge.

of each type of phage. The data of TABLE 1 are an analysis of windborne fallout of a mixed injection of T2 and T4 into the surf. The number of plaque forming units of T2, T4, and T2 + T4 are given for a single column of settling plates of the matrix on the beach. The data of TABLE 1 show that the fraction of all plaques containing only T4 was 0.67. Substituting this observed nonT2-containing fraction of the total into the zeroth term of the Poisson expansion we see that $e^{-m} = 0.67$ where m is the mean number of T2 particles per drop in the observed population. It follows that the population mean of all aerosol drops is 0.4 T2 phages per aerosol drop. In the same manner for zero counts of T4, we have $e^{-m} = 0.18$ and the mean number of T4 phages per drop in the population is 1.7. The combined dosage of T2 and T4 per drop is 2.1.

The total number of plaques counted on the day we collected the data of TABLE 1 was 3922, of which 722 were pure T2 and calculating from these additional data, we see the number of T4 per drop is 1.78 per drop in excellent agreement with the 1.7 T4 per drop calculated from a single row. Expanding the Poisson analysis to calculate the probability of more than one, more than two, and so on, phages per drop reveals excellent internal consistency of the data and excellent agreement of the calculated and observed numbers per drop. For example the Poisson expansion predicts that 45% of the plaques containing a T2 particle should also contain a T4 particle. In excellent agreement with the predicted number, the observed number was 45.2%.

We can now calculate the concentration factor which Blanchard and Syzdek[7] have found to be as high as 1000 in certain laboratory experiments with bacteria. We assume somewhat conservatively that there are two phages per drop and that the volume of each drop is 2×10^5 cubic micrometers of seawater. This gives a phage concentration in the drop of 1×10^8 per milliliter. Now, if we assume a phage concentration of 10^6 per milliliter in the surf, this gives us a concentration factor of 100 and is a very conservative estimate because actual measurements of phage concentration in the surf were 2×10^4 and 2×10^5 phages per milliliter of seawater. We have not used these observed surf phage concentrations in our calculations because we cannot be certain we have measured the phage in seawater where the phage was most concentrated.

Estimates of the concentration factor made from aerosol fallout into iced tryptone broth on three different releases of phage during one day gave average phage concentrations per drop of 500 which, if contained in a 2×10^4 cubic micrometer drop, gives a phage concentration of 2.5×10^{10} phages per milliliter and with an estimated surf concentration of 10^8 phages per milliliter gives a concentration factor of 250. In all cases our calculations of concentration factors suffer from the uncertainty of what the actual concentrations were, at their highest, in the surf. Therefore we think our calculated concentration factors are low and we know they are conservative.

In addition we employed an Andersen Viable Sampler. On some days we obtained less than 20 plaques on all six plates while the settling plates contained many hundreds. On two occasions we obtained approximately 500 plaques on the Andersen plates. We do not understand the high variability of the Andersen Sampler data.

The public health implications of our experiments are fairly simple. If you live occasionally exposed to a dilute cloud of potential pathogens, you may acquire a set of immunities without ever experiencing a full blown clinical infection. For example, neither enteric nor respiratory disease epidemics are

TABLE 1

AN ANALYSIS OF WINDBORNE FALLOUT OF T2 AND T4 INTO THE SURF*

Phage Type	Row Number			Row Total
	1	2	3	
T4	135	171	184	490
T2	36	68	27	131
T2 + T4	24	52	33	109
Total number of plaques counted				730

*T4 alone: $490/730 = 0.67 = e^{-m} = 0.4$ T2/drop; T2 alone: $131/730 = 0.18 = e^{-m} = 1.7$ T4/drop. The zeroth term of the Poisson expansion is given by $f(x) = m^x e^{-m}/x! = e^{-m}$ when $x = 0$ and m is the mean number of T2 or T4 virus particles per drop in the observed population. The table represents an analysis of the data from release No. 2 of 15 July 1976. Data show the windborne fallout from a mixed injection of T2 and T4 in the surf and are expressed as numbers of plaque-forming units. A single column of the collecting matrix was analyzed for the relative numbers of pure and mixed plaques present in rows 1, 2, and 3 at 1, 11, and 22 m, respectively, from the water's edge.

reported for the south shore of Long Island yet it is known that occasional untreated sewage intrusions occur there when several days of southwesterly winds blow the plume of the Hudson River as much as 100 km east along the shore of Fire Island. On such occasions, human cultural artifacts commonly associated with sewage litter the beaches but few coliform bacteria are found in the seawater. This apparent paradox is partly explainable by dilution of the New York Harbor bacterial count of 10^{12} per cubic meter[12] in the turbulent mixing of the surf. The greater portion of the bacteria adsorb to bubbles from white caps and from the surf from whence they are ejected into the wind. Blanchard and Woodcock[13] have shown that the surf produces 3×10^5 bubbles per square meter per second. Now, an area 25 meters wide and 100 km long emits 7.5×10^{11} bubbles per second and if each jet carries only one bacterium the removal rate is 7.5×10^{11} bacteria per second compared with the calculated[3] input rate of 5×10^{14} bacteria per second from the Hudson River plume. The difference between the Hudson River input and the aerosol losses of approximately 10^3 bacteria per second is easily accounted for by filter feeder predation, sedimentation, natural death rate and turbulent mixing.

We offer the tentative prediction that persons in residence down wind of the Hudson River plume will be found to have a broad spectrum of immunities to enteric and respiratory diseases. Yet such a broad spectrum of immunities offers little protection against a new suddenly appearing mutant for which no previously developed immunity exists. If that new mutant is sewage borne and produces an epidemic in New York City, the sea surf and white caps will certainly help spread it.

REFERENCES

1. SCHAEFFER, VINCENT. Atmospheric Sciences Research Center. State University of New York at Albany. Albany, N.Y. Personal communication.
2. MAYNARD, NANCY. 1968. Significance of airborne algae. Zeitschr. F. Allg. Mikrobiologie **8** (3); 225–226.
3. GRUFT, H., J. KATZ & D. C. BLANCHARD. 1975. Postulated source of *Mycobacterium intracellulare* (Battey Infection). Am. J. Epidem. **102**: 311–318.
4. FRASER, D. W. & J. E. McDADE. 1979. Legionellosis. Sci. Am. **241** (4): 82–99.
5. BAYLOR, E. R., M. B. BAYLOR, D. C. BLANCHARD, L. D. SYZDEK & C. APPEL. Virus transfer from surf to wind. Science **198**: 575–580.
6. BAYLOR, E. R., V. PETERS & M. B. BAYLOR 1977. Water-to-air transfer of virus. Science **197**: 763–764.
7. BLANCHARD, D. C. & L. SUZDEK. 1970. Mechanism of water-to-air transfer and concentration of bacteria. Science **170**: 626–628.
8. MACINTYRE, F. 1974. The top millimeter of the ocean. Sci. Am. **230**: 62–77.
9. WOODCOCK, A. H., C. F. KIENTZLER, A. B. AARONS & D. C. BLANCHARD. 1953. Giant condensation nuclei from bursting bubbles. Nature **172**: 1144.
10. PETERS, VIRGINIA. Peters Research. Woods Hole, Mass. 02543.
11. INMAN, D. L., R. J. TAIT & C. E. NORDSTROM. 1971. Mixing in the surf zone. J. Geophys. Resch. **76**: 3493–3514.
12. CASSIN, J., Biology Dept. Adelphi Univ. Garden City, N.Y.
13. BLANCHARD, D. C. & A. H. WOODCOCK. 1957. Bubble formation and modification in the sea and its meteorological significance. Tellus **9**: 145–148.

SPREAD OF MICROORGANISMS BY
AIR-CONDITIONING SYSTEMS—ESPECIALLY
IN HOSPITALS

K. O. Gundermann

Department for Hygiene and Public Health
University of Kiel
D2300 Kiel, Germany

It was the air-conditioning system in a new tuberculosis hospital, that, in 1965, first made us look into the problems connected with these systems in hospitals. Overpressure ventilation was applied in the ward corridors of this building to prevent room-to-room spread of microorganisms. The design of the air flow was as follows: initially blown into a cavity right above the suspended ceiling of a ward corridor, the air entered the corridor via several air inlets. With this sort of design, suction of the air from the corridor into the cavity could occur at several flaws. Examining this cavity, which could not be disinfected, we were able to find mycobacterium tuberculosis at several places. Familiar with the work of Riley[1] on the infectiousness of mycobacterium tuberculosis spread with the dust, we had to insist on a complete reconstruction of this air-conditioning system. Several cases of gas gangrene in a hospital in Hamburg, West Germany prompted us as well to our subsequent investigations. The investigations there indicated, that the air-conditioning system of this hospital also caused the presence of spores of *Clostridium welchii* in the operation theaters.[2]

To make comprehensible the hazard of microorganisms being spread via air-conditioning systems, I shall very shortly describe the more general structure of such a system (FIGURE 1). The outside air intake usually is placed at the external wall, upon the roof, or is separated from the corresponding building. After gross filtration, the air is worked up in a central unit by humidifying, heating and cooling it. A ventilator also is part of this central unit. After solitary or repeated filtration, the air is delivered to the room to be ventilated by means of a ductwork. Similarly, the exhaust air is removed from the room and is blown outdoors at an appropriate place of the building.

To humidify the air, two distinct techniques may be employed. Firstly, the air may be blown through so-called water wash units, where water is sprayed. Drops not taken up by the air fall down to be sprayed again, drops that are not evaporated but swept along by the air are precipitated in a drop-separator. The exact setting of humidity is done by additionally heating or cooling the humidified air. Another principle is to humidify the air by means of water-vapor. The exact setting of humidity is done here in much the same way. Water drops may thus precipitate on the cooling units as well.

The spread of microorganisms by means of air-conditioning systems may be effected by a variety of causes. The main ones, however, are the suction of microorganisms into and their growth within these systems. An inappropriate position of the outside air intake may cause the contamination of an air-conditioning system, provided it is run only with outside air. Since this outside air basically is not free of microorganisms, all these are sucked into the air-conditioning system. We were able to find particularly high numbers of microorganisms with air intakes near or below surface level. The high proportion of

0077-8923/80/0353-0209 $01.75/0 © 1980, NYAS

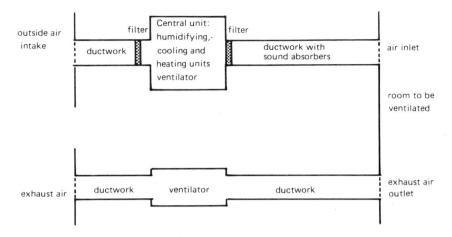

FIGURE 1. Structure of an air-conditioning system.

spores, amongst them spores of gas-gangrene as well, should be pointed out, but other classes of microorganisms were present as well. The presence of sources emitting microorganisms in the immediate surroundings of an air intake, as may be the case with exhaust air outlet ducts emitting microbially contaminated air, results in an increased suction of microorganisms into the air-conditioning system, a construction, which effectively is then quite similar to a return air system.

Growth of microorganisms may occur, wherever the air comes into contact with the water, respectively wherever water is present in the system or the relative air moisture is above 97%. According to our investigations, microbial growth does not occur below this level of air moisture. Water is present in the water wash units. Since the influx of water is coupled with its consumption, microorganisms may concentrate and grow in great numbers in these spray units. They may be found there in concentrations of 10^6 microorganisms per ml. On the inside walls of the humidifying boxes, microorganisms may grow very densely. Of course these microorganisms may be carried away by the air and thus reach the rooms to be ventilated. Microbial growth also may occur on the drop-separators or the cooling units. This is true as well if the air is humidified with water-vapor which initially is free of microorganisms. Growth of microorganisms may occur with the formation of condensing water on the cooling units or ductwork walls. Already in 1959, Anderson[3] reported the spread of *Pseudomonas pyocyanea* by means of an air-conditioning system. The cause of this spread has been water in the system's cooling unit, that has been highly contaminated with *Pseudomonas*. Taken up by the air, it has been spread by the system.

Microorganisms also may be spread by means of an air-conditioning system working with return air. In this system, the exhaust air is not blown outdoors but rather, after being worked up again, will say heated, cooled and humidified, returned to the rooms to be ventilated. In case this air is not all or only insufficiently filtered, every exhausted microorganism is returned to the rooms. The result is a more or less uniform distribution of microorganisms originating from one room over all the rooms supplied by the same system. Shaffer and McDade[4] reported in 1963 the spread of *Staphylococcus aureus* from patients of one ward to an empty ward. This ward has been disinfected, but after some time elapsed, Staphylococci could be found there. An air-conditioning system working with return air has been the cause for this. The main microorganisms spread by air-conditioning systems are firstly those found in normal outside air, such as *Staphylococcus albus*, other micrococci, and spore-forming bacteria, amongst which aerobic as well as anaerobic ones are to be found. In addition, so-called moist microorganisms occur, growing in the system, particularly Pseudomonas and Aeromonas species. In quite a few cases, Enterobacteriaceae, especially Klebsiella species, but also Coli, Proteus and Acinetobacter species are found. On top of this, fungi, including Aspergillus and Penicillium species are found regularly in abundant proportions in the wet areas.

Prompted by the fatal cases in Hamburg, where the responsibility of the air-conditioning system for an infection with *Clostridium welchii* and subsequent gas gangrene could not be excluded with certainty, we investigated a larger number of air-conditioning systems. All these systems were constructed according to specifications usually to be met by those systems, i.e. keeping the room temperature and the room humidity within prefixed limits and to remove exhaust air, particularly odorous substances and anesthetic vapors (TABLES 1a, 1b). The possibility of a spread of infection via those systems has not been seriously considered in constructing them. Out of ten air-conditioning systems we investigated in 1972,[5] none showed satisfactory results. Despite not being able to make quantitative investigations because the necessary equipment was lacking, we were able to find very high numbers of airborne microorganisms. On the Petri dishes exposed to the air-flow for some 30 minutes there was sometimes such a dense growth of microorganisms, that no count was possible at all. We found mainly gram-negative rods, including *Pseudomonas* and *Klebsiella* species, as well as aerobic and anaerobic spores and mold fungi. All of the examined humidifiers showed a heavy microbial burden. There was usually only insuffi-

TABLE 1A

GENERAL SPECIFICATIONS FOR AIR CONDITIONING SYSTEMS

1.   To keep physical parameters below certain limits
1.1. Fixed temperature
1.2. Fixed humidity
2.   To keep chemical parameters below certain limits
2.1. To remove exhaust air and thus CO_2 and odorous substances as well
2.2. To provide fresh air

TABLE 1B

SPECIFICATIONS FOR AIR CONDITIONING SYSTEMS IN HOSPITALS

1. To provide air free of microorganisms (or at harmless levels)
2. To purge the room of contaminants
3. To achieve defined air currents in rooms
4. To remove anesthetic vapors and gases

TABLE 2

EFFICIENCY OF FILTERS

Classification	Efficiency in % by fine dust (A) <5μ(A) (mid. 0,5-1μ) in concentration <5mg/m³	
A Gross-filter	1. normal	40 (30–50)
	2. good efficient	50 (40–60)
B Fine dust filter	1. normal	70 (60–80)
	2. good efficient	80 (70–90)
C Finest dust filter		95 (90–98)

cient filtration of the supplied air, with filters grade B, so-called fine-dust-filters. C-filters were employed only in one case. TABLE 2 illustrates the efficiency of these filters. Results similar to those of these ten hospitals were found in other air-conditioning systems as well. Particularly the heavy pollution of the duct-works attracted attention. This may be caused partly by creeping air movements in a shut-down system. However, these systems usually have not been cleaned sufficiently after having been mounted. On top of this, the sucked-in air not cleaned sufficiently brings in dust and thus microorganisms as well. In TABLE 3 the hygienic hazards are to be shown.

The results of investigations performed by ourselves and other authors led to the achievement of new specifications for air-conditioning systems in hospitals. In this standard,[6] figures for the air exchange are set for certain rooms as well as the design of such a system and the exact filtration is specified (TABLE 4). For all rooms with high requirements for freedom of microorganisms, a three-step filter arrangement is specified, the first and second stage being placed before and after the central unit of the air conditioning system and consisting of B- and C-grade filters, the third stage being placed at the end of the ductwork system close to the air inlets using HEPA-filters. The humidification of the intake air has to be performed in a way to secure the prevention of hazards of infection. Additional disinfection measures had to be taken for the spray humidifying units, because within these—although effecting a certain cleaning of the air by means of

TABLE 3

HYGIENIC HAZARDS IN AIR CONDITIONING SYSTEMS

1.	Suction of microorganisms together with the outside air connected to incorrect placing of the outside air intake;
2.a.	Using water-wash units: concentration of microorganisms in the washing water and thus contamination of the air;
2.b.	Using humidifiers working with water-vapor: precipitation of condensing water with possible concentration of microorganisms
3.	Insufficient air-filtration:
	3.a. Inappropriate filter quality
	3.b. Damaged or leaking filters
4.	Polluted air ducts:
	4.a. By construction
	4.b. By creeping air movements in a shutdown system
5.	Incorrect design of the air flow

sprayed water—microorganism may concentrate considerably. However, the continuing disinfection of such a unit has to be considered with certain toxicologic objections. Small amounts of the disinfectant may be blown into rooms and thus inhaled by those people present in such rooms. That is why preference usually is given to humidification by means of water vapor.

Investigations which we performed on air-conditioning systems constructed to these new German standards, showed always a clean ductwork free of microorganisms after the third filtration step; the incoming air, having ten microorganisms per m^3 (=cubicmeter) the most, could be considered free of microorganisms. Despite the high requirements for the filtration, return air systems are not approved in Germany. Only in connection with laminar airflow systems is the recirculation of air within the same room authorized.

To examine the effect air-conditioning systems have on the number of

TABLE 4

GERMAN STANDARDS FOR AIR CONDITIONING SYSTEMS IN HOSPITALS*

		Times per hour changes of air are necessary	Specification of filters
Rooms with especially high asepsis	Operating theaters for transplantation orthopedic surgery cardio vascular operations etc.	20	$B_2 + C + S$†
	Other rooms in these operating units	10	$B_2 + C + S$
Rooms with high asepsis	Other operating theaters	20	$B_2 + C + R$†
	Other rooms in these operating units	10	$B_2 + C + R$
	Units or wards for intensive care	10	$B_2 + C + R$
	Units for obstetrics	10	$B_2 + C + R$

*From DIN 1946 part 4, in rooms with high asepsis, air conditioning system is necessary.
†"S" and "R" are specifications of HEPA filters, "S" is the highest qualification.

microorganisms in the air of the room being ventilated, we examined the air not only at the air inlet but at several points of the room as well. We were able to find that, in general, the number of microorganisms in ventilated rooms is lower than in rooms not ventilated; however, these numbers rose considerably with the more intensive use of the room, i.e., with the presence of numerous persons and the degree to which they moved around. The number of microorganisms then usually were considerably higher than generally accepted for safe room usage (TABLE 5). The following figure illustrates the interdependence of the number of airborne microorganisms and the number of people working in a specific room (TABLE 6).

Lowering the numbers of airborne microorganisms in a room ventilated by a conventional system with turbulent ventilation only by increasing the air exchange per hour is no longer feasible, without causing new problems, such as draught. With specific systems of directing the air flow, such as blowing the air

TABLE 5

NUMBER OF MICRO ORGANISMS IN VENTILATED AND NONVENTILATED
OPERATION THEATERS*

		Number of microorganisms tested by filtration of air
1. Nonventilated	n	120
10 op.-units	$\bar{x}$	580 cfu/m³
(during work)	r	240-1100 cfu/m³
2. Ventilated	n	354
5 op.-units	$\bar{x}$	235 cfu/m³
(during work)	r	34-1398 cfu/m³

*n = number of tests (filtrations)
$\bar{x}$ = for all tests
r = range of $\bar{x}$ for each series
cfu/m³ = colony forming units per m³ of tested air

into the room over specially designed ceilings with the help of a so-called support stream the results improve considerably, but still do not seem sufficient for special operations with particular high requirements for freedom of microorganisms.

A system, with which the number of airborne microorganisms in a room may be lowered even further is the laminar airflow system.[7] The expenditure for such a system is very high indeed and the necessity may be questioned. In many cases, the results are not as clear-cut as initially expected. In addition, to prevent turbulances caused by persons working in the airflow may in turn cause problems for example with operations. Equally low numbers of airborne microorganisms may also be achieved in a cabin with conventional ventilation but with specific dresses and a special exhaust of the respiration.

Another system, having the advantage of a low expenditure for mounting it and low energy costs as well, is the clean field system developed by Esdorn and Nouri.[8] With this system (FIGURE 2), a pipe permeable to air is placed around the operation wound as well as all other areas to be kept particularly clean. Clean air is then blown through this pipe and an area of air relatively free of microorganisms is thus created above the operation area, which may not even be disturbed

TABLE 6

INTERDEPENDENCE OF THE NUMBER OF MICROORGANISMS AND THE NUMBER
OF PEOPLE IN AN OPERATION THEATER

Point of filtration	>10 persons	6-10 persons	2-5 persons	0-1 person
1 cfu/m³	660* cfu/m³	400 cfu/m³	380 cfu/m³	76 cfu/m³
2	700	480	270	68
3	620	250	250	60
4	540	240	210	144
M	630	350	280	81

*Colony forming units/m³, $\bar{x}$ from 3 tests.

by movements of the operating team. Investigations in a number of hospitals showed that this system is able to achieve especially low numbers of microorganisms in the area of the operation wound, numbers which are quite comparable to those produced with the laminar airflow systems. It may be pointed out that there was no relation between the number of microorganisms in the room and the

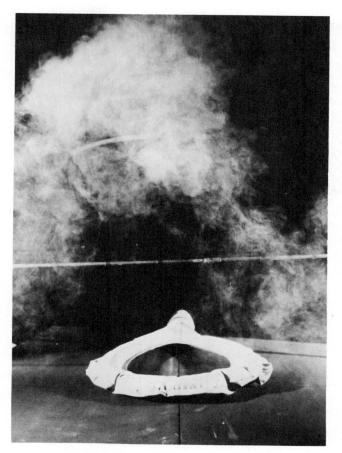

FIGURE 2. Model of the clean field system developed by Esdorn and Nouri. Air is blown out by a permeable pipe and the clean field is seen ahead of it. In use for operating, the pipe is placed around the wound.

number in the operating area, the latter ones being very low, no matter how high the number of airborne microorganisms were in other parts of the room (TABLE 7). If further bacteriologic and clinical investigations and tests confirm these favorable results, we herewith have a system at hand which is able to achieve optimal low figures in the operation area, without causing such a high technical expenditure as the laminar airflow system does. The ventilation of the remaining room may then be designed to specifications for the burden of heat, odorous substances and waste gases.

To summarize we may state that the spread of microorganisms by means of air-conditioning systems may be of importance whenever these systems are built too cheaply. Air-conditioning systems as far as the air intake, its working up and its filtration are concerned should be well-constructed in order to prevent the suction of considerable numbers of microorganisms into the system as well as their growth within the system. On top of this the remaining microorganisms are to be removed by filtration as far as possible. These principles are particularly relevant for air-conditioning systems in hospitals, but their are true basically for all other air-conditioning systems as well. A healthy individual is much less apt to acquire an infection than a sick person with a lowered resistance. However, an

TABLE 7

NUMBER OF MICROORGANISMS IN AN OPERATION AREA WITH A CLEAN FIELD SYSTEM

Hospital	Number of Series	Air in the Operation Room		Air in the Operation Area	
A	12	$\overline{x}$	366*	$\overline{x}$	9,9
		r	(155-1398)	r	(0-33)
B	10	$\overline{x}$	120	$\overline{x}$	13
		r	(34-275)	r	(4-30)
C	17	$\overline{x}$	273	$\overline{x}$	7,4
		r	(71-493)	r	(1-21)
D	6	$\overline{x}$	128	$\overline{x}$	5,8
		r	(46-212)	r	(1-17)
E	6	$\overline{x}$	163	$\overline{x}$	56,5
		r	(106-224)	r	(7-124)

*$\overline{x}$ for all tests in a hospital
r range of $\overline{x}$ for each series
Numbers = colony forming units/m^3

infection is not to be excluded with certainty in the presence of very high numbers of airborne microorganisms, nor should we forget possible sensitization through a heavy growth of fungi via the air-conditioner's air intake.

REFERENCES

1. RILEY, R. L. 1957. Aerial dissemination of pulmonary tuberculosis. Amer. Rev. Tuberc. **76:** 931-941.
2. THOMSEN, K. & D. KREBS. 1972. Fehlerhafte Klimaanlage infizierte Operationstrakt. Dtsch. Ärzteblatt **69:** 544-547.

3. ANDERSON, K. 1959. Ps. pyocyanea disseminated from an air cooling apparatus. Med. J. Austr., 529–532.
4. SHAFFER, J. G. & J. J. McDADE. 1963. Airborne *Staph. aureus*. A possible source in air control equipment. Arch. Environ. Health **5:** 547–551.
5. GUNDERMANN, K. O., 1972. Zum Problem der Hygiene von Belüftungsanlagen im Krankenhaus. Gesundheitswesen u. Desinfektion **64:** 58–62.
6. DIN 1946, part 4, Raumlufttechnische Anlagen im Krankenhaus (German standards for air conditioning systems in hospitals) 1978, Beuth Verlag, D-1000 Berlin 30.
7. CHARNLEY, J. 1973. Clean air in the operating room Clev. Clin. Quart. **40:** 99–114.
8. NOURI, Z. & H. ESDORN. 1978. The application of a new energy saving clean-field technique in operating theaters under clinical conditions. Proc. 4th Intern. Symp. on contamination control. Washington, D.C. 1978. ICCCS.

THE ROLE OF AIRBORNE BACTERIA IN THE CONTAMINATION OF FINE PARTICLE NEBULIZERS AND THE DEVELOPMENT OF NOSOCOMIAL PNEUMONIA

Steven G. Kelsen

Pulmonary Division, Department of Medicine
University Hospitals of Cleveland
Case Western Reserve University School of Medicine
Cleveland, Ohio 44106

Maryanne McGuckin

Infectious Disease Division
University of Pennsylvania
Philadelphia, Pennsylvania 19104

INTRODUCTION

Previous studies have shown that reservoir nebulizers are exceedingly vulnerable to bacterial contamination by gram negative organisms and produce aerosols containing large numbers of bacteria.[1,2] These contaminated aerosols have been shown to cause bacterial colonization of the respiratory tract and nosocomial pneumonia.[1-3] Several years ago, we studied the role of airborne bacteria in the contamination of fine particle nebulizers by comparing the incidence of contamination in groups of nebulizers placed in hospital locations whose airborne bacterial flora differed.[4] More recently, we have examined the relationship between airborne bacteria and nosocomial attack rates in a surgical intensive care unit. In this unit, both the incidence of nosocomial respiratory tract infections and the bacterial profile of the ambient air were determined serially over a 5-year period.

The data from these studies indicate that: 1) contamination of fine particle nebulizers can be produced by the airborne route; and 2) the incidence of nosocomial respiratory infections is significantly related to airborne bacterial levels.

Airborne Contamination of Fine Particle Nebulizers

Fine particle reservoir nebulizers utilizing the venturi principle are commonly used in medical practice to increase the water and oxygen content of inspired air. FIGURE 1 illustrates schematically the operating principles of this type of respiratory therapy equipment. A gas (usually 100% oxygen) under pressure and with a high linear velocity is directed across the mouth of a capillary tube whose lower end is submerged in the reservoir. The negative pressure produced at the mouth of the capillary tube by the rapidly flowing gas (Bernoulli effect) sucks water up from the reservoir into the gas stream. After entering the stream, the water is impacted against a baffle, dispersed into droplets, and carried out of the nebulizer in particulate form.

The oxygen concentration of the effluent is decreased below 100% by mixing

218

0077-8923/80/0353-0218 $01.75/0 © 1980, NYAS

the oxygen with room air. The volume of room air entering the nebulizer is regulated by a venturi valve in communication with the oxygen stream. At a given O_2 flow rate, the venturi valve determines the magnitude of the negative pressure inside the nebulizer and hence, the volume of room air entrained.

METHODS

Two areas of the hospital known to have different airborne bacterial flora on the basis of prior air sampling were chosen as test areas. These areas are the administrative offices of the respiratory therapy department (Area 1) and the surgical intensive care unit (Area 2). Area 1 (100 sq. m) is a nonpatient care area used for storage of records and light equipment. Ventilation of this room took place through a door communicating with a main corridor of the hospital. On the

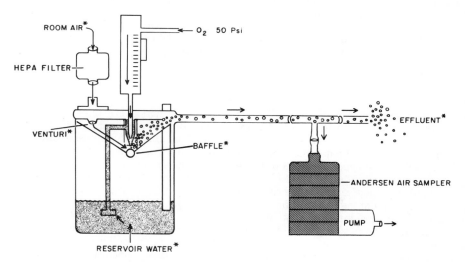

FIGURE 1. Fine-particle nebulizers. Asterisks indicate sites cultured and the direction of gas and water flow is indicated by arrows.

other hand, Area 2 (650 sq. m) is an undivided, 12-bed surgical intensive care unit in which, at the time of the study, a plenum system of ventilation that recirculated 80% of the vented air and exchanged it 7.5 times per hour was in use. The ventilation system in Area 2 will be described in more detail subsequently.

Twelve and 15 fine particle reservoir nebulizers were placed in Areas 1 and 2, respectively. All nebulizers were sterilized with ethylene oxide and vacuum-aerated prior to study. Nebulizers were filled with sterile water and were placed in continuous operation for 72 hours, propelled by oxygen at a pressure of 3.52 kg/sq cm from wall outlets. To avoid the possibility of exogenous contamination from patient sources, at no time were any nebulizers in patient use. The following operating conditions were controlled, 1) so that both groups of nebulizers would entrain the same volume of room air (30 liters/min), the flow rate of oxygen was set at 10 liters/min and the venturi attachment was set to deliver a gas mixture of

40% O_2 so that the final effluent volume was 40 liters/min; 2) to control temperature, a heating element placed in the nebulizer maintained the reservoir at 37°C.

Cultures were obtained ten minutes after operation was begun (0 hour) and then after 24, 48, and 72 hours of continuous operation from the following sites: nebulizer effluent, venturi, baffle, and reservoir water. At the same time intervals, cultures of background air were obtained. Cultures of nebulizer effluent and background air were obtained through use of an Andersen air sampler and were collected over a ten-minute period at a sampler flow rate of 28 liters/min (FIGURE 1).[5] Air sampler cultures were collected on 100 mm Petri dishes prefilled with sterile Navy blood agar, counted by the positive hole and microscope sector method, and expressed as colony forming units per cubic foot of air.[5]

The nebulizer venturi and baffle were cultured using a sterile swab, while reservoir water was obtained with a sterile pipette after the nebulizer had been opened by unscrewing the reservoir jar. Specimens were then inoculated into fluid thioglycollate medium. All cultures were incubated at 35.5°C and were examined after 24 and 48 hours. Organisms were identified by gram stain, colony morphology, biochemical characteristics, and antibiogram.[6]

ASSUMPTIONS

It seems possible that bacteria in the room air which are drawn into the nebulizer may come into contact with all parts of the nebulizer prior to being emitted as part of the aerosol. If this is the case, the ability to culture organisms from the interior of a nebulizer may not indicate that the device is contaminated. As a result, the usual concepts of bacterial contamination may not apply. It has been suggested by others that nebulizer contamination has occurred when the nebulizer effluent contains a greater concentration of organisms than are present in an equivalent volume of room air.[1,7-8] In this view, the nebulizer is considered a site of bacterial multiplication and transmission.

In the present study, conditions were adjusted so that 75% of the effluent volume was made up of room air circulated through the nebulizer. Knowing the bacterial concentration of room air allowed an "expected" bacterial count in the effluent aerosol to be determined (i.e., multiplying the simultaneously obtained background air value by 0.75).

These assumptions were tested in preliminary experiments by placing nebulizers in an enclosed chamber in which the bacterial concentration could be changed (FIGURE 2). Airborne bacterial counts in this chamber were altered by discharging the effluent of a nebulizer whose reservoir contained from 10^2 to 10^4 Pseudomonas aeruginosa per milliliter into the sealed chamber. Ten nebulizers were placed in this chamber and the effluent emitted by these exposed nebulizers was vented to the outside of the chamber where it was cultured with an Andersen air sampler ten minutes after operation was begun (0 hour). Aerosol concentrations were then related to the concentration of airborne bacteria inside the chamber (FIGURE 3). As may be seen (open circles), the number of bacteria actually present in the aerosol fell on the line of identity with the concentration predicted on the basis of the simultaneous background air sample (background air × 0.75).

In addition, six nebulizers placed in Area 2 were fitted with 0.3 μ pore-size, ultra-high-efficiency (HEPA) particulate air filters. This filter retains 99.9% of all

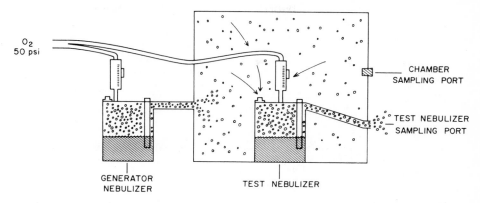

FIGURE 2. Chamber in which nebulizers were exposed to different levels of airborne bacteria.

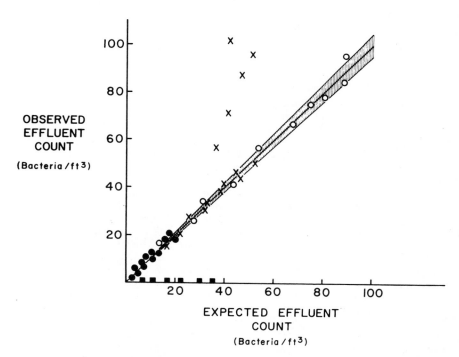

FIGURE 3. Relationship between expected bacterial count and bacterial count actually present in nebulizer effluent. Points represent the sample obtained from area 1 (dark circles), area 2 (crosses), zero time (0), and filtered nebulizers (dark boxes). Line represents the relationship of identity ±5% sampling error associated with Andersen air sampler.

TABLE 1

AIRBORNE BACTERIAL COUNTS (CFU/FT³)

	Area I	Area II	
Background Air	12.6 ± 2.3 S.E.	47.6 ± 2.9 S.E.	$P < 0.05$
Effluent	11.8 ± 2.3 S.E.	63.3 ± 10.4 S.E.	$p < 0.05$

particles 0.3 μ or greater at airflow rates up to 200 liters/sec. Filters were placed over the venturi intake valve so that all room air was bacterially filtered prior to entering the nebulizer (FIGURE 1).

As may be seen in FIGURE 3, the aerosols produced by these nebulizers contained almost no bacteria and the data points fell along the abscissa.

Nebulizer Surveillance Data (Based on 463 Cultures)

Both the number and type of bacteria present in Area 2 differed from those in Area 1 (TABLE 1). In Area 2, a signifcantly greater number of bacteria were present in background air and were predominantly gram negative in type. In Area 2, *Pseudomonas aeruginosa* was the most prevalent organism (45.6% of all isolates) while in Area 1, *Staphylococcus epidermidis* was most common (31.5% of all isolates).

Bacterial counts in effluent aerosols produced by Area 2 nebulizers were significantly greater than in Area 1 nebulizers (TABLE 1). However, this may have been due to the greater number of bacteria present in the entrained air of Area 2.

When the effluent bacterial count of each nebulizer was related to the concentration of bacteria present in a simultaneously obtained sample of room air (FIGURE 2), it became apparent that 5 (33%) Area 2 nebulizers deviated from the line of identity and numbers of bacteria than expected. In contrast, none of the 12 Area 1 nebulizers emitted more than the expected number of bacteria. This difference of Area 2 and 1 nebulizers (33% vs 0%) was significant statistically ($p < 0.05$).

Cultures of nebulizer parts were positive in 6 of the Area 2 and 1 of the Area 1 nebulizers. In contrast, bacteria were isolated from reservoir water only in the Area 2 nebulizers which emitted greater than expected concentrations of bacteria. The incidence of positive cultures in the 5 nebulizers producing contaminated aerosols were significantly greater than in the 22 which did not ($p < 0.05$).

The significantly greater incidence of contamination in nebulizers which were operated in identical fashion but differed only in the type of air entering the nebulizer suggests that airborne bacteria represent a pathway by which bacterial inoculation of fine particle reservoir nebulizers may take place. The isolation of bacteria from the internal parts of a nebulizer does not appear to discriminate between machines producing contaminated aerosols and those which do not, perhaps because the organisms present on nebulizer parts may simply be traversing the nebulizer. In contrast, the presence of bacteria in reservoir water is a significant finding and may be a clinically useful index of nebulizer contamination.

It may be expected then that nebulizers placed in environments in which large numbers of gram negative organisms are present in the background air will show a relatively high incidence of contamination. It should be pointed out that the levels of airborne bacteria observed in the intensive care area surveyed in the present study approximate those found in patient care areas in previous studies.[9] This suggests that large numbers of bacteria may be present in ambient air and find their way into the nebulizers operated in these locations. Nebulizer contamination and secondary nosocomial respiratory tract infection may be decreased, therefore, by decreasing the number of bacteria entering the nebulizer. This may be achieved by altering the airborne flora by frequent exchanges of room air or if air is recirculated by interposing a bacterial filter in the ventilation system. Alternatively, providing a barrier to bacteria at the level of individual units may be a more cost effective way of dealing with the problem. HEPA filters which can be attached to the nebulizer are now commercially available.

Relationship of Airborne Bacteria to Nosocomial Respiratory Tract Infection

In the past several years, prolonged bacteriological surveillance of both the patients and ambient environment of Area 2 (the intensive care unit) has allowed us to relate the incidence of nosocomial respiratory tract infection to airborne bacterial levels.

Ventilation of Area 2

A diagramatic representation of the ventilation system in Area 2 is shown in FIGURE 4. With the exception of a single enclosed isolation area, the 12 beds in the

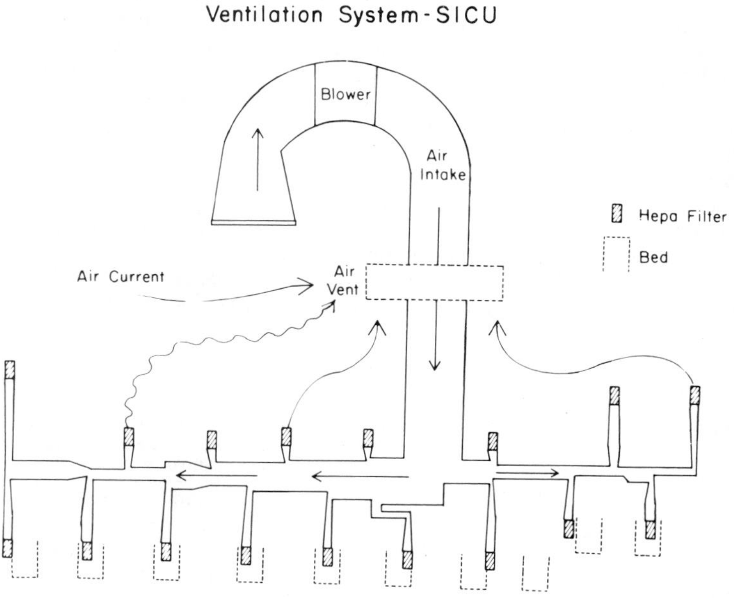

Ventilation System-SICU

FIGURE 4. Diagram of area 2. Ventilation return ducts are situated over each bed.

unit were arranged in Nightingale fashion around a large undivided space. Ventilation of the unit was accomplished by recirculating room air (80% recirculation, 20% fresh air) 7.5 times per hour. After temperature was adjusted by passage over either heating or cooling elements, the vented air was passed through a low efficiency filter to remove large dust particles (>250 μ) and returned to the unit by vents located over each bed. Ventilation of the isolation area was performed by the same system.

As a result of the high airborne bacterial counts observed in the preceding study, the ventilation system was modified in December 1974 by fitting the existing return vents with 0.3 micron-size ultra-high efficiency (HEPA) filters. Airflow was maintained constant despite the filters by installing a more powerful blower. Room pressure was made positive relative to the outside ($+2$ cm H_2O) by increasing the resistance of the inflow ducts.

Patient Population

The population of the unit consists primarily of patients on the cardiothoracic surgical service although general, genitourinary, and vascular surgical patients were present. Approximately 400 patients are admitted to this unit each year usually immediately post-operatively. The average length of stay is 5–7 days. A nonselective admissions policy allowed all "clean," "clean-contaminated," and "dirty" cases to be admitted.[10] Most patients (84%) had endotracheal or tracheostomy tubes in place at some time during their stay. Almost all patients were treated with fine particle nebulizers or intermittent positive pressure breathing (IPPB). Separate nursing and anesthesia personnel were assigned to this unit.

Surveillance of patients and environment in the unit consisted of routine sputum and urine cultures in all patients and periodic cultures of room air and nebulizer effluent. Intensive culturing was performed for several weeks at a time, at intermittent intervals over a 5-year period. During each month in which surveillance was performed, at least 12 air samples were obtained with the Andersen air sampler and at least 25 patients cultured. Data reported represent monthly averages (Table 2).

Nosocomial respiratory tract infections were considered to be present when the following criteria were met: 1) a new infiltrate was present on chest x-ray; 2) sputum gram stain revealed significant numbers of organisms and inflammatory cells; and 3) organism specific antibiotic therapy was begun. In addition, nonrespiratory nosocomial infections including bacteremias, urinary tract, skin, and wound infections were monitored according to standard surveillance criteria.[10]

TABLE 2

MONTHLY AVERAGES OF NOSOCOMIAL ATTACK RATES OVER A 5-YEAR PERIOD

	Respiratory	Nonrespiratory				
		UTI*	Bacteremia	Wound	Skin	Total
Mean	7.0%	4.2%	2.8	2.8	0.5	10.3
±1 S.E.	1.3	±0.6	±0.4	±0.7	±0.1	±1.7

*Urinary tract infections.

TABLE 3

NOSOCOMIAL ATTACK RATES OVER A 5-YEAR PERIOD

Time Period	Airborne Count (CFU/FT³)	Organism	% Airborne Count	Organism Specific Nosocomial Pneumonia Rates (%)
11/73–11/74	69.0 ± 5.6 S.E.	Pseudomonas aeruginosa	43.6	43
		Klebsiella	13.4	12
		Flavobacterium	0	0
		Staphylococcus epidermidis	15.3	0
		Bacillus	6.7	0
		Diphtheroids	6.0	0
			88%	
1/75–1/76	7.4 ± 1.0 S.E.	Pseudomonas aeruginosa	0	14
		Klebsiella	0	5
		Flavobacterium	0	0
		Staphylococcus epidermidis	60	0
		Bacillus	20	0
		Diphtheroids	10	0
			90%	
7/77	40.0 ± 4.8 S.E.	Pseudomonas aeruginosa	40	40
		Klebsiella	10	15
		Flavobacterium	0	0
		Staphylococcus epidermidis	15	0
		Bacillus	10	0
		Diphtheroids	5	0
			80%	
8/78	39.0 ± 5.2 S.E.	Pseudomonas aeruginosa	72	69
		Klebsiella	0	2
		Flavobacterium	9	0
		Staphylococcus epidermidis	10	0
		Bacillus	0	0
		Diphtheroids	0	0
			91%	

Nosocomial Infection Rates

Nosocomial attack rates are defined as the number of infected cases over the total number of patient exposed; nonrespiratory attack rates represent the sum of all nonrespiratory tract nosocomial infections and include bacteremias, wound, urinary tract, and skin infections. Average attack rates for the period of the study are shown in TABLE 3. Over the 5-year period from November 1973 to August 1978, the respiratory tract nosocomial attack rates varied from 0.7 to 17%. Over the same period, nonrespiratory attack rates varied from 1 to 25%.

Over the same time, monthly airborne bacterial counts varied from 1.0 ± 0.8 S.E. bacteria/ft³ to 96.0 ± 6.8 S.E. bacteria/ft.³ Counts represent the total number of colonies on all plates of the sampler.

The airborne bacterial counts and nosocomial attack rates present during each month of the study are shown in FIGURE 5. As may be seen, airborne bacterial counts were highest over the period of 11/73 to 11/74. During this time, the incidence of both respiratory and nonrespiratory nosocomial infections was

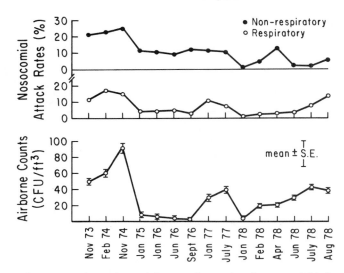

FIGURE 5. Change in airborne bacterial counts (bottom) and nosocomial infection attack rates (top) in area 2 during the 5-year period of surveillance. Nosocomial attack rates are divided into respiratory (O) and nonrespiratory (●) (i.e., all other nosocomial infections) groups.

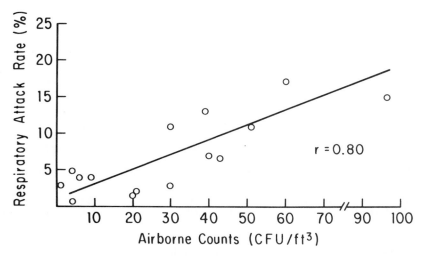

FIGURE 6. Relationship between airborne bacterial counts and respiratory tract attack rates. Correlation coefficient (r = 0.80) determined by least squares regression analysis (p < 0.05).

also highest. In 1/75, air filtering of the unit was instituted. This period was associated with a reduction in both airborne bacteria and the incidence of both respiratory and nonrespiratory infections. In 1/77, an increase in airborne counts was observed and simultaneously the incidence of respiratory tract infections also increased. Subsequent investigation of the ventilation system revealed the filters to be in need of cleaning and/or replacement. Airborne counts in 1/78 following maintenance procedures returned to the previously observed low levels, only to begin rising shortly thereafter (2/78 to 8/78).

FIGURE 6 relates the incidence of respiratory tract nosocomial infections occurring during each month of the study to the mean airborne bacterial count observed over that month. As may be seen, there was a reasonably close correlation between airborne bacterial levels and the incidence of nosocomial pneumonia ($r = 0.81$, $p < 0.05$).

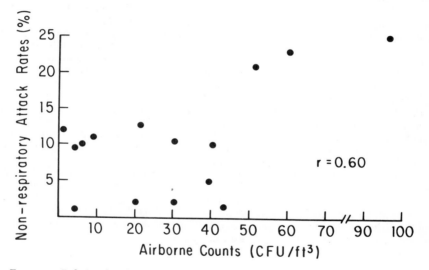

FIGURE 7. Relationship between airborne bacterial counts and nonrespiratory attack rates. Correlation coefficient ($r = 0.60$) was not significant statistically ($p > 0.05$).

The organism responsible for the respiratory nosocomial infections and the most common gram (+) and gram (−) organisms obtained during air sampling are shown for four representative periods in TABLE 3. As may be seen, *Pseudomonas aeruginosa* was the organism most frequently responsible for nosocomial pneumonia. It was also the most prevalent organism in air sampler cultures when the nosocomial attack rates were highest. Furthermore, when the relationship between *Pseudomonas aeruginosa* nosocomial attack rates were related to the number of colonies of *Pseudomonas* present in the air over the period of the study, a close correlation ($r = 0.88$, $p < 0.05$) was found.

FIGURE 7 shows the relationship between nonrespiratory nosocomial infection attack rates and airborne bacterial levels. In contrast to what was found for respiratory tract infections, there was no significant relationship between air counts and nonrespiratory attack rates ($r = 0.60$, $p > 0.05$).

The infection rate in surgical patients is influenced by a variety of factors which include: environmental factors both physical and bacteriological; personnel practices and procedures; host susceptibility; and the adequacy of infection control procedures.[11] Given these considerations, there appear to be at least three possible explanations for the significant relationship between nosocomial respiratory tract infections and the airborne bacterial levels. First, it is possible that direct inoculation of the airway by airborne bacteria explains the relationship observed. This is the simplest explanation, but there is no direct support for this mechanism in the present study. Indirect support comes from previous studies which have implicated an airborne route of spread for operating room acquired *Staphylococcus aureus* wound infections.[12]

Second, the airborne bacterial counts may simply be a reflection of the general level of "cleanliness" in the environment. That is, the airborne levels may relate to the degree of contamination of the environment (e.g., sinks, floors, hands, etc.). The more contaminated the environment, the greater the chance of inoculating the airway when breaks in technique occur (e.g., during tracheal suction). In this pathway, the airway is inoculated by direct contact and the airborne bacterial levels merely reflect the bacterial concentration on the surface of the environment. While we believe this mechanism to be likely, we would expect a close relationship between all forms of nosocomial infection and the airborne count. This was not the case, however.

Third, it is possible that the high airborne counts led to an increased incidence of contaminated nebulizers which, in turn, produced the high nosocomial attack rates. This would explain the lack of a significant relationship to other nosocomial infections since only the respiratory tract comes in contact with these devices. Unfortunately, intensive surveillance of nebulizers was not performed over the entire study and so this possibility could not be tested.

Regardless of the pathway(s) involved, it is of interest that over a prolonged period, the airborne bacterial level in an intensive care unit bears a significant relationship to the incidence of nosocomial respiratory tract but not other nosocomial infections. This suggests that on an empiric basis alone, surveillance of the airborne environment may prove to be a useful epidemiological tool in the study and control of nosocomial respiratory tract infections in certain high risk patient care areas.

REFERENCES

1. REINARZ, J. A., A. K. PIERCE & B. B. MAYS. 1965. The potential role of inhalation therapy equipment in nosocomial infection. J. Clin. Invest. **44:** 831–839.
2. GRIEBLE, H. G., F. R. COLTON & J. J. BIRD. 1970. Fine particle humidifiers: Source of *Pseudomonas aeruginosa* infections in a respiratory disease unit. N. Engl. J. Med. **282:** 531–535.
3. PIERCE, A. K., J. P. SANFORD & G. D. THOMAS. 1970. Long term evaluation of decontamination of inhalation therapy equipment and the occurrence of necrotizing pneumonia. N. Engl. J. Med. **282:** 528–531.
4. KELSEN, S. G., M. McGUCKIN, D. P. KELSEN & N. S. CHERNIACK. 1977. Airborne contamination of fine particle nebulizers. J. Am. Med. Assoc. **237:** 2311–2314.
5. ANDERSEN, A. A. 1958. New sampler for the collection, sizing, and enumeration of viable airborne particles. J. Bacteriol. **76:** 471–484.
6. EDWARDS, P. R. & W. EWING. Eds. 1972. Identification of *Enterobacteriaceae*, 3rd Edit., Minneapolis. Burgess Publishing Company.

7. NAZEMI, M. M., D. M. MUSHER & R. R. MARTIN. 1972. A practical method for monitoring bacterial contamination of inhalation therapy machines. Am. Rev. Resp. Dis. **106:** 920–922.

8. SCHULTZE, T., E. B. EDMONDSON & A. K. PIERCE. 1967. Studies of a new humidifying device as a potential source of bacterial aerosols. Am. Rev. Resp. Dis. **96:** 517–519.

9. GREENE, V. W., D. VESLEY & R. G. BOND. 1962. Microbiological contamination of hospital air. Appl. Microbiol. **10:** 561–567, 567–571.

10. GARNER, J. S., J. V. BENNETT, W. E. SCHECKLER, D. G. MAKI & P. S. BRACHMAN. 1971. Surveillance of nosocomial infections. American Hospital Association. Chicago.

11. ALTERMEIER, W. A., J. F. BURKE, B. A. PRUITT & W. R. SANDUSKY. Eds. 1976. Manual on Control of Infection in Surgical Patients. J. B. Lippincott. Philadelphia-Toronto.

12. WALTER, C. W., R. B. KUNDSIN & M. M. BRUBAKER. 1963. The incidence of airborne wound infection during operation. J. Am. Med. Assoc. **186:** 908–913.

AIR SAMPLING IN HOSPITALS

Dieter H. M. Gröschel

University of Virginia School of Medicine
Charlottesville, Virginia 22908

Introduction

In 1970, Brachman[1] introduced a historical review and discussion of the airborne transmission of nosocomial infection with the sentence, "The airborne route of infection exemplifies the pendular nature of the theory of infectious diseases." With the swings of the pendulum, we have seen also changes in the attitude toward sampling of hospital air for the detection of airborne microorganisms. They not only reflect our thinking about the transmission of nosocomial infectious diseases but also the change in spectrum of nosocomial organisms, the effectiveness and use of antimicrobial agents, and, last but not least, our personal bias. Several participants in the conference, especially Riley[2] and Walter and Kundsin,[3] have reminded us over the years to be conscious of the airborne mode of spread despite our preoccupation with endogenous and direct-contact infections.

Muir[4] mentioned in his excellent book on the clinical aspects of inhaled particles that the average human inhales about 10,000 liters of air daily and with it airborne particles which are deposited in different parts of the respiratory tract due to various physical parameters. It was the father of antisepsis, Lister,[5] who first noted the filtration efficiency of airways of the lung, and experiments by Tyndall[6] showed that air exhaled from the depths of the lung was free from suspended matter. The physiologist, Findeisen,[7] first studied the relations between particle mobility, caliber of airways and speed of air flow in each part of the respiratory tract.

After World War II the interest in the airborne route of transmission dwindled but was rekindled by the world-wide nosocomial epidemic with staphylococci and their spread by hospital air.[8] An excellent summary of reports on hospital air and infection in the English language literature between 1966–1976 was published by Wenzel et al.[9] These authors stated that most studies had considerable shortcomings, some of them due to the lack of standardization of techniques of air sampling and others due to doubtful interpretation of data. This leaves the clinical microbiologist and epidemiologist with a dilemma: Shall he study the microbial content of hospital air at all; do this routinely; at random; or only if the epidemiologic situation requires it? It is obvious that the question of air sampling is subjected to the same "pendular nature"[1] as the question of airborne transmission of infections. A few years ago the American Hospital Association[10] and the American Public Health Association[11] issued statements discouraging the routine culturing of the inanimate environment in hospitals. Neither routine nor even occasional nonoutbreak monitoring of bacterial shedders among hospital personnel was recommended by the Center for Disease Control.[12] The question arises whether or not there is any role left for the microbial air sampler in hospitals. The answer is yes, but with the qualification that its use is subjected to Kundsin's five criteria[13] for microbiological monitoring: The study must be purposeful, planned, scientifically accurate, properly analyzed, and effectively communicated.

0077-8923/80/0353-0230 $01.75/0 © 1980, NYAS

Based on the literature of the past years and on personal experience, I shall outline some of the reasons why clinical microbiologists and infection control specialists should be familiar with air-sampling apparatus and techniques. Also, I shall present air-sampling data from a personal study comparing the Casella slit-sampler with two newer air sampling devices.

REASONS FOR AIR SAMPLING IN HOSPITALS

Sampling of air may be performed in hospitals for epidemiologic, research, safety, or quality control purposes.

Epidemiologic Investigation of Nosocomial Infectious Diseases

The investigation of hospital-associated outbreaks of infections often includes the study of the inanimate environment, air. Brachman[1] quoted two recent outbreaks of nosocomial disease to emphasize the importance of purposeful, planned epidemiologic investigations, the smallpox outbreak in Meschede (Germany) and a nosocomial tuberculosis outbreak in Florida. On the other hand, numerous reports are found in which airborne transmission is implicated in hospital-acquired infections but the epidemiologic data provided make it impossible to accept them as scientifically accurate and properly analyzed.[9] During the Sixth International Symposium on Aerobiology,[14] Parker reviewed the airborne transmission of infections in hospitals. Two aerial routes of spread are recognized, by droplets and droplet nuclei and by dry particles from the body surface or, secondarily, from inanimate surfaces. Droplets play a role in the transmission of tuberculosis, Streptococcus pyogenes and in certain other respiratory infections. Squamae and other dry particles from the body surface are incriminated in the transfer of staphylococci and streptococci. Transfer of gram-negative bacilli by air has been shown with respiratory therapy equipment, in burn units and in Legionnaire's Disease and Pontiac Fever (see contributions elsewhere in this book by D.W. Fraser and G. F. Mallison). In investigations of nosocomial infectious disease microorganisms isolated from air samples need to be present in the immediate environment of the patient, must be identical to the patient isolate, have access to a susceptible site in the patient and must be capable numerically to colonize or infect the patient. In most hospital settings, the microbiology laboratory is not equipped to fulfill all these requirements, and data obtained by air sampling are analyzed by teleological assumptions rather than by scientific methods. Such erroneous interpretation of sampling data may lead either to unnecessary and expensive "remedial actions" with no benefit to the patient or to the assumption that airborne transmission does not exist. Due to the complex nature of this route of spread, considerable experience in epidemiological techniques is required and studies should be performed only by recognized experts.

Research of Airborne Microorganisms–Spread and Control

The research application of air-sampling in the hospital environment has mainly involved the establishment of baseline levels of microbial load, the influence of physical and chemical control systems, and the spread of microorganisms under various conditions. For time reason, only a few examples of the use of air sampling in studies of the hospital environment will be quoted. Gundermann[15] in Germany has studied the microbial contamination of air, the airborne contamination of surfaces and the influence of air currents and environmental control systems (see contribution elsewhere in this book). Walter and Kundsin[2] have conducted extensive studies of the airborne components of wound contamination and infection in operating theaters. In their investigations they tested carriers and "shedders," fall-out in the sterile field, clothings and drapes, floors, ventilation and other parameters using air- and surface-sampling as well as personnel cultures.

In the past few years the question of carpeting in patient care areas has generated considerable interest with hospital administrators and infection control specialists. Numerous techniques have been reported to sample carpeting such as impressions, suctioning, punch sampling, etc. Investigators in Europe (Rotter et al.[16]) and in New Zealand (Bakker and Faoagali[17]) have used air-samplers to assess the effect of carpets on the number of airborne microorganisms.

The investigation of transmission of Hepatitis B-virus in hemodialysis units has led to the study of air samples for the presence of HB_s antigen by Favero's group at the Center for Disease Control Phoenix Campus.[18]

Use of Air Sampling in Monitoring Biohazardous Procedures

Many procedures in hospitals are associated with the generation of potentially hazardous aerosols. Therefore, air sampling is an excellent tool to assess potential biohazards in various hospital departments and services. Dr. Mazzarella already discussed the airborne bacterial hazards in dental clinics. Stern et al.[19] studied the aerosol production associated with clinical laboratory procedures using an Andersen sieve sampler. The test aerosols contained coli phages which were sampled onto agar plates containing a feeder layer with susceptible E. coli. Aerosol of $<5\mu$ was generated when shaking liquids in a confined space, from spilling on the floor, from Oxford pipettes and during controlled pouring. Interestingly, centrifugation, Vortex mixing of closed containers, Pasteur pipetting and opening containers did not result in small aerosol particles. However, all procedures caused considerable surface contamination. Turner et al.[20] used a Reyniers slit air sampler to demonstrate that an ultrasonic device designed for cleaning surgical instruments produced a significant microbial aerosol. Like other microbiologists, we have used air samplers to assess bacterial aerosols generated by vaporizers, humidifiers and respirators, as well as effluent air from vacuum cleaners.

Air Sampling as a Quality Control Measure

Probably the greatest role for air sampling in today's hospital is assigned to the assessment of techniques and procedures aimed at the reduction of airborne microorganisms. It starts in the clinical laboratories, e.g., to monitor exhaust systems over specimen processing areas, the performance of aerosol-preventing devices in centrifuges or to find sources of contamination in controlled environments. Recently, air sampling helped us to trace the continued aspergillus contamination of tissue cultures in a research laboratory to a contaminated filter inside the air-CO_2 mixing unit of an incubator.

Air sampling has been used for many years to monitor the efficacy of disinfection procedures for respiratory therapy equipment. Ryan and Mihalyi[21] recently evaluated the Aerotest Sampler, a device used to test aerosols generated by respirators. It is similar to the funnel-tube method of Edmonton and Sanford[22] and the styrofoam cup method of Nazemi et al.[23]

The evaluation of air conditioning and air-filtering devices by air sampling is practiced widely. Unfortunately, no standards have been set that may be applied to all health care institutions. Shaffer's[24] experience suggests that in his hospital, using a slit sampler, average levels of 5-15 CFU/ft³ air can be achieved. Various studies have suggested that air in operating rooms should have not more than 1-3 CFU/ft³.[25] Whether or not such suggested levels have any influence on infection rate is unknown. If air sampling is used by an infection control committee to assess the quality of hospital air, one must develop individual, hospital-accepted standards. However, such studies should not lead to meaningless routine sampling schedules.[26] Once baseline values have been established, it is simple to assess the performance of air conditioning and air-filtering installations after major repairs or alterations.

Special considerations deserve clean rooms used for patient isolation during periods of high susceptibility to infection such as used in cancer, transplant and other specialty centers. Here routine air sampling is often performed to assess the effect of antimicrobial measures on the body surfaces and in the environment.

Methods of Air-Sampling in Hospitals

Over the years, a number of air-sampling methods have been applied to the study of airborne microorganisms in hospitals.

The average size of airborne viable microbial particles in hospital wards is 13 μ, about one-third are larger than 18 μ and 7% less than 4 μ.[27] Whereas the larger particles will settle out, very small droplet nuclei ($\sim 3\mu$) may be suspended indefinitely in dry air. Depending on the aims of a study, the investigator must select a collection device which will allow him the recovery of all particles of interest.

Four types of air-sampling have been useful for hospital studies: sedimentation, impaction, filtration, and precipitation. The ideal sampler of aerosols should count all living airborne particles per unit volume of air, the viable units per particle and the size of particles containing such units. Such an ideal unit would require 100% sampling efficiency, no loss of viability, and an ideal medium for recovery of damaged microorganisms.[28] As a general rule, sedimentation plates and solid phase impactors will rarely break up particles (with the possible exception of shearing forces of slits or sieves in vacuum aspirators), whereas liquid impactors or impingers may allow the dispersal and break up of larger particles. For practical use in hospitals, air samplers should have short collection times.

Sedimentation

The average particle in hospital air (13 μ) settles at a rate of about one foot per minute. Thus, an agar surface in a 100 mm petri dish (approximately $\frac{1}{15}$ ft²) will collect particles from 1 ft³ of stagnant air in 15 min by sedimentation due to normal gravity.[27] However, airflows in its immediate vicinity greatly influence the delivery of particles to the agar surface. This method of sampling is inexpensive, used widely, and gives information about particles containing viable microorganisms settling onto surfaces but it says little about smaller droplet nuclei.

Impaction

Centrifugal forces or vacuum have been used to impact smaller particles on solid, semisolid or liquid-film surfaces. Numerous instruments have been designed and only the most commonly used shall be mentioned here.

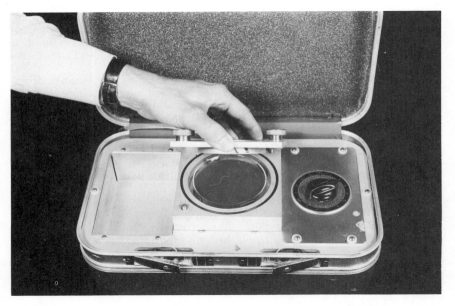

FIGURE 1. Microban Sieve Air Sampler, Ross Industries, Inc., Midland, Virginia.

Vacuum Aspiration–Impaction

The slit sampler (Reyniers, Casella and New Brunswick Scientific Co.) have been widely used in this country and abroad. In these devices, air is aspirated by vacuum through a slit and the airborne particles are impacted onto an agar surface. Each viable particle or droplet nucleus will form a colony which may contain one or more microorganisms. With large concentrations of airborne particles viable nuclei may be superimposed on one another.

The stacked sieve sampler of Andersen which is available in 8, 6 and 2-stage models is useful for low concentration in airborne bacteria and for determining the size distribution of airborne particles.[27-29] A recent study by Curtis et al.[30]

showed that the 2-stage disposable unit which is supposed to separate particles usually deposited in the upper or the lower respiratory tract generally gave lower counts than the 8-stage model.

The disadvantage of these units is the need for a separate vacuum unit and, if the vacuum pump is incorporated in the sampler, its size and weight.

A recent development by Ross Industries, the Microban sieve sampler, is less bulky and easily portable. Like the other vacuum impactors, the sampler is an electric safety hazard in operating rooms during inhalation anesthesia.

Centrifugal Force Impaction

The Wells Air Centrifuge was described almost 50 years ago and is rarely used today. A recently developed German device, the Reuter centrifugal air sampler (sold as Biotest RCS centrifugal sampler in this country) is of the size of a large flashlight and powered by batteries. A centrifugal impeller samples 1.4 ft³ per minute of air and impacts particles on an agar strip. This sampler has been studied in West Germany[31,32] and was found to compare well with other air-sampling methods.

Filtration

Collection of airborne particles by filtration may be achieved by the use of solid filters, soluble materials and liquids. For large volume collection, liquids

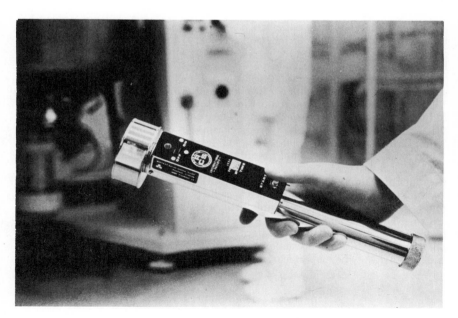

FIGURE 2. Biotest Reuter Centrifugal Sampler (RCS), Folex–Biotest–Schleussner, Inc., Moonachie, New Jersey.

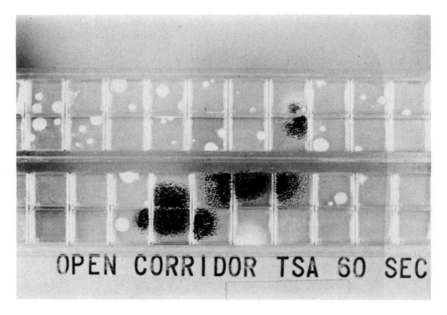

FIGURE 3. Biotest RCS Agar Strips with Microbial Colonies.

are most suitable. One may either use a bubbler at low air velocity, a high velocity impinger[33] or an air scrubber.[34] Except for special studies such as contamination of respiratory therapy equipment (Edmonton and Sanford[22]) filtration with liquids is rarely used in hospitals.

On the other hand, sampling of airborne bacteria and fungi with solid or soluble filters is quite popular, especially in Europe. Rotter and colleagues of Vienna reported on the use of gelatine air filters[35,36] and the development of a fully-automated sampling apparatus.[37] The previously mentioned studies with the Reuter centrifugal sampler were performed in comparison with the German Sartorius filter sampler.[31,32] Fields et al.[38] in this country tested the performance of a membrane filter (0.45 μ) field monitor for microbiological air sampling and found that it detected about 79% of the colony-forming units obtained with the Reyniers air sampler. Johnston et al.[39] described their studies of settling plates and Nucleopore filters contained in a Casella personal dust sampler in comparison with a six-stage Andersen sampler in a closed room housing experimental animals. The filter and sieve samplers gave comparable results with the settling plates being less sensitive. Filter samplers may influence the survival of airborne microorganisms due to impaction and drying-out. Also, pore sizes commonly used (4-4.5 μ) may be too large to retain certain viable particles.

Precipitation

Except for research projects, precipitation samplers using thermal or electrostatic forces are not useful for hospitals. For the recovery of rare pathogens from natural aerosols, large volume samplers have been used such as the Litton sampler which collects up to 10,000 liters of air per minute and electrostatically precipitates particles onto a thin-flowing film of collecting fluid.[28]

Example of Comparative Air-Sampling

During 1976 and 1977, the Infection Control Service of the University of Texas System Cancer Center, Houston, conducted studies of airborne microorganisms with two new air-samplers, the Reuter centrifugal sampler (Biotest RCS) and the Ross Microban sieve sampler, comparing them to the Casella slit sampler. Air samples were obtained in wards, operating rooms, intensive care units, support areas, laboratories and animal quarters. The following volumes of air were collected per minute: 1 ft^3 with the Casella; 0.7 ft^3 with the Ross; and 1.4 ft^3 with the Reuter samplers. The air intake areas of the samplers were positioned on a cart at the same height above the floor about 2–3 ft apart. Data obtained from 131 parallel 2 min sampling periods were analyzed.

TABLE 1 shows that the overall performance of the samplers was comparable. However, when individual test samples were compared, often considerable differences were noted. Some of the more obvious differences are shown in TABLE 2. For example, in areas with counts in the lower range (<20 CFU/ft^3) the centrifugal sampler often showed higher counts than the vacuum samplers. On the other hand, the vacuum sampler counts were higher in areas of high microbial load. This could be explained by the assumption that larger particles are broken up in passing through the slit or hole. Beck and Wille[31] found that in areas of low microbial load (<20 CFU/ft^3) the centrifugal sampler showed higher counts than the Sartorius filter sampler. They speculated that the Reuter sampler may have a more constant air flow than a sampler connected to a vacuum pump. Sequential sampling with the centrifugal sampler in areas served by the same air-handling unit and with a similar activity showed reproducible results and clear changes with any procedure known to generate airborne particles. For example, air samples were obtained in the post-operative care unit before and during the change of bed linen. Before changing the bedding, the count was 4.5 CFU/ft^3; when the linen was removed, 33 CFU/ft,^{3} and when the new linen was applied, 15 CFU/ft.^{3}

TABLE 1

COMPARISON OF DATA OBTAINED FROM 131 PARALLEL AIR SAMPLES USING THE CASELLA SLIT SAMPLER, THE ROSS MICROBAN SIEVE SAMPLER AND THE BIOTEST REUTER CENTRIFUGAL SAMPLER

	Colony Forming Units per ft^3‡		Standard Error*	Significance of Differences†
	Mean	Range		
Casella	11.1	O-TNTC‡ (>64)	±1.96	N.S.
Ross	10.7	O-TNTC (>91)	±2.72	N.S.
Reuter	11.4	0-109	±2.41	N.S.

*95% confidence limit.
†N.S. = Not significant.
‡TNTC = Too numerous to count.

TABLE 2

SAMPLE DATA OBTAINED IN VARIOUS AREAS (IN CFU/FT^3)

Area	Room	Activity	Samples	Casella	Ross	Reuter
Exp. Surgery	I	None	2	4	1.9	0.7
	II	None	2	1.5	2	1.7
P.O.C.U.	M.I.	Pt. care	8	8.5	4.5	10
		Pt. transfer	4	4.2	5.5	12
Pt. Rooms	W315	None	3	9	8	15
		Cleaning	3	19	12	16
	W308	Empty	2	9	9	8
		Dry mopping	1	50	71	34
	E205	Bedding changed	1	14	13	27
	E207	Dry mopping	1	47	40	70
Clinic	10/11	Very active	2	8.5	4.5	13
	50	Active	2	7.5	5.5	13
Kitchen	Dishes	Active	2	7.7	9.5	6.2
Nurses Stations	L5	Quiet	2	1.4	4.2	2.5
Animal Area	Hall	Normal	4	38	20	28
	Hall	Cage cleaning	4	32	42	22.5

Differences were also noted between the counts obtained by the Casella and Ross samplers. A detailed analysis of discrepancies between sampling devices was beyond the scope of our study. With the absence of standards for airborne viable microorganisms in hospitals small differences in efficacy of air-sampling devices are acceptable. In the hospital setting, versatility and practicability of a sampler are of greatest importance. The Ross Microban sampler is much lighter and smaller than the slit samplers. However, it requires an electric power source. In contrast, the Biotest RCS centrifugal sampler is independent of an electric outlet, is easy to use, almost noiseless and allows sampling in hard-to-reach areas. My colleagues and I have used this instrument over a three-year period and consider it to be the most useful for epidemiologic and quality control studies of hospital air.

SUMMARY

Air sampling in hospitals is performed for the epidemiologic investigation of nosocomial infections, for the elucidation of spread and control of airborne microorganisms, for assessing biohazards associated with instruments, equipment and procedures and for controlling the performance of devices and techniques used for the reduction of airborne contaminants. Many different air-sampling devices are available but only a few have found use in hospitals. Certain samplers are used for special studies such as the Andersen stacked-sieve impactor or the liquid impingers. Lately, samplers have been developed which due to their size and weight are more useful to the hospital microbiologist and epidemiologist than the older slit samplers. The Ross Microban sieve sampler and the Biotest Reuter Centrifugal Sampler were tested in comparison with the Casella slit sampler and found to show comparable results. The hand-held, battery-operated Biotest RCS sample is the most versatile for general sampling of hospital air.

REFERENCES

1. BRACHMAN, P. S. 1971. Nosocomial infection—airborne or not? Proceedings of the International Conference on Nosocomial Infection. Center for Disease Control. August 3-6, 1970. American Hospital Association, Chicago.
2. RILEY, R. L. 1972. Editorial. The ecology of indoor atmosphere: Airborne infection in hospitals. J. Chron. Dis. 25: 421-423.
3. WALTER, C. W. & R. B. KUNDSIN. 1973. The airborne component of wound contamination and infection. Arch. Surg. 107: 588-595.
4. MUIR, D. C. F., 1972. Clinical Aspects of Inhaled Particles. F. A. Davis. Philadelphia.
5. LISTER, J. 1868. An address on the antiseptic system of treatment in surgery. Brit. Med. J. 2: 53.
6. TYNDALL, J. 1882. Essays on the Floating Matter of the Air in Relation to Putrefaction and Infection. D. Appleton & Co., New York.
7. FINDEISEN, W. 1935. Über das Absetzen kleiner, in der Luft suspendierter Teilchen in der menschlichen Lunge bei der Atmung. Pflüger's Arch. ges. Physiol. 236: 367.
8. NOBLE, W. C. & R. R. DAVIES. 1965. Studies on the dispersal of staphylococci. J. Clin. Path. 18: 16-19.
9. WENZEL, R. P., J. M. VEAZEY & T. R. TOWNSEND. 1977. Role of the environment in hospital-acquired infections. In Infection Control in Health Care Facilities: Microbiological Surveillance. K. R. Cundy & W. Ball, Eds. University Park Press. Baltimore.
10. AMERICAN HOSPITAL ASSOCIATION. 1974. Statement on microbiologic sampling in the hospital. Hospitals 48: 125-126.
11. AMERICAN PUBLIC HEALTH ASSOCIATION. 1975. Environmental microbiologic sampling in the hospital. Health Lab. Sci. 12: 234-235.
12. MALLISON, G. F. 1977. Monitoring of sterility and environmental sampling in programs for control of nosocomial infections. In Infection Control in Health Care Facilities: Microbiological Surveillance. K. R. Cundy & W. Ball, Eds. University Park Press. Baltimore.
13. KUNDSIN, R. B. 1977. Microbiological monitoring of the hospital environment. In Infection Control in Health Care Facilities: Microbiological Surveillance. K. R. Cundy & W. Ball, Eds. University Park Press. Baltimore.
14. HERS, J. F. Ph. & K. C. WINKLER, Eds. 1973. Airborne Transmission and Airborne Infection. John Wiley & Sons. New York.
15. GUNDERMANN, K. O. 1974. Die Keimbelastung in verschiedenen Krankenhausbereichen. Zentralbl. Bakt. Org. B 159: 231-243.
16. ROTTER, M., M. KUNZE & A. A. MESCHKAT. 1974. Der Einfluss von Teppichböden auf den Keimgehalt der Luft. Zentralbl. Bakt. Org. A 227: 532-541.
17. BAKKER, P. G. H. & J. L. FAOAGALI. 1977. The effect of carpet on the number of microbes in the hospital environment. N. Z. Med. J. 85: 88-92.
18. PETERSON, N. J., W. W. BOND, J. H. MARSHALL, M. S. FAVERO & L. RAIJ. 1976. An air sampling technique for hepatitis B surface antigen. Health Lab. Sci. 13: 233-237.
19. STERN, E. L., J. W. JOHNSON, D. VESLEY, M. M. HALBERT, L. E. WILLIAMS & P. BLUME. 1974. Aerosol production associated with clinical laboratory procedures. Am. J. Clin. Pathol. 62: 591-600.
20. TURNER, A. G., J. R. WILKINS & J. G. CRADDOCK. 1975. Bacterial aerosolization from an ultrasonic cleaner. J. Clin. Microbiol. 1: 289-293.
21. RYAN, K. J. & S. F. MIHALYI. 1977. Evaluation of a simple device for bacteriological sampling of respirator-generated aerosols. J. Clin. Microbiol. 5: 178-183.
22. EDMONSON, E. B. & J. P. SANFORD. 1966. Simple method of bacteriologic sampling of nebulization equipment. Am. Rev. Respir. Dis. 94: 450-453.
23. NAZEMI, M. M., D. M. MUSHER & R. R. MARTIN. 1972. A practical method for monitoring bacterial contamination of inhalation therapy machines. Am. Rev. Respir. Dis. 106: 920-922.
24. SHAFFER, T. G. 1974. Environmental monitoring in a community hospital. Health Lab. Sci. 11: 293-298.

25. GALSON, E. & K. R. GODDARD. 1968. Hospital air conditioning and sepsis control. Am. Soc. Heating, Refrigerating and Air Conditioning Engineers J. **10:** 33–41.
26. EICKHOFF, T. C. 1974. Microbiologic sampling of the hospital environment. Health Lab. Sci. **11:** 73–75.
27. BARTLETT, R. C., J. V. BENNETT, R. A. WEISTEIN & G. F. MALLISON. 1979. The microbiology laboratory: Its role in surveillance, investigation, and control. *In* Hospital Infections. J. V. Bennett & P. S. Brachman, Eds., Little, Brown & Co. Boston, Mass.
28. AKERS, A. B. & W. D. WON. 1969. Assay of living, airborne microorganisms. *In* An Introduction to Experimental Aerobiology. R. L. Dimmick & A. B. Akers, Eds. Wiley-Interscience. New York, N.Y.
29. AMERICAN CONFERENCE OF GOVERNMENTAL INDUSTRIAL HYGIENISTS. 1962. Air Sampling Instruments. 2nd Edit., ACGIC. Cincinnati, O.
30. CURTIS, S. E., R. K. BALSBAUGH & J. G. DRUMMOND. 1978. Comparison of Andersen 8-stage and 2-stage viable air samplers. Appl. Environ. Microbiol. **35:** 208–209.
31. BECK, E. G. & B. WILLE. 1977. Vergleichende Untersuchungen an zwei Luftkeimsammelgeräten. Hyg. & Med. **2:** 361–364.
32. SONNTAG, G. H., V. HINGST & H. GÄRTNER. 1979. Luftkeimmessungen im Krankenhaus. Hyg. & Med. **4:** 177–181.
33. LIPSCOMB, B. & K. E. AVIS. 1979. Aerobiological model for assessing microbial contamination. J. Parent. Drug Assoc. **33:** 3–16.
34. WHITE, L. A., D. J. HADLEY, D. E. DAVIDS & R. NAYLOR. 1975. Improved large-volume sampler for the collection of bacterial cells from aerosol. Appl. Microbiol. **29:** 335–339.
35. ROTTER, M. & W. KOLLER. 1973. Sammlung von Luftkeimen mit Gelatinefiltern. Zentralbl. Bakt. Orig. B **157:** 257–270.
36. KOLLER, W. & M. ROTTER. 1974. Weitere Untersuchunger über die Eignung von Gelatinefiltern zur Sammlung von Luftkeimen. Zentralbl. Bakt. Orig. B **159:** 546–559.
37. RESCH, W., J. SCHEDLING, J. WANIEK, H. FLAMM & M. ROTTER. 1973. Vollautomatische Sammlung von Luftkeimen mittels eines Filtergeräts. Zeutralbl. Bakt. Orig. B **158:** 206–218.
38. FIELDS, N. B., G. S. O. X. BORROW, J. R. PULEO & C. M. HERRING. 1974. Evaluation of membrane filter field monitors for microbiological air sampling. Appl. Microbiol. **27:** 517–520.
39. JOHNSTON, J. R., A. M. BUTCHART & S. J. KGAMPHE. 1978. A comparison of sampling methods for airborne bacteria. Environ. Res. **16:** 279–284.

TECHNIQUES USED FOR SAMPLING AIRBORNE
MICROORGANISMS ASSOCIATED WITH INDUSTRIAL
CLEAN ROOMS AND SPACECRAFT ASSEMBLY AREAS

Martin S. Favero

Hepatitis Laboratories Division
Bureau of Epidemiology Center for Disease Control
U.S. Public Health Service
Phoenix, Arizona 85014

John R. Puleo

Planetary Protection Laboratory
Jet Propulsion Laboratory
Cape Canaveral, Florida

Introduction

For the past 20 years one of the principal objectives of the space science programs of the National Aeronautics and Space Administration (NASA) has been to determine whether life exists or has existed on other planets. In the 1960s the NASA decided in conjunction with other space-launching countries[1,2] that spacecraft destined to impact planets of biological interest, such as Mars, should not introduce viable terrestrial microorganisms. In those years there was a scientific consensus that the introduction of terrestrial microorganisms might result in devastating growth that would profoundly alter indigenous extraterrestrial environments. Further, contamination with terrestrial microorganisms could preclude demonstration of the existence of extraterrestrial life by confusing sensitive life detection equipment on automated spacecraft.

Although a number of physical and chemical decontaminating procedures were considered for reducing or eliminating microbial contamination associated with spacecraft and their components,[2] it was decided early on that the most applicable procedure was dry heat. Since this sterilization procedure was to be employed it was reasoned that the probability of obtaining a sterile spacecraft was enhanced significantly if the level of microbial contamination, especially bacterial spores, was relatively low prior to the sterilization process. Accordingly, it was decided that spacecraft requiring sterilization should be assembled and tested in areas where microbial contamination could be maintained at an extremely low level.

The purpose of this paper is to discuss: 1) the various techniques which were used to establish levels of airborne microorganisms in a variety of spacecraft assembly areas; 2) the comparative levels of airborne contamination in these areas from both quantitative and qualitative standpoints; 3) the unique application of some of these procedures for predicting the level of microbial contamination on surfaces of space hardware; and 4) techniques which were used to collect naturally occurring airborne spores to determine their dry heat resistance and ultimately to verify the proposed sterilization cycles.

0077–8923/80/0353–0241 $01.75/0 © 1980, NYAS

Microbiologic Profiles of Spacecraft Assembly Areas

Since a primary objective for spacecraft requiring sterilization was to maintain levels of microbial contamination on and in space hardware at a level as low as possible, it was initially thought techniques used for elimination of particulate contamination in industrial clean rooms and airborne microorganisms in surgical suites might apply to spacecraft assembly areas. It soon became apparent that from a microbiologic standpoint the use of existing technology for controlling airborne contamination in surgical suites had little application to spacecraft contamination requirements since surgical suites contained much higher levels of particulate, as well as microbiologic airborne contamination than some of the more sophisticated industrial clean rooms.

Starting in 1965, investigators at the Jet Propulsion Laboratory, Pasadena, California; the University of Minnesota, Minneapolis, Minnesota; and the United States Public Health Service's Center for Disease Control, Phoenix, Arizona began a coordinated study to determine the levels of microbial contamination present in the intramural environments of 17 different spacecraft facilities located in three geographical areas in the United States. Volumetric air sampling was performed using slit samplers (Reyniers and Sons, Chicago, Illinois) which were loaded with tryptic soy agar. Cultures were incubated at 32°C for 72 hours. Colonies were counted and in some instances picked and identified. Data were expressed as the number of viable particles per cubic foot of air.

A simple but unique technique was devised by workers at the United States Army Biological Laboratories at Fort Detrick, Maryland[3] for determining the level of airborne microorganisms which accumulated on surfaces. The technique consisted of placing a series of 1 by 2 inch sterile, stainless steel strips in an area for relatively long periods of time, i.e., several weeks to one year. At intervals, a number of stainless steel strips were retrieved, subjected to a rinse procedure[4] and assayed for viable microorganisms as well as bacterial spores.[5-7] There were several interesting characteristics associated with this particular assay technique. First, all investigators noted the existence of a "plateau phenomenon." This meant that the levels of microbial contamination resulting from fallout of airborne microorganisms onto stainless steel surfaces did not increase significantly during the relatively long exposure periods of up to 21 weeks. After 1–2 weeks the level of microorganisms per square foot of surface for a particular intramural environment would remain the same. In fact, one study showed that stainless steel surfaces exposed to the intramural air of an industrial clean room for one week contained the same level of microorganisms per square foot as those exposed for 52 weeks.[3] It is emphasized that this plateau phenomenon is most likely the result of a dynamic rather than a static system and one that is influenced by multiple factors. The most plausible explanation for the plateau is that the number of microorganisms deposited on or surviving on surfaces is balanced by the number of microorganisms dying or being removed by physical forces from the same surface. In any event this assay system was used to determine significant differences in microbial contamination levels between industrial clean rooms whose personnel practices and air handling practices differed greatly. Further, it was shown that the stainless steel collecting technique was a much more sensitive and reliable method for assessing airborne microbial contamination in an industrial clean room than was the use of volumetric air samplers.[5]

Some of the typical data that were obtained in these studies are shown in

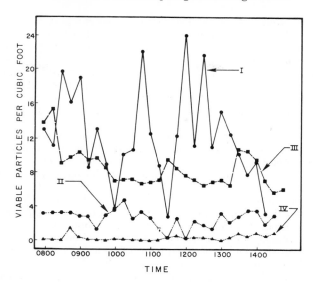

FIGURE 1. Typical comparative levels of airborne contamination among a surgical suite (I), a conventional industrial clean room (II), a manufacturing-factory area (III), and a horizontal laminar flow clean room (IV).

FIGURE 1. These were data obtained by the use of volumetric air samplers and represent the comparative levels of airborne microbial contamination in a conventional hospital surgical suite (I), a conventional industrial clean room (II), a manufacturing area where personnel, clothing, and efficient air handling constraints were not practiced (III), and a horizontal laminar flow clean room (IV). As can be seen, much higher levels of airborne microorganisms were obtained in the surgical suite than in the industrial clean rooms. In some cases the number of airborne viable particles per cubic foot of air was higher in the surgical suites than in a conventional manufacturing area and other controlled areas such as hospital corridors. Lowest levels occurred in the horizontal laminar flow clean room–an observation which was confirmed many times in the succeeding years. In laminar or unidirectional flow clean rooms whether the airflow be horizontal or vertical the variables of personnel activity and density had considerably less effect than in conventional industrial clean rooms and surgical suites. In the latter areas highest levels of airborn contamination were directly associated with high personnel density and activity. Further, in surgical suites or industrial clean rooms personnel density practices as well as the use of protective clothing significantly determine the types of microorganisms found in air as determined by volumetric slit samplers. For example in manufacturing areas and most of the hospital surgical suites studied approximately 60–75% of the microorganisms detected were those associated with soil and dust, such as bacterial sporeformers, fungi, and actinomycetes. The remainder were vegetative microorganisms which are normally associated with humans (i.e., from human hair, skin, or the respiratory tract). In contrast these microbiologic profiles were significantly different in those industrial clean rooms where personnel access, density and clothing were rigorously controlled. In these area 70–90% of the microorganisms detected in air were vegetative microorganisms, normally associated with humans and the remaining group were microorganisms associated with dust and soil (TABLE 1). In the case of laminar flow clean rooms there were so few microorganisms detected that one could not reliably establish a microbiologic profile; however, almost all of the microorganisms detected in the air of laminar flow clean rooms were vegetative bacteria normally considered to be of human origin.

FIGURE 2 shows typical data obtained by the use of stainless steel collecting surfaces. These particular data[8] were obtained in spacecraft assembly-areas located at Cape Kennedy, Florida and used for the assembly of the Surveyor and Apollo spacecrafts. After two weeks of exposure the levels of microorganisms per square foot of surface do not differ, from a statistically significant standpoint, from levels obtained from after as long as 10 weeks and in other studies 21 weeks or longer. When the types of microorganisms which accumulated on stainless steel surfaces were identified it was found that environments which were strictly controlled in terms of personnel density, clothing and access not only had less organisms per square foot but also the types of organisms were primarily those (approximately 70%) associated with humans rather than dust and soil. On the other hand, in manufacturing areas, hospital surgical suites, and industrial clean rooms where minimal constraints on personnel density and clothing were practiced the vast majority of microorganisms found were fungi, bacterial sporeformers and other organisms associated with soil, and levels of microorganisms accumulating per square foot were high. It was concluded that the fallout assay procedure was able to detect gross differences in environmental contamination, for example between manufacturing areas and highly controlled industrial clean rooms. In fact, the sensitivity and reliability of this assay procedure was reported to be best in an ultraclean environment.[5] In this study, it was shown that stainless steel colleting strips placed in a horizontal laminar flow clean room for several weeks showed no microorganisms until there was a failure of the air handling system for several hours. In all probability volumetric air samplers would not have adequately detected this failure.

TABLE 1

TYPES OF AEROBIC MESOPHILIC MICROORGANISMS DETECTED IN THE INTRAMURAL AIR OF TWO HOSPITAL SURGICAL SUITES AND TWO INDUSTRIAL CLEAN ROOMS

Site	Vegetative Microorganisms Associated with Humans* (%)	Bacterial Sporeformers, Fungi, Actinomycetes, and Other Microorganisms Associated with Soil and Dust (%)
Hospital A	26	74
Hospital B	36	64
Clean room A	69	28
Clean room B	92	6

*Staphylococcus spp., Micrococcus spp., Corynebacterium-Brevibacterium group, and Streptococcus spp.

Laminar Flow Systems

Since it was the space program that basically was responsible for the use of laminar flow systems in conjunction with the control of microbial contamination, brief mention will be made of the use of this system in spacecraft sterilization and its application to the general field of microbiology. The evolution of design and operational concepts of laminar or unidirectional flow systems has been multi-faceted and was influenced initially by contamination problems associated with certain industrial processes. The aerospace and electronics industries became aware of the need to eliminate airborne contaminants such as dust, lint and fibers from many different types of instruments. As miniaturized electronics and precisioned instrumentation developed, need for contamination control in many cases became an absolute requirement. The first environmentally controlled areas were referred to as "white rooms" and/or "clean rooms" and were defined as enclosed areas employing control over the particulate matter of air with temperature, humidity and pressure control as required. For some assembly operations these conventional clean rooms were adequate. However, the major problem of eliminating air contaminants to a degree sufficient to assure continuous surface cleanliness was still not solved because air flow patterns in many clean room areas were nonuniform and turbulent. As a result eddy currents and static areas developed which often caused an increase in contamination due to an accumulation of particulates and recycling turbulent air on exposed surfaces.

In 1962 Willis Whitfield at the Sandia Corporation, Albuquerque, New Mexico developed the first laminar air flow clean room. His principle, although quite simple, was extremely effective. Large volumes of air were introduced into

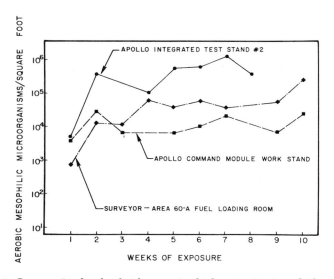

FIGURE 2. Comparative levels of airborne microbial contamination which accumulated on stainless steel surfaces exposed to the intramural environment of two Apollo spacecraft assembly areas and the fuel loading room used for the Surveyor spacecraft.

a room through a bank of ultra-high efficiency filters,[9] commonly referred to as HEPA filters. Since this filter bank acted as a large diffuser, it reduced the velocity of supply air considerably and produced a uniform air flow which travelled with a minimum of turbulence. The exhaust system consisted of a series of grills equal in size to the inlet diffuser. Air flow could be from wall to the opposite wall, ceiling to floor, or wall to floor. The air made one uniform pass through the room travelling at approximately 100 feet per minute. Airborne contaminants were removed almost as fast as they were produced. In addition, clean items kept upstream from the source of contamination remained free of contaminants. As a result, personnel restrictions with respect to clothing and clean room access could be markedly reduced as were maintenance costs.

Since this first operational implementation by Whitfield,[10] laminar flow air systems have been incorporated into a variety of configurations to meet the demands of specific contamination control requirements. For example,there are: 1) vertical laminar flow clean rooms (ceiling to floor), 2) horizontal laminar flow (wall to wall or wall to floor), 3) laminar flow tunnels (wall to open end of tunnel), 4) vertical laminar flow curtain units (portable units, ceiling to ungrilled floor to surrounding area, 5) laminar flow cabinets (horizontal or vertical flow, both designed for product protection), 6) laminar flow biologically safety cabinets (usually incorporates vertical flow and a filtered exhaust and is designed for both product and personnel protection).

As early as 1964 it was recognized that laminar flow systems might be used effectively in the control of airborne microbial contamination. As mentioned earlier, the Planetary Quarantine Office at NASA was in the process of evaluating by means of its research groups at Jet Propulsion Laboratory, University of Minnesota and Center for Disease Control, Phoenix, a variety of conventional clean rooms for possible use in the assembly and testing of spacecraft required to be dry heat sterilized. Early investigations[3,5,7,11] showed that very few viable microorganisms could be detected in any type of laminar flow clean room. Indeed the air was so devoid of microorganisms that the assay techniques associated with these studies had to be significantly modified. For example, air and surface samples taken in laminar flow clean rooms could not be processed in conventional microbiology laboratories because the level of background contamination was significantly higher than that of the clean room. Consequently, the probability of airborne microorganisms contaminating the assay medium to a significant degree was relatively high. Subsequently, it was shown that these types of assays could be done reliably only when all tests and manipulations were performed themselves in a laminar air flow system.[12-14] It was further shown that the level of microbial contamination which accumulated on surfaces as determined by stainless steel collecting surfaces usually never exceeded 10^2 microorganisms per square foot and was usually less then 50 organisms per square foot when microorganisms were detected at all. Virtually, no airborne microorganisms could be detected in vertical and horizontal laminar flow rooms when samplers were placed upstream from personnel. Even when personnel and density activity were high and samplers were placed downstream from personnel the maximum level of viable particles per cubic foot of air was about 1–2 in horizontal laminar flow clean rooms. Under similar circumstances in vertical laminar flow clean rooms it was not uncommon to detect less than 5–10 viable particles per 100 cubic feet of air. These contamination levels were several orders of magnitude lower than those obtained in conventional clean rooms and surgical suites.

At the same time of this development in the field of spacecraft sterilization, the pharmaceutical industries in the United States began to investigate the use of laminar flow cabinets as a clean environment in which sterility tests and aseptic filling operations could be performed. The occurrence of false positive sterility tests due to background contamination had often necessitated resterilization of entire batches of commercial products.[15] It was found that by using the laminar flow concept either on a cabinet or room system the problem of background microbial contamination was virtually eliminated and as a result sterility testing and aseptic fill operations were revolutionized, the result being that today virtually all of these types of operations, not only in the United States but also in many countries of the world, are performed using laminar flow systems. In addition, laminar flow cabinets designed for product protection or laminar flow biological safety cabinets have become commonplace in laboratories throughout the world. It was predicted in 1970[14] that history would view the use of laminar air flow systems for microbiologists as a fairly significant development in the field of biological contamination control. But there was a caution offered: it would be unfortunate if this advancement was accompanied by a period of confusion due to a misunderstanding of the principals of laminar air flow. This has happened in the past with the indiscriminate use of antibiotics and certain disinfectants. The laminar air flow system when designed and operated properly will either protect a product or personnel or both. It obviously will not sterilize, decontaminate or disinfect surfaces or liquids nor will it eliminate microbial contamination that is due to direct contact.

Methods for Determining the Thermal Resistance of Naturally Occurring Bacterial Spores

As was previously mentioned, the sterilization procedure that was chosen for spacecraft was dry heat. The temperature ranges were quite different than are used in hospitals and laboratories (i.e., 170–190°C) and due to the relative heat sensitivity of spacecraft parts temperatures of 110–125°C were considered for the dry heat sterilization cycles. Initially the various dry heat sterilization cycles for spacecraft were based on the thermal inactivation characteristics of *Bacillus subtilis* var. *niger* (*B. globgii*) spores. The assumption was made that this organism could be used as an index of the dry heat resistance of spores found on spacecraft. However, the existing data in the literature pointed out that *B. subtilis* var. *niger* spores had never been detected on spacecraft.[8,16-18] In fact, it had been shown[16,19] that naturally occurring bacterial spores in soil are significantly more resistant to dry heat than *B. subtilis* var. *niger* and that subcultured spores are often more sensitive to dry heat than naturally occurring spores. In addition, it was found that bacterial spores isolated from the surfaces of actual flight spacecraft can be significantly more heat resistant than *B. subtilis* var. *niger* spores even when these isolates are subcultured. It was finally suggested[16,19] that naturally occurring airborne spores associated with spacecraft and their assembly areas should constitute the index population rather than *B. subtilis* var. *niger*.

We found that it was virtually impossible to collect spores directly from spacecraft surfaces in sufficient numbers to be used for dry heat resistance studies. Several methods had been evaluated for collecting large numbers of spores from air: membrane filters, large volume air samplers, vacuum cleaner dust, and extraction from prefilters in ventilation systems. These techniques proved to be unsuccessful. In 1975 we reported on a study which described the evaluation of a method developed by M. Wardle of the Jet Propulsion Laboratory, by which large numbers of naturally occurring airborne spores were collected on Teflon ribbon surfaces and subsequently exposed to a thermal treatment to determine the resistance of the heterogenous airborne spores population. The basic technique involved exposing three-inch (17.8 cm) wide and six-foot (188 cm) long Teflon ribbons to pertinent spacecraft assembly areas at the Kennedy Space Center, Florida in the same manner that was used for stainless steel collecting services described earlier. It was determined that within 1–2 weeks a "plateau" of airborne microbial contaminants accumulating on these Teflon surfaces was achieved. After a suitable period of exposure the ribbons were aseptically collected, exposed to a controlled dry heat environment at various temperatures, and subsequently assayed.

This technique for the first time offered a method by which the actual dry heat inactivation rates of naturally occurring airborne spores could be determined and directly applied to a sterilization cycle of an item which constituted a real indicator of resistance rather than one that was artificial or based on an index organism. These results prompted further studies which culminated in a procedure that could be used to verify the actual sterilization cycle utilized for the terminal dry heat decontamination of the Mars bound Viking spacecraft.[21]

We suspect that this method could be used to great advantage by the pharmaceutical industry who in the last few years are required by the Food and Drug Administration to verify various sterilization cycles and to take into consideration the level of microbial contamination on the products prior to sterilization.

Other Air Sampling Techniques

One of the continuing goals of microbiologists involved in determining levels of microbial contamination on spacecraft as well as the environments in which they were assembled was the development of tests which could almost instantaneously determine gross levels of contamination. For example, it was thought that if one could document a consistent and predictable relationship between the concentration of total versus viable particles suspended in intramural air one could then instantaneously and reliably predict the level of viable particulate contamination. Such a study was reported in 1974.[22] The numbers of viable and total particles in a microbiology laboratory and in the Manned Spacecraft Operations Building (MSOP) at Kennedy Space Center were examined for a predictable relationship to aid in the monitoring of airborne microbial contamination. Six-stage Andersen air samplers were used to enumerate and size airborne viable particles and a modified Royco total particle counter was used to enumerate total particles. It was found that over 99% of the total particles present in both environmental areas were less than one micrometer in size. However, only 1 in 10,000 of the particles in this size range were viable. At the other end of the particle size scale, it was found that less than 0.1% of the total particles were greater than 5.4 micrometers in size, but only 4.5% of these particles were viable. These data are illustrated in FIGURE 3 and 4. It was apparent that viable particles make up only a very small portion of the total particles making any correlation undetectable. An analysis of the combined data from both environmental areas using only total and viable particles over 5.4 micrometers tended to show a positive correlation. However, analysis of the data from each area individually showed no correlation. Consequently, it was concluded that although the estima-

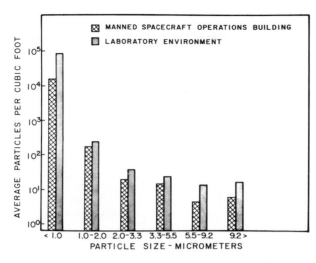

FIGURE 3. Particle size distribution for total particles in two test areas.

tion of viable particulates from enumeration of total particulates in the relatively larger particle ranges is possible under limited conditions, the method could not be recommended for areas where large numbers of non-viable particles are being generated by processes not directly related to personnel activity.

Another air sampling innovation that was developed for use in spacecraft assembly areas was the use of conventional membrane filters for sampling

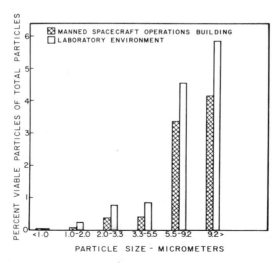

FIGURE 4. Viable particle concentration expressed as percentages of total particle concentrations.

naturally occurring airborne microorganisms. As mentioned previously, most of the volumetric air sampling done by the various research groups was performed using the Reyniers slit air sampler. However, it was quickly realized that certain engineering constraints restricted the use of this relatively large sampler and its associated ancillary equipment so that it could not be used, for example, inside of spacecraft (i.e. the Apollo Command Module) or in certain areas surrounding the spacecraft. In 1974 we reported on a study which was conducted to test the feasibility of using membrane filter field monitors in lieu of the Reyniers air sampler so that more sites in spacecraft-associated environments could be sampled for airborne microbial contamination.[23] The study was conducted over a two-year period in two different types of environments: an uncontrolled laboratory area and a clean room in the Manned Spacecraft Operations Building where Apollo spacecraft were assembled and tested. The comparative testing procedure basically consisted of running a manifold holding six membrane filter (.45 micrometers) field monitors in parallel with two Reyniers slit air samplers at contiguous sites. TABLE 2 shows the differences in the recovery of microorganisms from air between the two sampling procedures. In the laboratory environment even though the Reyniers sampler had a slightly higher mean recovery than the membrane filter technique, the difference was not statistically significant. In the MSOB clean room the recovery of microorganisms on the membrane filter was about 60% of the slit sampler, a statistically significant difference. This difference in recovery in the clean room of the MSOB was thought to be due to two reasons. First, it was shown that large airborne particles are broken into smaller particles by passing through the slit of the Reyniers air sampler. This would result in more viable particles on colony forming units being produced giving the impression of more efficient recovery. Second, the slit air sampler recovered a greater percentage of microorganisms in the *Corynebacterium-Brevibacterium* groups (TABLE 3). Interestingly, however, the other types of microorganisms recovered by both sampling methods were similar. At the time it had been assumed by many environmental microbiologists that the membrane filter technique could not be used for sampling airborne microorganisms because vegetative bacteria would become desiccated on the membrane filter, and recovery would be significantly lower as compared to the more conventional types of air sampling such as the Reyniers slit sampler or the all glass impinger. This did not appear to be the case. The reason that it had been assumed that the membrane

TABLE 2

COMPARISON OF VIABLE AIRBORNE PARTICLES COLLECTED BY REYNIERS SLIT AIR SAMPLERS AND 0.45-μM MEMBRANE FILTER FIELD MONITORS*

		Mean No. of Viable Particles Per Ft^3	
Location	No. of Days Samples	Reyniers Sampler†	Membrane Filters‡
Laboratory	20	2.80	2.55
MSOB§	13	0.92	0.58

*Laboratory: T = 0.735; T.05 = 2.093; difference is not significant. MSOB: T = 12.414; T.05 = 2.179; difference is significant.
†Six samples per day.
‡Nine filters per day.
§Manned Spacecraft Operations Building.

TABLE 3

COMPARISON OF TYPES OF MICROORGANISMS COLLECTED WITH THE REYNIERS SLIT
SAMPLER AND MEMBRANE FILTERS

Microorganisms	Organisms (%) Collected at Laboratory		Organisms (%) Collected at MSOB	
	Reyniers	MF	Reyniers	MF
Corynebacterium-Brevi-bacterium spp	35.2	24.1	39.4	16.5
Gram-positive cocci	42.2	41.2	51.7	71.3
Gram-negative rods	0.0	0.7	0.4	0.0
Gram-negative cocci	0.2	0.2	0.0	0.0
Actinomycetes	3.5	5.2	0.0	0.5
Yeasts	4.9	5.2	1.5	2.1
Molds	4.4	4.8	4.3	6.4
Bacillus spp.	9.6	18.6	2.7	3.2

filter could not be used, most probably was due to testing of the membrane filters for this purpose using laboratory grown cultures of vegetative bacteria. It is emphasized that microorganisms that are found in the natural environment are relatively resistant to death by desiccation since organisms that are the most susceptible to environment stresses having already been eliminated.

A total of 60 paired measurements were made in evaluating the qualitative and quantitative microbial recovery abilities of the Reyniers slit air sampler and the membrane filter field monitors. The differences between the mean values obtained with the slit sampler and the mean values obtained with the membrane filter were tested statistically for each set of data with the results being that the membrane filter usually recovered significantly fewer viable particles than did the slit sampler. To determine whether the difference between the two sampling methods were consistent and the membrane filter values could be used to estimate the slit sampler values, the data were subjected to regression analysis. The data points regression line and equation for the regression lines are presented in FIGURE 5. The data demonstrated consistent relative agreement as evidenced by the line passing very near the origin and a high correlation coefficient ($r = 0.93$). It was found that in general, membrane filter samplers detected 79% of the concentration of airborne viable particles measured by the slit samplers. Consequently, it was apparent that the membrane filter technique is applicable in the field of environmental microbiology due largely to its consistency in estimating the number of microorganisms in the air and its ability to detect accurately the types of microorganisms found in the environment. The small amount of equipment needed, the economy and ease of handling membrane filters could make an air sampling apparatus available to every laboratory that needs to perform environmental microbiologic sampling.

The Use of Air Samplers for Predicting Microbial Contamination on Surfaces of Spacecraft

In this paper we have discussed only air sampling and airborne contamination in relationship to spacecraft sterilization. However, we also point out that by the 1970's there had been a variety of techniques developed for sampling surfaces of space hardware in order to estimate the total microbiologic load.[2,24] These types of data were needed to set certain parameters of the sterilization process. Obviously, these techniques required contact with the surface that was to be sampled. Unfortunately, there were certain surfaces on spacecraft such as optical equipment, thermal blankets, solar panels, and certain electronic components that could not be sampled by any contact or handling method. Consequently, our laboratories studied the feasibility of estimating the level of microbial contamination on a spacecraft surface without actually sampling the surface per se. In 1972 a set of mathemetical models was designed for this purpose.[25] In 1974 we reported on the use of this mathematical model with actual air and surface sampling data.[26]

The primary objective of this study was to determine if volumetric air sampling, in conjunction with a mathematical model,[24] could be used instead of the conventional contact or swab rinse methods for estimating the numbers of microorganisms deposited on surfaces by natural airborne fallout. Among the significant parameters necessary for the mathematical model were the effect that angled surfaces would have on the quantitative level of viable particle collection and the determination of the number of viable cells per viable particle. The deposition of viable particles on angled surfaces was determined by the use of stainless steel fallout strips inclined at various angles ranging from 0–90° to the horizontal. The number of viable microorganisms per viable particle was determined by using stainless steel fallout strips and comparing the data obtained to that of membrane field monitors. It was found that the number of viable cells per viable particle remained constant for a particular environment. Comparisons between the actual level of surface contamination resulting from airborne fallout and the volumetric air sampling—mathematical model technique was performed

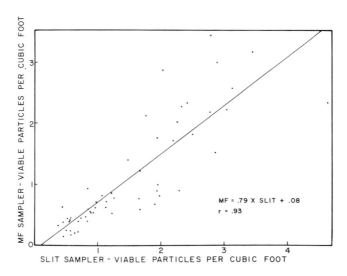

FIGURE 5. Relationship between membrane filter and volumetric slit air sampler results with regression line and equation.

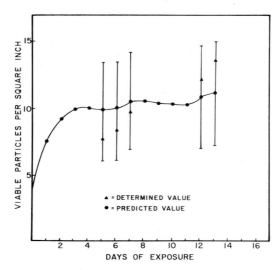

FIGURE 6. Comparison of microbial fallout on stainless steel surfaces and predicted fallout based on Reyniers air sampling in the Manned Spacecraft Operations Building.

in a relatively dirty, uncontrolled area as well as in the clean room of the MSOB. Typical data are shown in FIGURE 6. As can be seen, there was a close nonlinear correlation between volumetric air sampling and airborne microbial fallout on surfaces and all of the surface contamination data points falling within the 95% confidence limits as predicted by the mathematical model.

In addition to the application this basic technique has to the field of spacecraft sterilization, we believe that there is a much more tangible application to current problems facing the United States pharmaceutical industries. As mentioned previously, under regulations pertaining to good manufacturing practices, the Food and Drug Administration requires that the microbiologic burden of items requiring sterilization be determined. We would suggest that by the use of air sampling and a mathematical model specifically tailored to the pharmaceutical environment that the required quantitative data could be obtained in a much more cost effective manner.

REFERENCES

1. HALL, L. B. & C. W. BRUCH. 1964. Procedures necessary for the prevention of planetary contamination. Life Sci. Space Res. **3:** 48–62.
2. HALL, L. B., M. S. FAVERO & R. G. LYLE. 1977. Spacecraft sterilization. *In* Disinfection, Sterilization and Preservation. 2nd Edit. Seymour S. Block, Ed.: 611–638. Lea & Febiger. Philadelphia, Pa.
3. PORTNER, D. M., R. K. HOFFMAN & C. R. PHILLIPS. 1965. Microbial control in assembly areas needed for spacecraft. Air Eng. **7:** 46–49.
4. FAVERO, M. S., J. J. MCDADE, J. A. ROBERTSEN, R. K. HOFFMAN & R. W. EDWARDS. 1968. Microbiological sampling of surfaces. J. Appl. Bacteriol. **31:** 336–343.
5. FAVERO, M. S. , J. R. PULEO, J. H. MARSHALL & G. OXBORROW. 1966. Comparative levels

and types of microbial contamination detected in industrial clean rooms. Appl. Microbiol. **14:** 539–551.

6. FAVERO, M. S., J. R. PULEO, J. H. MARSHALL & G. S. OXBORROW. 1968. Comparison of microbial contamination levels among hospital operating rooms and industrial clean rooms. Appl. Microbiol. **16:** 480–486.

7. MCDADE, J. J., M. S. FAVERO & G. S. MICHAELSEN. 1966. Environmental microbiology and the control of microbial contamination. Proc. Natl. Conf. Spacecraft Sterilization Technol. Natl. Aeronautics Space Admin., Washington, D.C.

8. PULEO, J. R., N. D. FIELDS, B. MOORE & R. C. GRAVES. 1970a. Microbial contamination associated with Apollo 6 spacecraft during final assembly and testing. Space Life Sci. **2:** 48–56.

9. DECKER, H. M., L. M. BUCHANAN, L. B. HALL & K. R. GODDARD. 1963. Air filtration of microbial particles. Amer. J. Pub. Hlth. **53:** 1982–1988.

10. WHITFIELD, W. J. 1963. State of the art (contamination control) and laminar air-flow concept. Conference on Clean Room Specifications. Tech. Report No. SCR-652. Sandia Corp. Albuquerque, N.M.

11. POWERS, E. M. 1967. Microbiological burden on the surfaces of Explorer XXXIII spacecraft. Appl Microbiol. **15:** 1045–1048.

12. FAVERO, M. S. & K. R. BERQUIST. 1968. Use of laminar air-flow equipment in microbiology. Appl, Microbiol. **16:** 182–183.

13. MCDADE, J. J., M. S. FAVERO & L. B. HALL. 1967. Sterilization requirements for space exploration. J. Milk Food Technol. **30:** 179–185.

14. FAVERO, M. S. 1970. Industrial applications of laminar airflow. *In* Developments in Industrial Microbiology. **11:** 65–77. Am. Insti. Biol. Sci., Washington, D.C.

15. BREWER, J. H. & R. G. SCHMITT. 1967. Laminar air flow for sterility testing procedures (abstract). Bacteriol. Proc., Am. Soc. Microbiol.: 7.

16. BOND, W. W., M. S. FAVERO, N. J. PETERSEN & J. H. MARSHALL. 1971. Relative frequency distribution of D_{125C} values for spore isolates from the Mariner-Mars 1969 spacecraft. Appl. Microbiol. **21:** 832–836.

17. PULEO, J. R., G. S. OXBORROW, N. D. FIELDS & H. E. HALL. 1970. Quantitative and qualitative microbiological profiles of the Apollo 10 and 11 spacecraft. Appl Microbiol. **20:** 384–389.

18. PULEO, J. R., G. S. OXBORROW, N. D. FIELDS, C. M. HERRING & L. S. SMITH. 1973. Microbiological profiles of four Apollo spacecraft. Appl. Microbiol. **26:** 838–845.

19. BOND, W. W., M. S. FAVERO, N. J. PETERSEN & J. H. MARSHALL. 1970. Dry heat inactivation kinetics of naturally occurring spore populations. Appl. Microbiol. **20:** 573–578.

20. PUELO, J. R., M. S. FAVERO, G. S. OXBORROW & C. M. HERRING. 1975. Method for collecting naturally occurring airborne bacterial spores for determining their thermal resistance. Appl. Microbiol. **30:** 786–790.

21. PULEO, J. R., S. L. BERGSTROM, J. T. PEELER & G. S. OXBORROW. 1978. Thermal resistance of naturally occurring airborne bacterial spores. Appl. Environ. Microbiol. **36:** 473–479.

22. OXBORROW, G. S., N. D. FIELDS, J. R. PULEO & C. M. HERRING. 1975. Quantitative relationship between airborne viable and total particles. Health Lab. Sci. **12:** 47–51.

23. FIELDS, N. D., G. S. OXBORROW, J. R. PUELO & C. M. HERRING. 1974. Evaluation of membrane filter field monitors for microbiological air sampling. Appl. Microbiol. **27:** 517–520.

24. FAVERO, M. S. 1971. Microbiologic assay of space hardware. Environ. Biol. Med. **1:** 27–36.

25. ROARK, A. L. 1972. A stochastic bioburden model for spacecraft sterilization. Space Life Sci. **3:** 239–254.

26. OXBORROW, G. S., A. L. ROARK, N. D. FIELDS & J. R. PUELO. 1974. Mathematical estimation of the level of microbial contamination on spacecraft surfaces by volumetric air sampling. Appl. Microbiol. **27:** 706–712.

DOCUMENTATION OF AIRBORNE INFECTION DURING SURGERY

Ruth B. Kundsin

Harvard Medical School
Brigham and Women's Hospital
Boston, Massachusetts 02115

William Firth Wells described airborne contagion as the transmission of droplet nuclei, 2 to 10 micrometers in size, from one person's respiratory tract to the respiratory tract of another.[1] Wells' original description of dust, droplets and droplet nuclei is shown in TABLE 1. Surgical wound infections do not fit this traditional concept of airborne contagion. Particles from personnel, such as skin squames, lint, as well as droplet nuclei, bearing microorganisms, can be carried distances to be deposited on susceptible tissue in the wound. These particles may be larger than 2 to 10 micrometers with a settling velocity greater than one foot per minute.

The first documentation of airborne wound infection during surgical procedures was reported by our laboratory at the Peter Bent Brigham Hospital in 1963.[2] An intensive study of the bacteriology of personnel, patients and environment associated with 250 surgical procedures made it possible to identify the sources of microorganisms isolated from the wounds of post-operative wound infections. The presence of a disseminating carrier in the periphery of the room resulted in two wound infections among the 169 procedures he attended. The carrier had a *Staphylococcus aureus* with a phage type: 52 / 52A / 79 / 42D / 7 / 70 / 73 / 80 / 81 / 82 / 47C / in his nasopharynx. At no time was this same phage type isolated from either personnel or patients prior to surgery. The massive contamination of the environment during the 169 procedures during which he was present demonstrated the environmental contamination that occurred when a disseminating carrier, conventionally masked, gowned, and shod was present in the room. FIGURE 1 illustrates the areas where viable particles were sampled. Five settling plates were placed as indicated on the diagram, three on the floor and one on each of the instrument tables. Air samples were taken by the Wells air centrifuge with the intake six feet above the floor.

S. aureus with a phage type identical to that of the carrier could be recovered during 33% of the procedures on the aseptic field, during 25% of the procedures on settling plates on the floor, and during 11% of the procedures in volumetric air samples. Overall, *S. aureus* was recovered in 82 (49%) of the 169 procedures during which the carrier was present. This data is shown in TABLE 2. Counts were not high as shown in TABLE 3. The mean counts were well within the guidelines of a clean environment.

Sampling was not extensive. The five settling plates and three volumetric air samples (15 ft³) taken during each procedure represented only a miniscule fraction of contamination in the whole room. It was nevertheless established unequivocally that a disseminating carrier need not be a member of the surgical team in close proximity to the patient to successfully contaminate the environment and inoculate the patient's wound.

Twenty post operative wound infections occurred among the 250 patients (8%). Of these, 16 or 6.1% were endogenous and 4 or 2% were exogenous. The

255

0077-8923/80/0353-0255 $01.75/0 © 1980, NYAS

TABLE 1

COMPARISON OF DUST, DROPLETS, AND DROPLET NUCLEI*

	Sources of Material	Production	Mode of Suspension
Dust	solid matter, cellulose, etc.	attrition	air wafted
Droplets	fluid from nose & throat	atomization of fluids	projected into air by sneezing, etc.
Droplet nuclei	solid residues of evaporated droplets	evaporation of droplets	caught in air by evaporation

	Particle Diameter	Settling Velocity
Dust	10–100 micrometers	1 ft/min to 1 ft/sec
Droplets	>100 micrometers	>1 ft/sec
Droplet nuclei	2–10 micrometers	<1 ft/min

*Based on William Firth Wells' Comparison of Dust, Droplets, and Droplet Nuclei.[1]

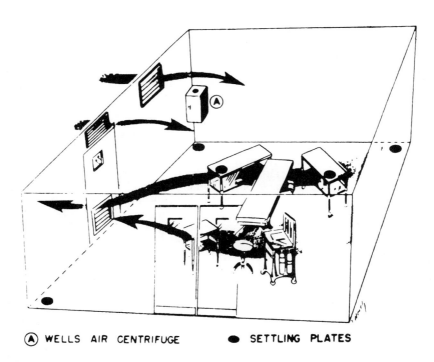

Ⓐ WELLS AIR CENTRIFUGE   ● SETTLING PLATES

FIGURE 1. Areas where microbial sampling was done in the operating room to determine bacterial content of the environment. Arrows indicate inflow and outflow of air.

TABLE 2

ENVIRONMENTAL ISOLATIONS OF
STAPHYLOCOCCUS AUREUS, PHAGE TYPE:
52 / 52A / 79 / 42D / 7 / 70 / 73 / 80 / 81 / 82 / 47C
FROM CARRIER DURING 169 OPERATIONS

	Number of Operations	Percent
Settling plates on aseptic field	56/169	33%
Settling plates on floors	42/169	25%
Volumetric air samples	19/169	11%
Total operations	82/169	49%
Two wound infections with S. aureus phage type identical to that of carrier	2/169	1%

exogenous infections could be traced to specific individuals in the operating room. Because of the small increment (2%) due to exogenous sources during the procedure, it is difficult to document significant decreases or increases in infections due to changes made in the operating room. It would take over 2000 operations to significantly evaluate a change in infections from 2% to 1%. Many of the remaining endogenous infections (6%), while not actually acquired during the procedure could be hospital associated. Evidence exists that length of hospital stay prior to surgery plays an important role in subsequent infections.[3] The use of devices such as urinary tract catheters, inhalation therapy equipment, and a remote site acquired infection may also be related to the frequency and type of post operative wound infections.[4]

Patients can also contaminate the operating room environment. A burned patient whose skin surfaces were heavily colonized with *Pseudomonas aeruginosa* of a specific pyocine type was debrided; during debridement, *Ps. aeruginosa* of his particular type was recovered in volumetric air samples, on fallout plates and on Rodac plates taken of the shelves. Even though the procedure did not deliberately create obvious aerosols, the prevalence of the patient's microorganisms in the room attested to the ease with which microorganisms could be disseminated in the environment from the patient on the operating table. (FIGURE 2). Open shelves where equipment and supplies were stored were contaminated and created a hazard for the next patient.

Because all horizontal surfaces were shown to be readily contaminated by

TABLE 3

SUMMARY OF TOTAL COUNTS OF BACTERIA CULTURED FROM THE ENVIRONMENT
IN 169 OPERATIONS

Type of Culture	Mean
Settling plates on aseptic field	3.3 ($\pm$1.9) VP/ft^2/min.
Settling plates on floor	4.3 ($\pm$1.9) VP/ft^2/min.
Volume air samples	3.7 ($\pm$2.7) VP/ft^3
Floor cultures	2.6 ($\pm$2.6)* VP/cm^2

*Geometric mean.

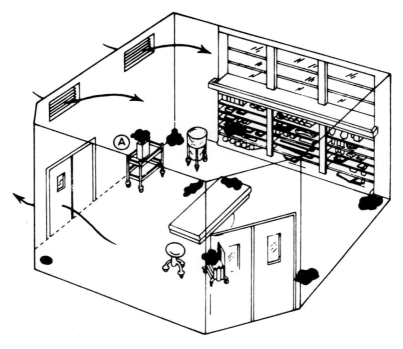

FIGURE 2. Black splotches indicate areas where *Pseudomonas aeruginosa* of the same pyocine type as the patient's were recovered in the operating room during debridement.

patients and personnel, disinfection between procedures with a freshly made up germicide, usually a synthetic phenolic, was established as an urgent priority.

Epidemiologic studies conducted in our hospital over several years have confirmed the proportion of post-operative wound infections acquired during surgery. Fifty-five epidemiologic consultations resulted in the detection of 13 (24%) infections which could be traced to a specific individual in the operating room. The remaining 42 (76%) were deemed to be either endogenous or due to the presence of a carrier who was not listed as a member of the team and consequently was not cultured. Matching of microorganisms from the carrier and the isolate from the wound could only be done with microorganisms that were typable by bacteriophages, serology, or pyocines. Nontypable organisms could

TABLE 4

55 POST OPERATIVE WOUND INFECTIONS

Source unidentified	42 (76%)
Source identified	13* (24%)
Total	55

* 5—4 surgeons
  6—3 anesthesiologists
  <u>2</u>—2 nurses
  13

not be traced. Antibiograms or biotypes have not been reliable indicators of bacterial identity. TABLE 4 shows the individuals who were identified as carriers of the strain identical to that isolated from the infections. Three were surgeons, four anesthesiologists, and two were nurses. One surgeon was implicated in two infections and one anesthesiologist in four infections.

Epidemiologic studies have also yielded information on calculations of probability that a disseminating carrier will infect a patient. Because several carriers have been studied who have had exposure to large numbers of patients during surgery, it has been possible to actually calculate the risk of infection as shown in TABLE 5. Two anesthesiologists, one a disseminating nasopharyngeal carrier of S. aureus, the other a disseminating anal carrier of Group A hemolytic streptoccocci were each implicated in 7% of infections. Apparently close proximity to the OR table resulted in a higher infection rate due to a shedding carrier than to the same shedding carrier in the periphery of the room.

Based on the observations in TABLE 5, the hazard to each patient can be mathematically predicted depending on the number of disseminating carriers in the operating room. If the probability of not becoming infected for each dissemi-

TABLE 5
THE DISSEMINATING CARRIER IN THE OPERATING ROOM

Organism	Carrier	Number of Procedures	Number of Documented Post Operative Infections
S. aureus*	Technician	169	2 (1.2%)
S aureus†	Anesthesiologist	55	4 (7.3%)
Beta-hemolytic‡ streptococcus, Group A	Anesthesiologist	183	13 (7.1%)

*52 / 52A / 79 / 42D / 7 / 70 / 73 / 80 / 81 / 82 / 47C.
†29 / 52 / 83A / 81 / 80 / 47C / 82 and 81 / 80 / 47C / 82.
‡T type 12.

nating carrier is known, the probability that any patient will be infected is equal to

$$p^I = 1 - q^{c_1} \cdot q^{c_2} \ldots q^{c_n}$$

Where:

p^I = probability that a patient will be infected.
p^{c_i} = probability that the ith carrier is an infector.
q^{c_i} = probability that the ith carrier is not an infector.
$q^{c_i} = 1 - p^{c_i}$.

$$i = 1, 2, \ldots n.$$

Assuming all three carriers described in TABLE 5 were in an operating room together during a procedure, the probability of the patient's being infected, p^I, can be calculated as follows:

$$p^I = 1 - (.93 \times .93 \times .99)$$
$$p^I = .144 \text{ or } 14.4\%$$

The airborne component of postoperative wound infections is not a fixed rate but varies from hospital to hospital, from operating room to operating room, and from surgical team to surgical team. The rate is directly proportioned to the number of disseminating carriers in the operating room. The disseminating carrier can be anywhere in the room. He does not necessarily have to be a member of the surgical team. He can be a casual visitor near the operative site, or a transient technician just inside the door, but each disseminating carrier in the room contributes to the cumulative risk incurred by the patient.

The emphasis on air supply to the surgical suite is important but assuming filters are changed on a regular basis and air intake is monitored, the micro-biology of the incoming air will easily fall within the recommended guidelines. The critical factor in our experience is the commensal flora of the people who are present. They can be scrubbed, masked, capped, gowned, and appropriately shod, but the disseminating carrier, whether nasopharyngeal or anal, will still have the capability of projecting his microorganisms into space.

Because disseminating carriers are the demonstrable cause of airborne infection during surgery, interception of transmission in the room is the only means of prevention. Even a clean environment such as the operating room has a consistent fallout on all horizontal surfaces. Approximately five viable particles

TABLE 6

ENVIRONMENTAL SAMPLING METHODS

Technique	Viable Particles (VP)* Information Obtained	Method of Detection	Method of Destruction
Volumetric air sampling	VP/ft^3	air sampler, such as Anderson, slit sampler, Reuter centrifugal sampler	ultraviolet irradiation, ventilation
Fallout	VP/ft^2/min	settling plate	surface germicides, such as synthetic phenolics
Accumulation	VP/25 cm^2	Rodac plate	surface germicides, such as synthetic phenolics

*Brigham and Women's Hospital's OR guidelines for each technique are ≤5 VP in each category.

fall out per square foot per minute. In our experience, the only effective method of interception has been ultraviolet irradiation during surgery. Not only is the wound irradiated, but the fallout on instruments, lamps, shelves and all horizontal surfaces can be intercepted.

The three basic types of environmental sampling are: 1) volumetric air sampling, 2) fallout of viable particles on surfaces, and 3) accumulation of viable particles. The techniques for detecting the three types of viable particles are different as are the methods for their destruction. Guidelines are shown in TABLE 6. The number of viable particles recovered and the types of microorganisms recovered are equally important. If any one organism predominates and is implicated in patient infections, it is an important finding. Guidelines for viable particles in the operating room have been established at the Peter Bent Brigham Hospital. They have been found helpful in evaluating environmental contamination. The three values are: 5 VP/ft^3 (volumetric air sampling), 5 VP/ft^2/min (fallout plates), and 5 VP/Rodac plate (accumulation).

If the three types of samples are taken simultaneously, a very precise definition of the quality of the environment can be secured. Settling velocity of viable particles can also be calculated by dividing area count by volume count. Particle size in turn can be calculated from the settling velocity. The types of microorganisms recovered are also useful in ascertaining the source. Thus, both the quantity and quality of isolations are basic to evaluation of the environment. TABLE 6 also shows the standards we have used for over 20 years at the Peter Bent Brigham Hospital.

Assuming the standards represent the average number of particles on the settling plate and in the volumetric air samples, the settling velocity or Vg can be calculated as one foot per minute:

$$Vg = \frac{5\ VP/ft^2/min}{5\ VP/ft^3}$$

From the Vg, equivalent diameter can be calculated using the formula $13.3\ \sqrt{Vg}$ which gives the equivalent diameter of water droplets settling at the same rate. In the operating room, the average viable particles would be 13 micrometers. The droplet nuclei described by Wells had a settling velocity or Vg of $.03$–$.04$ feet per minute and equivalent diameter of 2–3 micrometers. The operating room particle is larger and heavier than the droplet nucleus and is probably associated with particulate matter.

In conclusion, there is no longer any doubt that the airborne component represents 20%–24% of all postoperative wound infections. The percent of these airborne infections is directly related to the number of disseminating carriers in the operating room and can be mathematically calculated. Methods for intercepting the transmission of organisms from source to patient are available and have been documented. They are either ultraviolet irradiation or laminar air flow.

Post operative wound infections due to carriers in the operating room should no longer be tolerated or permitted by patients, surgeons, or hospital administrators.

ACKNOWLEDGMENT

The author gratefully acknowledges the help of Dr. Margaret Drolette, Professor of Biostatistics, Department of Biostatistics, Harvard University School of Public Health, for the calculations of probability of infection due to carriers.

REFERENCES

1. WELLS, W. F. 1955. Essay on dust-borne infection. *In* Airborne Contagion and Air Hygiene. An Ecological Study of Droplet Infections: 269–299. Harvard University Press. Cambridge, Mass.
2. WALTER, C. W., R. B. KUNDSIN & M. D. BRUBAKER. 1963. The incidence of airborne infection during operation. J. Am. Med. Assoc. **186**(10): 908–913.
3. ALTEMEIER, W. A., J. F. BURKE, B. A. PRUITT & W. R. SANDUSKY. 1976. Preoperative preparation of the patient. *In* Manual on Control of Infection in Surgical Patients: 70. J. B. Lippincott Company. Philadelphia, Pa.
4. EDWARDS, L. D. 1976. The epidemiology of 2056 remote site infections and 1966 surgical wound infections occurring in 1965 patients. Ann. Surg. **184**: 758–766.

REDUCTION OF DEEP SEPSIS FOLLOWING
TOTAL HIP ARTHROPLASTY

Robert H. Fitzgerald, Jr.

Department of Orthopedics
Mayo Clinic and Mayo Foundation
Rochester, Minnesota 55901

The clinicians' initial fears of an unusually high incidence of wound sepsis after the implantation of a large foreign body during total hip arthroplasty have not been substantiated.[5,9,10,15,16,20] However, Charnley and Eftekhar[4] were rightly concerned when they noted a 9.8% incidence of deep sepsis among the first 190 patients who had had total hip arthroplasty. Although the initial report of deep sepsis after total hip arthroplasties in a large series from the United States noted an incidence of 8%, subsequent experience demonstrated that the incidence of deep sepsis after this procedure was approximately 1.0%. Even though some physicians consider this level of sepsis to be acceptable, a lower incidence of deep sepsis should be achievable.

Reduction in the incidence of deep sepsis after total hip arthroplasty necessitates the identification of the potential and documented sources of contamination of the operative wound. When the natural history of deep sepsis after total hip arthroplasty is analyzed, further reduction in the incidence of deep sepsis appears to be possible by a careful preoperative evaluation of patients who have painful hip implants and by a reduction in the sources of contamination of the operative wound, both in the operating and in the hospital room.

Three distinct stages of deep sepsis after total hip arthroplasty can be identified on the basis of the clinical course and time of onset: stage I, an acute fulminating infection which is seen as an infected hematoma or as a superficial infection that progresses to deep sepsis and occurs within the first month; stage II, delayed, deep sepsis which develops as a creeping, indolent infection within the first 24 months; and stage III, a new hematogenous infection which develops in a previously asymptomatic hip 2 years or more after arthroplasty.[10]

In our experience at the Mayo Clinic, deep wound sepsis compromised the results of 42 of 3,215 total hip arthroplasties for which follow-up ranged from 2 to 5 years. Forty percent of the infections were stage I,[10] and half of these were infected hematomas that drained spontaneously within the first 3 weeks after arthroplasty. Forty-three percent of the deep infections were stage II. In retrospect, a third of the patients with stage II infections probably had low-grade sepsis about a painful hip implant before arthroplasty. Seventeen percent of the deep infections were stage III.

Although the prophylactic administration of antimicrobial agents to patients undergoing elective surgical procedures has been controversial, prospective studies have demonstrated a reduction in the incidence of deep sepsis when large foreign bodies—inert materials and bone grafts—are implanted during the procedure.[1,11] At this time, the administration of an antimicrobial agent during and for a brief period after total hip arthroplasty is indicated. The topical application of antimicrobials to irrigate the wound during the operative procedure appears to be of questionable value. Buchholz and Gartmann have

0077-8923/80/0353-0262 $01.75/0 © 1980, NYAS

suggested that the incidence of deep sepsis can be reduced by the introduction of antimicrobials into the bone cement.[2]

Preoperative Evaluation of the Patient

A thorough medical history and physical examination is mandatory, as is an effort to delineate any possible sources of remote sepsis before arthroplasty of the hip. A carefully taken history of the genitourinary system frequently can identify patients who have low-grade bacteriuria that can become troublesome during the postoperative course. Irvine and coworkers reported that, in their experience, most deep infections after total hip arthroplasty originate with a bladder infection that hematogenously seeded the arthroplasty.[14] The prostate should be examined in elderly male patients. If the prostate is enlarged or nodules are palpated, urologic consultation should be obtained before arthroplasty. When a prostatic biopsy specimen is required, hip surgery should be postponed until a negative midstream urine culture is obtained. If transurethral prostatic resection is performed, reconstructive hip surgery should be postponed for 12 weeks in order to allow reepithelialization of the prostate. With this routine, we have not encountered any deep infections of a total hip arthroplasty after prostatic surgery.

In any patient who has leukocytes noted on routine urinalysis, Gram staining should be done. If bacteria are present on Gram staining, a culture should be taken. Because total hip arthroplasty is an elective procedure, surgery should be postponed in patients with bacteriuria until the organism is identified and treated and the urine culture is negative.

During the physical examination, a careful examination of the skin, not only at the proposed surgical site but also in remote areas, such as the feet and back, is necessary. Only in this way can ingrown toenails or infected hair follicles, which can secondarily infect the arthroplasty, be identified.

Patients with a painful hip implant can be difficult to evaluate. A loose bone-prosthesis interface, metal articulating with eroded articular cartilage, or low-grade sepsis may account for the pain. Unfortunately, no single laboratory test can differentiate the aseptic from the septic hip. Although the erythrocyte sedimentation rate usually will be elevated before operation in patients with low-grade sepsis, a low or normal value has been obtained frequently enough to render the finding of a normal erythrocyte sedimentation rate equivocal. Bone scans—using technetium or gallium or both—have been equally unreliable in identifying the presence of a low-grade infection about the implant. Aspiration of the hip joint has been helpful, but false-negative cultures of the aspirate have been found in 25% of our patients. Frequently, the clinical and laboratory evaluations described are inconclusive.[7] In my experience, frozen-section histologic examination of tissue specimens obtained at surgery have been diagnostic and have correlated with the results of aerobic and anaerobic cultures of deep-tissue specimens.

The Operating Room

Several sources of potential bacterial contamination of the wound have been implicated in the conventional operating room. Airborne contamination of the operative wound is a distinct possibility in any operating room in which there is turbulent airflow.[4,6,15,18] Contamination can occur with direct fallout into the wound or onto the instrument table.[6,8,16] The wound suction system can lead to bacterial contamination of the surgical wound.[8] The patient's gown and the gurney are heavily contaminated with gram-negative bacillary organisms. Thus, when the patient is brought into the operating room, a new potential source of contamination is introduced. The gowns and masks worn by the surgical team and the drapes used to isolate the surgical site can lead to wound contamination either through direct contact if they are permeable to liquids or through airborne contamination.[3,6,12]

Airborne Bacterial Contamination

Air introduced into the operating room is essentially sterile unless there is a malfunction of the filtration system. The operating room personnel and patients introduce bacteria into the air. Although the use of surgical masks reduces this contamination, movement by personnel leads to shedding of skin scales, some of which carry bacteria.

In any operating room without a unidirectional airflow system, there is turbulent airflow.[8] The modern conventional operating room will have 25 to 30 room air exchanges per hour. The air provided to these operating rooms will have been filtered by an industrial filter, which removes gross dirt and contamination before final filtration by a high-intermediate efficiency filter that removes 97% of particles 0.5 μm in size or larger. Older operating rooms may have similar filtration systems, but the room air exchanges will be lower, that is, about 10 per hour.[6] These older rooms exhibit greater turbulence of airflow and an increased risk of airborne bacterial contamination of the wound. Airborne bacterial monitoring with a slit sampler of both types of conventional operating rooms reveals similar levels of contamination, with slightly lower levels in those rooms that have higher rates of room air exchange. However, the differences are not statistically significant. In general, the level of airborne contamination in the conventional operating room increases as the number of personnel in the operating room increases. Although there is variation based on the activity level of the personnel, this relationship is more apparent in operating rooms with low rates of room air exchange.

A rather consistent pattern of airborne bacterial contamination is obtained by the chronologic recording of slit-sampler contamination levels during total hip arthroplasty (FIGURE 1). With the arrival of the patient in the operating room, the level of airborne bacterial contamination increases over that observed when the circulatory and scrub nurses are organizing the sterile instruments. As the activity of the anesthesia and surgical team increases, there is a concomitant increase in the level of airborne contamination. However, by the time the incision is made, the level gradually decreases to between four and six viable particles per cubic foot of air. Subsequent increases in the level of airborne bacterial contamination are noted when the surgical team is physically active in removing a failed endoprosthesis, nails, or plates, in preparing the acetabulum, and in reaming the femoral canal. We have observed less airborne bacterial contamination in the operating room when the doors were kept closed, thereby reducing the traffic into and out of the room by the circulatory nurse and anesthesia team, and when the number of personnel in the operating room was limited to 10.[8,16]

The level of airborne bacterial contamination in the hallways and outpatient cast facilities can be considerably higher than that observed in the operating room. We have observed a onefold to fourfold higher level of airborne bacterial contamination in the hallways adjacent to the orthopedic operating rooms. Thus, it is important to keep the operating room doors closed and operating room traffic to a minimum. The airflow should be from the operating room into adjacent rooms and hallways.

The operating rooms should be monitored to ensure that they have a positive-pressure relationship to adjacent workrooms, hallways, and scrub rooms. This can be easily achieved by using a commercially available smoke bomb or smoke stick.

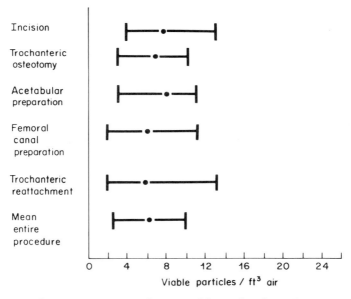

FIGURE 1. Airborne contamination during total hip arthroplasty. Room air exchanges were 12 to 14 per hour.

Although the use of a back table for the storage of instruments throughout the operating day reduces the delay between operative procedures and improves utilization of the operating room, the level of contamination on the surface of such tables varies from 48 to 121 colony-forming units per square foot per hour. Thus, an appreciable level of contamination of the instruments can occur. Likewise, it seems incongruous for the scrub nurse to organize all of the instruments for the procedure before bringing the patient into the operating room and then to expose the instruments to high levels of airborne bacterial contamination during the induction of anesthesia, the surgical scrub, and draping of the operative site. The instruments should be covered before the patient is brought into the operating room, or individual trays of instruments for the various portions of the operation should be used unless a unidirectional airflow back table is available.[4,8]

Wound Suction System

The use of a sterile sucker tip and suction hosing attached to a clean but unsterile glass receptacle is unsatisfactory. The clean glass receptacle can harbor many organisms, *Pseudomonas maltophilia* and *Pseudomonas aeruginosa* in particular. If the sucker tip or suction hosing becomes clogged during the procedure, retrograde contamination of the hosing or tip (or both) is possible. Because blockage of the hosing frequently occurs with musculoskeletal surgery, a sterile receptacle is necessary. Many of the glass receptacles will not tolerate sterilization in the autoclave. However, there are numerous disposable containers commercially available.

Patient's Gown and the Gurney

Additional sources of contamination of the operative wound with gram-negative bacillary organisms include the patient's gown and the gurney.[8] Although each patient is given a clean gown, we have noted heavy contamination, 80 to 100 colony-forming units per square foot, primarily with gram-negative bacilli. All too frequently, the patient's gown is only moved aside during the operative procedure to allow preparation of the operative site. Gurneys for transporting patients in the operative suite should be cleaned if they are used to transport patients to and from the surgical wards. When a cleaning procedure is not utilized after each trip from the operating suite, we have noted more than 1,000 colony-forming units per square foot on the wheels and top of the gurney. The organisms isolated have been predominately gram-negative bacilli, for example, *Escherichia coli, Enterobacter aerogenes,* and *P. aeruginosa.* Thus, the patient should be provided with a clean gown just before entering the operating room and should be transferred in a holding area adjacent to the operating suite to a gurney that remains within the operating suite. If this is not possible, the patient should be transferred onto the operating table at the door of the operating room.

Hoods, Gowns, and Drapes

The use of the head hood, an extension of the aseptic technique, which was fashionable in earlier years of surgery at the Mayo Clinic, fell into disrepute as surgeons desired more comfort and freedom. Little thought was given to control of bacterial fallout from the head and neck of the surgical team. There is much bacterial contamination of the skin at the angle of the jaw. Because most masks move up and down, the shedding of skin scales and bacteria occurs. We have been able to reduce the level of bacterial contamination at the orifice of the wound by 68% and on the instrument table by 30% with the use of an impermeable hood and large mask that cover the entire face, except for the areas about the eyes.[8]

Repellent drapes should be used, especially in orthopedic surgery, where wounds are frequently irrigated. The repellent drapes and gowns should be monitored to ensure that their repellent quality has not been lost through modern laundry techniques.[3]

In a recent study of the operative wound contamination using microspheres, Ha'eri and Wiley demonstrated contamination from the surgeon's scrub suit, undersurface of the surgeon's mask, and the patient's chest in the conventional operating room.[12] These data suggest that current draping and gowning procedures, even with impermeable materials, are inadequate.

In a recent study of total hip arthroplasty performed in four different institutions utilizing different types of operating rooms but incorporating the features discussed above, the lowest rate of sepsis was noted in a vertical unidirectional airflow facility in association with the use of a personnel-isolator system[9] (TABLE 1). However, in that same study, a similar level of sepsis was noted

TABLE 1

THE ROLE OF THE OPERATING ROOM IN DEEP SEPSIS AFTER TOTAL HIP ARTHROPLASTY

Operating Room Type	Total Procedures	Procedures Associated With Deep Sepsis	
		Number	(%)
Vertical unidirectional (personnel isolators)	518	3	0.6
Horizontal	580	6	1.0
Horizontal (personnel isolators)	337	2	0.6
Conventional and vertical unidirectional	1,421	7	0.5
Conventional	3,215	42	1.3

when a horizontal, unidirectional airflow facility and a personnel-isolator system were used. Although that study was neither prospective nor randomized, the findings suggest that a lower incidence of deep sepsis may be achieved with a unidirectional airflow facility and that there is a need for a controlled, prospective study of such facilities.

The Hospital Room

In addition to the usual measures for preventing cross contamination and nosocomial infections, certain precautions are necessary in the hospital room on the surgical ward for the management of patients who have undergone total hip arthroplasty. We have encountered deep wound infection after intramuscular injection into the ipsilateral buttock.[10] Thus, injections must be avoided into soft tissues that are near total joints. If drains are inserted during wound closure, they should be attached to a sterile portable suction receptacle in the operating room. This receptacle should have a reflux valve so that it can be emptied through a separate portal without the need for separating the drainage tube; this eliminates a potential source of contamination.

If a superficial or deep hematoma begins to drain after the operation, it should be treated in the operating room by prompt debridement and closure under sterile conditions. With this approach, we have successfully treated six of eight patients who had infected hematomas and who were followed up for 5 years after surgery.

Antimicrobial Agents and Total Hip Arthroplasty

Although the use of antimicrobial agents can be associated with adverse side effects, Boyd et al.[1] demonstrated that the prophylactic application of these agents in high-risk operative procedures, such as total hip arthroplasty, was associated with a reduction in the incidence of deep sepsis. Because staphylococci are the predominant causal organisms in the development of deep sepsis, a semisynthetic penicillinase-resistant penicillin or a cephalosporin agent seems to be the agent of choice. Methicillin was the agent used during the early total joint procedures performed at the Mayo Clinic. However, nephrotoxicity developed in three patients from the brief (72 hours) exposure. Studies comparing the osseous levels of methicillin, oxacillin, and cephalothin have demonstrated greater osseous penetration by cephalothin. Thus, at the present time, a cephalosporin is the agent used in nonallergic patients undergoing total joint arthroplasty.

Buchholz and Gartmann[2] introduced antibiotic-impregnated bone cement to achieve high local concentrations and to avoid the adverse side effects associated with elevated systemic concentrations. Wahlig et al.[19] demonstrated that several of the agents could be leached from the methylmethacrylate but believed that gentamicin would be the drug of choice. Using a radioactive label on either penicillin or gentamicin, Hoff et al.[13] demonstrated that concentrations of more than 140 $\mu g/g$ of bone can be achieved at the endosteal surface of the dog femora in the laboratory. Simultaneously, the highest concentration in the serum and urine was far below toxic levels. Hoff et al. demonstrated that gentamicin is released in bactericidal concentrations for at least six months after implantation.

Buchholz and Gartmann[2] demonstrated a significant reduction in the incidence of deep sepsis, utilizing gentamicin-impregnated cement prophylactically during total joint arthroplasty. Although none of their patients has had an allergic reaction, if a patient were to have one, treatment would require removal of the prosthetic components and the bone cement. It would appear that the parenteral administration of antibiotics is superior for the prophylactic use of antibiotics during total joint arthroplasty.

Because new hematogenous infections do occur in patients with total hip arthroplasty, this group of patients should receive antimicrobials prophylactically when other types of surgical procedures or dental manipulations are performed.[17]

CONCLUSIONS

A careful preoperative evaluation of the patient can identify remote sites of infection and can prevent the hematogenous seeding of the arthroplasty during the postoperative course. The patient with a painful hip should be thoroughly evaluated for the presence of low-grade sepsis about the implant. Only with a high index of suspicion can these infections be identified before hip reconstruction with an arthroplasty that would otherwise become infected.

We have not been able to relate the level of airborne bacterial contamination during an operative procedure to the development of deep wound sepsis. However, we have noted that, in the older operating rooms with low rates of room air exchange, the overall infection rate after total joint arthroplasty is statistically higher than the newer operating rooms with higher rates of room air exchange. When the more difficult operative procedures are performed in such rooms, especially when these are done by less experienced surgeons, this relationship is more obvious. Procedures performed later in the day in such rooms are also associated with a higher rate of postoperative wound sepsis.

When older operating rooms with low rates of room air exchange are used for high-risk orthopedic procedures, careful monotoring of the operating room, control of traffic, and the other techniques outlined are mandatory.

The prophylactic administration of one of the antistaphylococcal cephalosporins during and for a short time after total hip arthroplasty will help to maintain a low incidence of deep sepsis.

REFERENCES

1. BOYD, R. J., J. F. BURKE & T. COLTON. 1973. A double-blind clinical trial of prophylactic antibiotics in hip fractures. J. Bone Joint Surg. [Am.] 55: 1251–1258.
2. BUCHHOLZ, H. W. & H.-D. GARTMANN. 1972. Infektions-prophylaxe und operative Behandlung der schleichenden tiefen Infektion bei der totalen Endoprothese. Chirurg 43: 446–453.
3. CHARNLEY, J. & N. EFTEKHAR. 1969. Penetration of gown material by organisms from the surgeon's body. Lancet 1: 172–174.
4. CHARNLEY, J. & N. EFTEKHAR. 1969. Postoperative infection in total prosthetic replacement arthroplasty of the hip joint: with special reference to the bacterial content of the air of the operating room. Br. J. Surg. 56: 641–649.
5. EFTEKHAR, N. S., H. A. KIERNAN, Jr. & F. E. STINCHFIELD. 1976. Systemic and local complications following low-friction arthroplasty of the hip joint: a study of 800 consecutive operations. Arch. Surg. 111: 150–155.
6. FITZGERALD, R. H., Jr. 1977. Contamination of the surgical wound in the operating room. Instructional Course Lectures, Am. Acad. Orthop. Surg. 26: 41–46.
7. FITZGERALD, R. H., Jr. 1979. Laboratory diagnosis of postoperative sepsis of the musculoskeletal system. Orthop. Clin. North Am. 10 No. 2: 361–374.
8. FITZGERALD, R. H., Jr. 1979. Microbiologic environment of the conventional operating room. Arch. Surg. 114: 772–775.
9. FITZGERALD, R. H., Jr., C. O. BECHTOL, N. EFTEKHAR & J. P. NELSON. 1979. Reduction of deep sepsis after total hip arthroplasty. Arch. Surg. 114: 803–804.
10. FITZGERALD, R. H., Jr., D. R. NOLAN, D. M. ILSTRUP, R. E. VAN SCOY, J. A. WASHINGTON II & M. B. COVENTRY. 1977. Deep wound sepsis following total hip arthroplasty. J. Bone Joint Surg. [Am.] 59: 847–855.
11. FOGELBERG, E. V., E. K. ZITZMANN & F. E. STINCHFIELD. 1970. Prophylactic penicillin in orthopaedic surgery. J. Bone Joint Surg. [Am.] 52: 95–98.
12. HA'ERI, G. B. & A. M. WILEY. 1979. The role of drapes and gowns in wound contamination: a study using tracer particles (abstract). Orthop. Tr. 3 No. 2: 131–132.
13. HOFF, S. F., R. H. FITZGERALD, Jr., P. J. KELLY & J. A. WASHINGTON II. 1978. Penicillin and gentamicin cortical bone penetration from Palacos R bone cement (abstract). Orthop. Tr. 2 No. 1: 174–175.
14. IRVINE, R., B. L. JOHNSON, Jr. & H. C. AMSTUTZ. 1974. The relationship of genitourinary tract procedures and deep sepsis after total hip replacements. Surg. Gynecol. Obstet. 139: 701–706.
15. MEDICAL RESEARCH COUNCIL. 1968. Aseptic methods in the operating suite. I. Prepara-

tion of the surgical team. II. The operating suite and equipment. III. Preparation of the patient and performance of the operation. Lancet **1:** 705–709; 763–768; 831–839.

16. NELSON, J. P. 1977. The operating room environment and its influence on deep wound infection. Proc. Sci. Meet. Hip Soc. **6:** 129–147.

17. RUBIN, R., E. A. SALVATI & R. LEWIS. 1976. Infected total hip replacement after dental procedures. Oral Surg. **41:** 18–23.

18. SYMPOSIUM. 1965. The prevention of hospital infection by design. J. R. Coll. Surg. Edinb. **11:** 260–315.

19. WAHLIG, H., H.-J. SCHLIEP, R. BERGMANN, W. HAMEISTER & A. GRIEBEN. 1972. Über die Freisetzung von Gentamycin aus Polymethylmethacrylat: II. Experimentelle Untersuchungen *in vivo*. [Release of gentamicin from polymethyl methacrylate: II. Experimental *in vivo* tests.] Langenbecks Arch. Chir. **331:** 193–212.

20. WILSON, P. D., Jr., H. C. AMSTUTZ, A. CZERNIECKI, E. A. SALVATI & D. G. MENDES. 1972. Total hip replacement with fixation by acrylic cement: a preliminary study of 100 consecutive McKee-Farrar prosthetic replacements. J. Bone Joint Surg. [Am.] **54:** 207–236.

ULTRAVIOLET LIGHT FOR THE CONTROL OF AIRBORNE BACTERIA IN THE OPERATING ROOM

J. Leonard Goldner, Mary Moggio, Stephen F. Beissinger,
and Donald E. McCollum

*Division of Orthopaedic Surgery
Duke University Medical Center
Durham, North Carolina 27710*

In 1881 surgical asepsis was initiated by Semmelweis, who showed that improved personal hygiene could diminish contact contamination. Lister subsequently championed antiseptic techniques in the operating room and was a proponent of the "germ theory" of Koch as the cause of infection. Airborne infection was recognized as an entity but the application of aseptic techniques in operating on patients delayed the development of provisions for adequate ventilation in the operating room.[1,2] In 1933, Meleney[3] reemphasized the importance of airborne bacteria as a cause of wound sepsis. The first significant investigation of the relationship between airborne bacteria and sepsis in burns was completed in 1946 and 1948.[4,5] This study showed that the use of "extract ventilation" brought bacteria contaminated air from outside into the operating room. The number of airborne bacteria was effected to the shedding from textiles, hair, skin and the upper respiratory tract of the operating room personnel.[5] These observers influence the design of ventilation systems where clean air was brought in under positive pressure and the volume of air was sufficient to rapidly remove airborne microorganisms originating from operating room personnel. The aerospace industry introduced laminar flow with high-efficiency particulate air (HEPA) filters in the early 1960s. The unidirectional airflow (UAF) systems were used in the medical field in 1969.[6,7] Charnley and others have indicated that reduction of wound infection was primarily related to UAF rooms even though UAF systems provided clean air relating to particles, but standards of biologic clean air are not yet defined, nor has the actual effectiveness of UAF in the reduction of wound infection been documented by controlled clinical trials. The airborne spread of infection has been documented, but precise data as to the number of operative wound infections resulting from airborne transmission alone versus other endogenous and exogenous routes are still lacking.[4,5,8–19]

In the operating room, air is the only unsterile material with access to the wound and to other objects that may be placed in the wound.[20] Airborne bacteria do effect the incidence of wound infection as the number of individuals in the operating room at any given moment increases the chance of wound infection also increases.

Traditional methods of reducing airborne bacteria are: (1) air conditioning systems that maintain 12 air exchanges per hour, air inflow near the ceiling with air exit near the floor, mechanical filtration of air prior to entering the operating room, regular cleaning of filters, humidity control at about 50%, and temperature control at approximately 21.1°C; (2) minimal number of personnel in the operating room; (3) minimal personnel talking and movement; (4) detection and elimination of personnel with infection;[21,22] (5) adequate nose and face mask and head cover. Many systems have air conditioning now available for airflow control, for the entire room or for local control.

271

0077–8923/80/0353–0271 $01.75/0 © 1980, NYAS

The orthopaedic operating rooms at Duke University Medical Center have used ultraviolet light since 1934. The air exchange in the original operating rooms was seven to 12 times per hour and the necessity for a supplementary system to diminish bacteria in the air was essential.[15] Currently and for the past 15 years the modern air conditioning system provides air exchanges of 32 times per hour and we continue to complement this with UV irradiation. The incidence of wound infection of refined clean cases since 1940 has been less than 0.5%.[14] The incidence of wound infection in total hip arthroplasty in patients defined as refined clean cases (no prior operation on the involved hip) is approximately 0.6%. These patients are analyzed and the actual relationship with airborne contamination to infection was negligible. The combination of the current system of air conditioning and ultraviolet light virtually elminate airborne infection based on a nine year experience with total hip replacements with the operative procedures being performed by eight senior surgeons and 72 different senior residents operating with the senior surgeons. (TABLE 1)

During the winter of the early 1930s there was a 10% postoperative wound infection rate with Staphyloccoccus aureus. Hart[1,2] initiated procedures that are emphasized now such as exclusion of visitors from the operating room, limited number of operating room personnel; the use of masks during and between operative procedures; detection of nasopharyngeal carriers of S aureus; and frequent washing and painting of the operating room as well as use of filtered air, isolation helmets and suction devices. These procedures did not reduce wound infection to an acceptable level at that time of 5% to 7%. Hart[1] and his colleagues demonstrated in 1934 that UV irradiation (25 uW/cm²/s) destroyed pathogenic bacteria. Sterilization of Petri dishes of blood agar sprayed with S aureus placed at the operative site and exposed to UV irradiation were sterilized within one to three minutes. These observations were confirmed during the next thirty years.[16]

TABLE 1

DUKE NINE YEAR EXPERIENCE TOTAL

Year	1969	1970	1971	1972	1973
Number of Patients	67	123	175	178	168
Annual Infection Totals	2 / 2.9%	2 / 1.6%	4 / 2.2%	2 / 1.1%	2 / 1.1%
Refined Clean Cases Infected	0	1 / 0.8%	1 / 0.57%	1 / 0.56%	1 / 0.9%
Deep Infection	2	1	4	1	2
Superficial Infection	0	1	0	1	0
Primary Organism	Proteus M. Enterococcus	Clostridia perfringes { E. Coli Enterobacter Proteus M.	Staph. epid. E. Coil Enterobacter Proteus	Staph. aureus { Enterobacter Proteus M. Staph. aureus	Staph. aureus Enterococcus

*This Table provides the number of patients operated upon each year, the number of patients determined to have superficial or deep infection each year, those with deep infection, those with

A protocol was prepared in 1973 to examine the extent and kind of airborne contamination directly over the wound during total hip arthroplasty both with and without UV irradiation.

SUBJECTS AND METHODS

Experience in the Duke Orthopaedic Operating Rooms

All sampling during total hip arthroplasty was conducted in either operating room 3 or 4. Sampling was done only when the total hip arthroplasty was the first scheduled procedure of the day. Operating rooms 3 and 4 are serviced by an air-handling unit located on the fifth floor of the 1957 hospital addition. The fresh air intake and exhaust are located in the east wall of the mechanical room of the observation suite. The fresh air passes through medium-efficiency filters, 90% downstream filters, preheat coil, air washer, cooling coils, a reheat coil, and a fan unit. After leaving the fan, the filtered air enters individual ducts leading to rooms 3 and 4 and passes through a final reheat coil. Air enters from the ceiling directly over the operating room table. There are no provisions for air recirculation. Air exchange rate in rooms 3 and 4 was measured at 36 and 34, respectively.

The placement and arrangement of UV lights in these two rooms are different. Room 4 has a high-vaulted ceiling, which allows for the installation of eight unshielded UV ceiling lights. There are 12 wall lights. Room 3 has no overhead well. The UV lights[15] are installed within ceiling pans. The UV light is toward the ceiling, which is painted with aluminum paint, allowing for reflected light. There are, in addition, 12 sidelights. Measurement of UV intensities was

HIP REPLACEMENT-INFECTIONS*

Year	1974	1975	1976	1977	Totals Numbers Percent
Number of Patients	195	150	134	132	1,322 100%
Annual Infection Totals	2 1.0%	2 1.3%	1 0.6%	1 0.6%	18 1.36%
Refined Clean Cases Infected	2 1.0%	1 0.65%	1 0.6%	1 0.6%	9 0.68%
Deep Infection	0	2	1	0	
Superficial Infection	2	0	0	1	
Primary Organism	Pseudomonas Pseudomonas	Staph. aureus Enterococcus Proteus mirabilis	Microaerophilic strep.	E. Coli, Enterococcus, Pseudomonas	

superficial infection and some indication concerning the organisms predominating in the infections each year.[5]

done weekly. The intensity of light at the operating tabletop was inversely proportionate to the square of distance.

Before initiation of the study, background or baseline volumetric air sampling was conducted with and without UV irradiation (TABLE 2). Sampling was conducted with volumetric air sampler at what approximated the level of the operating table. In addition, the time-death relationship of a known number of *S aureus* to UV irradiation was conducted in these two rooms. An appropriate *S aureus* sample was made as follows: A lyophilized disk of *S aureus* was aseptically placed in digested casein-soy peptone-dextrose broth and incubated at 37°C for 24 hours. After 24 hours of incubation, serial dilutions of the original broth culture were made and spread onto a blood agar Petri dish (15 x 150 mm). The surfaces of the blood agar plates were allowed to dry at room temperature and then incubated at 37°C for about 48 hours.

After incubation, the dilution (10^6) that produced approximately 200 colony-forming units (CFUs) on the Petri dish was chosen. One milliliter of this 10^6

TABLE 2

UV LIGHT-PERCENT REDUCTION-STAPHYLOCOCCUS AUREUS

	Room 4 (17 mw/cm²/sec)*		Room 3 (12 mw/cm²/sec)*	
	Number of Colonies (10^6)	% Reduction/Time	Number of Colonies (10^6)	% Reduction/Time
Control	170	0	130	0
5 min.	29	83	45	65
10 min.	15	91	6	95
15 min.	8	95	5	96
20 min.	0	100	0	100
30 min.	0	100	0	100
60 min.	0	100	0	100
120 min.	0	100	0	100

*The microwatt reading is calibrated to a standard light source. The actual reading of the monitor will vary according to the calibration. The readings listed here are equivalent to 25 mw/cm²/sec. readings on the original indicator.[37,38] (Dr. Gordon Sharp)

dilution was spread onto 16 blood agar plates and allowed to dry at room temperature. The plates were then taken to operating rooms 3 and 4 and exposed to UV irradiation for 5, 10, 15, 20, 30, 60, and 120 minutes. The blood agar plates, including the control plates (no UV exposure) were incubated at 37°C for about 48 hours. The number of CFUs of *S aureus* was counted and recorded.

Total Hip Procedure

All volumetric air sampling (with/without UV lights) was done at the operative site with an air sampler.[15] The decision to turn off UV lights or to leave them on during the operation was made by the attending surgeon the day before the procedure. The environmentalist operating the sampler asked the surgeon in each instance whether the lights could be turned off or left on. Modification of the intake port of the sampler with a sterile, 180-cm (6-ft), corrugated plastic tubing allowed for air sampling at the operative site and allowed the investigator to be outside the sterile field. Petri dishes with digested casein-soy peptone-dextose agar were changed at 30-minute intervals. Volumetric sampling was conducted at the rate of 1 cu ft of air per minute and was accomplished by the use of a remote sampler cabinet containing the pump, flowmeter, and timer. This cabinet was located in the hallway adjacent to the operating room.

Sampling began at the time of the incision and ended at wound closure. The total hip arthroplasty procedure consisted of the following seven steps: (1) preparation and incision; (2) removal of femoral head with a high-pressure nitrogen saw; (3) reaming of the acetabulum-hand or nitrogen-driven reamer and placement of the prosthesis using the Duke external guide; (4) application of methylmethacrylate to acetabular prosthesis; (5) reaming of the femoral shaft; (6) trial reduction with femoral prosthesis and application of methylmethacrylate to femur; and (7) closure of wound incision.

During steps 3 through 6, a settle plate containing digested casein-soy peptone-dextrose agar was placed on the sterile instrument table. Cultures (swab) of the hip joint were taken before the use of irrigating fluid (sterile saline solution) with bacitracin, and before closure of the wound site. In addition, samples of each packet of methylmethacrylate were submitted for microbial analysis. Temperature and humidity of the respective rooms were recorded each time.

One additional procedure was initiated after the study was in process. During step 5 of one total hip arthroplasty operation, we recovered more than 300 colonies of a Gram-negative rod (100 colonies/cu ft/min of *Vibrio extorquens*). Contamination of water, sterile fluids, and intravenous liner caps with this bacteria has been documented. After consultation, we decided to submit a sample of the sterile water and saline (before the addition of bacitracin) at the time the containers were opened.

The sampling plots used in the volumetric air sampler were marked off in five-minute intervals. Results would later be expressed as the number of CFUs per cubic foot of air per minute. Settle plates were incubated at 37°C for about 48 hours and all CFUs were identified and counted. Results would later be expressed as the number of CFUs per square foot of air per minute. Any bacterial growth from the hip cultures, methylmethacrylate, sterile water, or saline solution were identified.

RESULTS

Forty-seven total hip arthroplasty operations were performed in this study (January 1974 to August 1975). Of this total, 23 total hip arthroplasty operations were performed in operating room 3, and 24 were performed in operating room 4. Twenty-eight of the total hip arthroplasties were performed with UV light; 19 without UV light. Results were subjected to both parametric (F test) and nonparametric (Wilcoxon rank) tests to ascertain significance (Dr. G. G. Koch, University of North Carolina at Chapel Hill performed this analysis).

TABLE 3 gives the average number of CFUs recovered by volumetric air sampling when both operating rooms were unoccupied. *Few, if any, bacteria are present in an unoccupied operating room.*

There were a total of 12,166 microorganisms recovered during 5,561 minutes of air sampling (47 procedures). The average number of CFUs with and without UV irradiation and in rooms 3 and 4 is given in TABLE 4. With the use of the F test

TABLE 3

AIRBORNE BACTERIA IN UNOCCUPIED OPERATING ROOMS 3 AND 4

	Room 3			Room 4		
	(Time) min	CFU	Av. CFU/ft.^{3}/min.	Time (min.)	CFU	CFU/ft^3/min
UV On	240	2	0.01	240	0	0.0
UV Off	240	0	0.0	240	0	0.0

(regression equation), the difference between rooms 3 and 4 is significant at the .05 level.

The difference in means, however, with and without the UV irradiation was significant at the .01 level. Parametric analysis of the cases done with or without UV light in room 3 and cases done with or without UV light in room 4 were compatible but not significant. Nonparametric analysis (Wilcoxon rank test) was performed to confirm the parametric tests of significance. When minutes were controlled, there were significant differences ($x^2 = 0.01$) in the rooms together with UV light on vs off, in room 3 with UV lights off vs on ($x^2 = 0.01$), and in room 4 with UV light on vs off ($x^2 = 0.01$). Results indicate that the number of airborne bacteria collected at the operative site in each conventional operating room without UV irradiation was quite low. The use of UV irradiation significantly reduces the average number of airborne bacteria over the operative site from that found without UV irradiation (TABLE 4).

The numbers and types of bacteria recovered at the operative site are given in TABLE 5. Analysis of the mean ranks (no room distribution) of bacteria recovered was performed. When minutes were controlled, there was a substantial difference only in the number of *Bacillus* sp ($x^2 = 0.01$) with UV lights on vs UV lights off. This data confirm the fact that airborne bacteria are a reflection of operating room personnel and their activities.

The V extorquens was recovered only during the step 5 of the total hip arthroplasty operation. We thought that this was a contaminant possibly introduced by contaminated irrigating fluid. Steps were instituted to locate the source but none was found.

All organisms recovered on the settle plates were less than 1 CFU/sq ft/min (TABLE 6). Although our technique to ascertain wound contamination was not quantitative, only two wounds were contaminated with one colony of *Staphylococcus* (coagulase negative) at the time of closure (TABLE 5).

The figures in Table 6 and the other data imply that the number of bacteria entering the wound from the air was negligible in all hips monitored with the UV lights on. Settle plates reflect the degree of air contamination. The air condi-

TABLE 4

AVERAGE NUMBER AIRBORNE BACTERIA IN ROOMS 3,4; CASES WITH/WITHOUT UV LIGHT

	THR	Time (min.)	CFU	Ave. CFU/ft^3/min.
Room 3	23	2,597	6,685	2.6 F = F 0.05
Room 4	24	2,964	5,481	1.9 Wilcoxan $x^2 = 0.01$
UV On	28	3,088	4,271	1.4 F = F 0.01
UV Off	19	2,473	7,895	3.2 Wilcoxan $x^2 = 0.01$

TABLE 5

REYNIERS AIR SAMPLER NUMBER, PERCENTAGE AND TYPES OF BACTERIA RECOVERED

	All THR (%)	Room 4	Room 3	UV On	UV Off
Total	12,166	5,481 (45.1)	6,685 (54.9)	4,271 (35.1)	7,895 (64.9)
Fungi, yeast	721 (5.9)	280 (5.1)	441 (6.6)	388 (9.1)	333 (4.2)
Bacillus sp.	2,241 (18.4)	1,499 (27.4)	742 (11.1)	457 (10.7)	1,784 (22.6)
Micrococcus sp.	4,407 (36.2)	1,575 (28.7)	2,832 (42.4)	1,643 (38.5)	2,764 (35.0)
Diphtheroids	2,744 (22.6)	870 (15.9)	1,874 (28.0)	1,143 (26.8)	1,601 (20.3)
Staph. (−)	1,661 (13.7)	914 (16.7)	747 (11.2)	617 (14.5)	1,044 (13.2)
Mima polymorpha	13 (0.1)	—	13 (0.2)	11 (0.3)	2 (0.03)
Klebsiella sp.	1 (0.01)	—	—	1 (0.02)	—
Staphylococcus aureus	36 (0.3)	1 (0.02)	35 (0.5)	11 (0.3)	25 (0.3)
Pseudomonas sp.	5 (0.04)	5 (0.09)	—	—	5 (0.06)
Neisseria sp.	1 (0.01)	1 (0.02)	—	—	1 (0.01)
B. anitratum	24 (0.2)	24 (0.4)	—	—	24 (0.3)
*Vibrio extorquens**	310 (2.6)	310 (5.7)	—	—	310 (3.9)
Serratia sp.	2 (0.02)	2 (0.04)	—	—	2 (0.03)

*The *Vibrio extorquens* was recovered only during step 5 of THR. It was felt that this was a contaminant possibly introduced by contaminated irrigating fluid. Steps were instituted to locate the source, but none was found.

tioning system in rooms 3 and 4 was sufficient to maintain airborne bacteria at a relatively low level. The addition of UV light diminished this level even more.

Clinical Analysis and Review of Patients

Altemeier and Levenson[8] (TABLE 7) provided data on the incidence of infection, although they wrote, "There is evidence that this incidence is much greater than generally suspected." They indicate that the 7.4% wound infection rate was determined for all types of operative wounds as determined during a 2 1/2-year collaborative study of UV light used in 15,613 consecutive operative procedures done in five American university centers, under the National Research Council. The operative wounds studied were of the following types: clean, clean/contaminated, contaminated, and dirty.

The incidence of postoperative wound infection was directly related to the type of operation; for herniorrhaphy the wound infection rate was 1.9%; for thyroidectomy it was 2.2%, and for radical mastectomy it was 18.9% (consider the axilla, hematoma, and so forth). Altemeier and Levenson[8] classified the infections according to the basis of source or base of infection, with the following three

TABLE 6

BACTERIAL SETTLE PLATES AND WOUND CONTAMINATION

	Total	UV on	UV off	Room 3	Room 4
CFU/ft²/min.	0.08	0.03	0.11	0.08	0.08
Contaminated wounds	2	1	1	2	—

general types: community or home-based infections, operating room-based infections, and hospital-based infections.

Infections that occur in patients during their hospitalization are designated as hospital-acquired or nosocomial infections. They are the result of microbial invasion, most often by antibiotic-resistant and virulent microorganisms of the hospital environment.

In the definition as agreed on by the surgeons at Duke and described by Altemeier and Levenson, a clean wound is considered to be a nontraumatic, uninfected operative wound in which none of the respiratory, alimentary, or genitourinary tracts or the oropharyngeal cavities are entered. Clean wounds are elective, primarily closed, and undrained wounds (Hemovac is currently used in most total hip replacements and this does add another element to the definition). There is an open hole present for as long as 24 to 48 hours after the tubes are removed, and the tubes, in themselves, can become contaminated from surrounding tissue.

Contaminated wounds include open, fresh, traumatic wounds, operations with a major break in sterile technique (e.g., open cardiac massage and incisions

TABLE 7

INCIDENCE OF OPERATIVE WOUNDS AND INFECTION*

Type of Operative Wound	Number	Incidence Number	Infection Percent
Clean	11,690	594	5.1
Clean contaminated	2,589	280	10.8
Contaminated, dirty	1,262	277	21.9
Not reported	72	6	8.3

*From Altemeier and Levenson.[8]

encountering acute, nonpurulent inflammation). Dirty wounds include old traumatic wounds and those involving abscesses or perforated viscera. The very definition of this classification suggests that the organisms causing postoperative infection are present in the operative field before operation. According to Altemeier and Levenson,[8] the controversy over the relative importance of aerial microbial contamination in the incidence of postoperative infection has continued since the last part of the 19th century to the present. Experimental evidence and clinical experience have emphasized the greater importance of contamination from endogenous and exogenous sources through contact. It is generally agreed, however, that there have been proven examples of infection from aerial contamination in hospital practice, but that additional research is needed to further define its importance and to develop appropriate methods of control.

Coventry said, "At Mayo Clinic in 1973, orthopedic surgical infections totaled 1.33%, both deep and superficial, including trauma as well as elective surgery."[26]

UV irradiation does sanitize the air and objects in the operating room. If the patient and operating room personnel are protected by appropriate skin covering and commercially available glasses, no harmful effects occur from UV light. The tissues exposed in various kinds of wounds are not effected adversely other than in ophthalmologic surgery. Airborne bacteria are the most important cause of wound infection although other etiologic factors such as urinary tract, abscessed teeth, wound drainage, skin openings, contamination of the operative site from adjacent areas such as the perineum, contamination of hematoma from adjacent skin, or involvement of a wound hematoma by bacteremia may account for wound infection. The consistently low incidence of wound infection on the Duke Orthopaedic Service without routine use of antibiotics, without special skin preparations, and without the initial limitation of traffic indicates that UV light has been a reliable method of maintaining a low incidence of airborne bacteria and in turn preventing S aureus from causing wound infection. Although we use prophylactic antibiotics (on call dose and for 48 hours postoperative) the purpose of this is to protect the patient from endogenous bacteremia rather than airborne contamination. Bacteria attached to implants may not be susceptible to antibiotics.[42,43]

We do not agree with the conclusions of the National Research Council's study of 1964.[29,30] We believe that study indicated that whenever UV light was used, the incidence of operating room infection when refined clean cases were involved was significantly diminished. Our experience with total hip arthroplasty is the same as our experience with all other refined clean orthopaedic cases with regards to incidence of infection.

Advantages of UV Light in the Operating Room

(1) There is a high output of irradiation in the bactericidal range and low output in the erythemic range; (2) the production of ozone is negligible even when 16 tubes are active; (3) negligible production of heat; (4) low cost of the irradiation unit, which is made up of high transmission glass instead of quartz and averages about $5,000 per room which includes equipment and installation; and (5) low operating cost and less energy used. The estimated life of a tube is 4,000 to 5,000 hours and 10 to 16 tubes are operated with as little current as is required to light a 150-W electric bulb.[15]

The pathologic shedder or carrier is the major target of our efforts in maintaining clean air, whether this be done with air conditioning and high-efficiency filters, unidirectional airflow, antibiotics, or UV light. Gryska and O'Dea[21] emphasized that even with prophylactic antibiotics, the streptococci carried on the anal verge of an anesthesiologist caused a severe bacterial epidemic in the operating room. In that epidemic the organism recovered from the carrier was also recovered from the settle plate within the room and from the wound indicating that the bacteria was primarily airborne.[21,31] Kundsin[17] indicated that the hazard to each patient can be mathematically predicted and this depends on the number of disseminating carriers in the operating room. She noted that in an epidemic involving 13 documented postoperative infections (7.1%) involving operations in 183 patients, an anesthesiologist known to be a B-hemolytic streptococci group A carrier participated in all of these operations. Kundsin[17] also noted that a technician carrying S aureus participated in 169 procedures in which a 1.2% postoperative infection occurred.

If all three carriers described in TABLE 5 were in the same operating room during an operative procedure, the probability of the patient being infected was calculated as 14.4%. The airborne aspect of postoperative wound infection does not occur at a fixed incidence but varies according to the environment in the operating room, the members of the surgical team, resistance of the patient, and the condition of the wound. However, all other factors being equal, *the rate of infection is directly proportional to the number of disseminating carriers in the operating room.* The disseminating carrier may be anywhere in the room, is not necessarily a member of the operating team, and may be in the periphery of the room. Each disseminating carrier contributes to the accumulative risk. Although limiting the traffic would hypothetically limit the number of potential pathologic shedders, that factor is not absolute protection on a day-to-day basis. Also, the air supply to the operative suite is important, but not the critical factor unless exogenous microorganisms are involved due to a faulty air intake system. The critical factor is the commensal flow of people who are present and *even when properly scrubbed, masked, capped, gowned, and shod, the disseminating carrier will still have the capability of projecting microorganisms into space.*

Total Hip Arthroplasty—Incidence of Infection

A review of all total hip arthroplasties done at Duke Hospital has been done annually and recently each patient with infection was identified and analyzed as to the circumstances occurring with each infection. A computer review of all medical records of patients having had total hip replacement was performed and those designated as having infection were reviewed. A second method of retrieval is a punch card system maintained by the Orthopaedic Division at Duke. This system was used to detect any hip arthroplasty infections that may have been missed by the computer review. Furthermore, information on all patients reported as having infection at a monthly complications conference was reviewed and to this was added an independent review which included each member of the attending staff who was asked to recall any patient with whom he had been involved who had a hip infection since 1969. Also, a nurse epidemiologist reviewed all infections from 1969 through 1977. Between these dates, 1,322 total hip replacements were performed by several senior surgeons assisted by many more resident staff members. *There were 18 patients with infections, a total raw infection rate of 1.35%.* These patients were classified both as early and late infections resulting from several different causes. Ten of the total 18 were defined as refined clean cases although the definition was not exact as all of these patients did have postoperative Hemovac drainage, which temporarily provides an exit to the outside from within the wound. *The infection rate for the refined clean cases was 0.68%. This was equivalent to nine of 1,322 patients. Of these nine refined clean cases, seven were readily explained on the basis of bacterial source other than the operating room.* Two of the nine cases of early infected hematomas could not be clearly categorized as to the source of the wound bacteria. Hence, the operating room infection rate when considering these two cases as possible airborne would then be 0.15%. These two patients, as well as two others in the total nine considered as refined clean cases, did not require removal of the prosthesis early or late (TABLE 8).

Conclusions—Clinical Wound Infections

Our view of these 1,322 total hip replacements and a review of the characteristics that effected the development of wound infection indicate that the *source of the bacteria causing the wound infection was usually not airborne.* There was a substantial difference in the number of *Bacillus* sp with UV lights on and with UV lights off. This data confirmed the fact that airborne bacteria are a reflection of the operating room personnel and their activities.

The number of bacteria entering the wound from the air was negligible in all hips monitored with UV lights on. Settle plates were monitored and showed that the air conditioning systems were sufficient to maintain airborne bacteria at a relatively low level, but that the addition of UV light diminished this level even more.

The assumption that auto infection occurred several times is justified. Nosocomial infection occurred on a few occasions in spite of antibiotics. We believe that the highly effective air conditioning system cools and dehumidifies the air in the orthopaedic operating rooms at Duke and provides adequate air exchange in cooling.[32] *The supplementary use of UV light during the time when the patient and the operating team are functioning will diminish airborne bacteria to an acceptable level.*[21,22,31]

TABLE 8

INFECTIONS IN REFINED CLEAN CASES

Patient Infection Refined Clean Case	Prosthesis Left In or Out	Operating Room Source?	Probable Source of Infection
Patient 3	Out	Yes	Methacrylate
Patient 5	Out	No	Urinary tract
Patient 10	In	No	Hematoma, external contamination
Patient 11	Out	No	Septecemia, 3 years
Patient 13	In	?	Hematoma
Patient 14	In	?	Hematoma
Patient 15	Out	No	1½ years respiratory infection
Patient 17	Out	No	1½ years, source ?
Patient 18	In	No	Urinary tract

The evidence provided by the air sampling study, both with and without the UV lights on, documents the effectiveness of UV lights in killing bacteria quickly on exposed surfaces.

Other Factors Contributing to Development of Wound Infection in Total Hip Arthroplasty

Factors other than airborne bacteria to be considered in analyzing the occurrence of wound infection in patients receiving total hip arthroplasty include the following: (1) drapes, gowns, scrub suits; comparative studies between various weaves, liquid repellents, and different kinds of wristlets, neck covers, and wraparounds;[33] (2) preparation of the perineum from the operative site with special draping techniques and avoidance of soilage during the procedure; (3) coverage of the operating room personnel, ie, the surgeon, with particular attention to the exposed or unexposed neck area, and head or facial hair. Fallout from pant legs, exposed back, and shedding from other sites;[34] (4) skin preparation, reanalyze immediate bacterial kill vs slow kill, and prolonged action of the skin antiseptic; (5) where to anesthetize the patient to decrease particle activity and bacterial concentrations—anesthetic room or in the main room with all instruments and prostheses covered?; (6) urinary tract infection-detect by urinalysis and, if necessary, preoperative culture; (7) aspiration and culture of previously operated hip, aerobic, anaerobic, L forms?; (8) catheterization—avoid before, during, and after the operation; (9) intravenous lines-eliminate as soon as possible: (10) anticoagulation monitored carefully. Avoid excess, even in high-risk patients; (11) postoperative wound management for Hemovac holes, wound compression, and management of persistent drainage or frank hematoma; (12) prophylactic antibiotics—initiate preoperatively, use intraoperatively, and minimal period of time postoperatively;[35] (13) sterility of implants including methacrylate, high-density polyethylene, and metallic components. Avoid exposure while waiting for insertion; (14) patient assessment as to high risk, e.g., rheumatoid arthritis (immune system), patient receiving short-term steroid therapy, or patient with chronic pulmonary obstructive disease; (15) epidemiologic studies of operating room personnel for skin contamination, respiratory infection, and hand cleansing during scrubbing; (16) anesthesiology personnel entering and leaving the room; coverage of hair; locus minoris resistance at site of intubation or other invasive procedures; and (17) wound management in regard to the following: excision of necrotic muscle and fat, nonabsorbable sutures deep or nonreactive, minimal reactive absorbable sutures subcutaneously, dead space closure, adequate Hemovac drainage, compression to absorb hematoma, and monitoring of anticoagulation.

REFERENCES

1. HART, D. 1936. Sterilization of the air in the operating rooms by special bactericidal radiant energy. J Thorac. Cardiovasc. Surg. **6**: 45–81.
2. HART, D. 1938. Pathogenic bacteria in the air of operating rooms: Their widespread distribution and the methods of control. Arch. Surg. **37**: 521–530.
3. MELENEY, F. L. 1933. The control of wound infection. Ann. Surg. **98**: 151–153.
4. BOURDILLON, R. B. & L. COLEBROOK. 1946. Air hygiene in dressing rooms for burns or major wounds. Lancet **1**: 561–565, 601–605.
5. BOURDILLON, R. B., A. M. MCFARLAN & J. C. THOMAS. 1948. Airborne Bacteria in Operating Theaters. In Studies of Air Hygiene. Medical Research Council, Special Report Series No. 262: 241–253. London. Her Majesty's Stationary Office.
6. CHARNLEY, J. & N. EFTAKHAR. 1972. Postoperative infection after total hip replacement with special reference to air contamination in the operating room. Clin. Orthop. **87**: 167–187.
7. LIDWELL, O. M. & A. G. TOWERS. 1969. Protection from microbial contamination in a room ventilated by unidirectional flow. J. Hyg **67**: 95–106.
8. ALTEMEIER, W. A. & S. LEVENSON. 1970. Trauma workshop report: Infections, immunology, and gnotobiosis. J. Trauma **10**: 1084–1086.
9. BOND, R. G., M. M. HALBERT & H. D. PUTNAM. 1964. Survey of Microbial Contamination in the Surgical Suites of 23 hospitals. University Health Service and School of Public Health. University of Minnesota. Minneapolis.
10. FEAGIN J. A., JR. 1976. The case for clean air. Workshop on Control of Operating Room Airborne Bacteria. Committee on Prosthetics Research and Development. Committee on Prosthetic Orthotic Education. Assembly of Life Sciences: 86–92. National Research Council. National Academy of Sciences.

11. FITZGERALD R. H. 1976. Airborne bacterial contamination in the conventional operating room. Committee on Prosthetics Research and Development. Committee on Prosthetic Orthotic Education. Assembly of Life Sciences: 93–103. National Research Council. National Academy of Sciences.

12. FITZGERALD, R. H., D. R. NOLAN & D. M. RALSTRUP, 1977. Deep wound sepsis following total hip arthroplasty. J Bone Joint Surg (Am) **59**(7): 847–855.

13. GOLDNER, J. L. 1975. Ultraviolet light in the orthopedic operating room. Read before the American Academy of Orthopedic Surgeons.

14. GOLDNER, J. L. & B. L. ALLEN. 1973. Ultraviolet light in orthopedic operating rooms at Duke University: 35 years' experience, 1937–1973. Clin. Ortho. **96**: 195–205.

15. GOLDNER, J. L., R. W. GAINES & M. HIGGINS. 1976. Ultraviolet light in the orthopedic operating rooms at Duke University: Thirty-seven Years' Experience, 1937–1974. Committee on Prosthetics Research and Development. Committee on Prosthetic Orthotic Education. Assembly of Life Sciences: 104–149. National Research Council. National Academy of Sciences.

16. HART, D., H. M. SCHIEBEL & D. G. SHARP. 1960. Bactericidal ultraviolet radiation in the operating room: Twenty-nine year study for control of infections. J. Am. Med. Assoc. **172**: 1019–1028.

17. KUNDSIN, R. B. 1976. Operating room as a source of wound contamination and infection. Workshop on Control of Operating Room Airborne Bacteria. Committee on Prosthetics Research and Development. Committee on Prosthetic Orthotic Education. Assembly of Life Sciences: 167–172. National Research Council. National Academy of Sciences.

18. LOWELL, J. D. 1976. Experiences with ultraviolet light in operating rooms. Workshop on Control of Operating Room Airborne Bacteria. Committee on Prosthetics Research and Development. Committee on Prosthetic Orthotic Education. Assembly of Life Sciences. 203–206. National Research Council. National Academy of Sciences.

19. WALTER, C. W., R. B. KUNDSEN & M. D. BRUBAKER. 1963. The incidence of airborne infection during operation. J. Am. Med. Assoc. **186**: 908–913.

20. WRIGHT, R. L. 1970. Septic Complications of Neurosurgical Spinal Procedures. Springfield, Ill. Charles C Thomas.

21. GRYSKA, P. F. & A. G. O'DEA. 1970. Postoperative streptococcal wound infection: The anatomy of an epidemic. J. Am. Med. Assoc. **213**: 1189–1191.

22. MCKEE, W. M., J. M. DECAPRIO & C. E. ROBERTS. 1966. Anal carriage as the probable source of a streptococcal epidemic. Lancet **2**: 1007–1009.

23. WHYTE, W. & B. H. SHAW. 1973. A bacteriologic evaluation of laminar air flow systems for orthopedic surgery. J. Hyg. **71**: 1–6.

24. SHARP, D. G. 1938. A quantitative method of determining the lethal effect of ultraviolet light on bacteria suspended in air. J. Bacteriol. **35**: 589–599.

25. SHARP, D. G. 1940. Effect of ultraviolet light on bacteria suspended in air. J. Bacteriol. **39**: 535–547.

26. KOCH, G. G. 1978. Department of Biostatistics. School of Public Health. University of North Carolina at Chapel Hill.

27. FITZGERALD, R. H., L. D. PETERSON & J. A. WASHINGTON, II. 1973. Bacterial colonization of wounds and sepsis in total hip arthroplasty. J. Bone Joint Surg. (Am) **55**: 1242–1250.

28. HART, D., J. NICKS. 1961. Ultraviolet radiation in the operating room: Intensities used and bactericidal effects. Arch. Surg. **82**: 449–465.

29. REUTSCHLER, H. C., R. NAGY & G. MONROMSEFF. 1941. Bactericidal effect of ultraviolet radiation. J Bacteriol. **41**: 745–775.

30. HART, D., R. W. POSTLETHWAIT & I. W. BROWN. 1968. Postoperative wound infections: A further report on ultraviolet irradiation with comments on the recent (1964) National Research Council Cooperative Study Report. Ann. Surg. **167**: 728–743.

31. National Research Council Study: Postoperative wound infections: the influence of ultraviolet irradiation in the operating rooms and of various other factors. 1964. Ann. Surg. **160**: 1–192.

32. MCINTYRE, D. M. 1968. An epidemic of *Streptococcus pyogenes* puerperal and

postoperative sepsis with an unusual carrier site—the anus. Am. J. Obstet. Gynecol. **101**: 308–314.

33. LIDWELL, O. M. 1973. The Ventilation of Surgical Operating Rooms: The Last 50 Years: Airborne Transmissions and Airborne Infection: 561–568. John Wiley & Sons. New York.

34. LAUFMAN, H. 1976. What is the hard evidence on the role of airborne bacteria in wound infection? Workshop on Control of Operating Room Airborne Bacteria. Committee on Prosthetics Research and Development. Committee on Prosthetic Orthotic Education. Assembly of Life Sciences. 173–182. National Research Council. National Academy of Sciences.

35. SCHAFFNER, W., L. B. LEFKOWITZ & J. S. GOODMAN. 1969. Hospital outbreak of infections with group A streptococci traced to an asymptomatic and carrier. N. Engl. J. Med. **280**: 1224–1225.

36. OGDEN, W. S., & J. L. GOLDNER. 1971. Antibiotics in Orthopedic Surgery: Changing Concepts. Duke University and Affiliated Institutions—Orthopedic Training Program Papers, No. 4, Durham, N. C.

37. MOODY, W. R. 1971. Suggested protocol for monitoring, maintaining, and insuring safe usage of ultraviolet germicidal lamps in the hospital. Thesis. The University of North Carolina at Chapel Hill.

38. GAGE, A. A., D. C. DEAN & G. SCHIMERT. 1970. *Aspergillus* infection after cardiac surgery. Arch. Surg. **101**: 384–387.

39. HUNTER, G. 1977. The natural history of the patient with an infected total hip replacement. J. Bone Joint Surg. (Br) **59**(3): 293–297.

40. KOLLER, L. D. 1952. Ultraviolet Radiation. John Wiley & Sons. New York.

41. LAWRENCE, C. A. & S. S. BLOCK. 1968. Disinfection, Sterilization, and Preservation: 761–773. Philadelphia. Lea & Febiger.

42. MOGGIO, M., J. L. GOLDNER, D. E. McCOLLUM & S. F. BEISSINGER. 1979. Wound infections in patients undergoing total hip arthroplasty—ultraviolet light for the control of airborne bacteria. Arch. Surg. **114**: 815–823.

43. GRISTINA, A. 1979. Personal Communication.

ULTRAVIOLET RADIATION AND REDUCTION OF DEEP WOUND INFECTION FOLLOWING HIP AND KNEE ARTHROPLASTY

J. Drennan Lowell, Ruth B. Kundsin, Charles M. Schwartz
and Deborah Pozin

Harvard Medical School
Brigham and Women's Hospital
Boston, Massachusetts 02115

Deep wound infection as a complication of clean surgery is not a new problem and it is not a problem solely limited to the specialty of orthopaedic surgery. It has been a concern of surgeons since the beginning of the surgical era and although tremendous strides have been made in prevention and treatment, the problem is still with us and will remain.

The issue forced itself upon the orthopaedic surgeon with renewed vigor in the late 1960s and early 1970s with the advent of total joint replacement surgery and its unique success in dealing with the problems imposed by arthritis of the weight-bearing joints. In a very few years, surgeons all over the world learned the techniques and applied them to thousands of patients. By the mid-1970s, it is estimated that in the United States, 100,000 patients annually were undergoing total hip replacement arthroplasty, with many more thousands having replacement surgery of the knee, ankle, shoulder, elbow, wrist, and hand. If we assume a deep wound infection rate of 1 percent, an exceedingly conservative figure, the number of patients developing wound infection of the hip would be 1,000 per year and the best evidence suggests that the infection rate is at least twice this. With the price of a hospital bed in many major medical institutions in excess of $200 per day and the length of hospitalization for treatment of these infections running from 4 weeks to 6 months, the cost of dealing with them, let alone the misery and suffering accruing to the patients, is staggering, averaging over $20,000 per patient and often exceeding $100,000.[1] The patient whose joint replacement prosthesis must be removed in order to control infection is often left worse off than prior to surgery.

The term 'refined clean surgery' is usually applicable to joint replacement procedures. The joints rarely have been the site of previous surgery or infection and contrary to the situation in general surgery, regions such as the gastrointestinal, genitourinary, and respiratory tracts are not entered. Endogenous bacteriologic soiling is an unlikely accompaniment of the procedure. Contamination must, therefore, come from without, the possible exception being a bacteremia from manipulations of the mouth and respiratory tract that accompany intubation as a necessary part of anesthetic management. The procedure is elective. Historically the orthopaedic community came by its concern quite naturally. The first uniformly successful method of managing the painful arthritic hip was developed by M. N. Smith-Petersen in the late 1930s and called mold arthroplasty. The femoral head and acetabulum were reshaped from deformed contours to round, matching, congruous surfaces. Between these, a nonperishable barrier was interposed of chrome-cobalt-molybdenum alloy to guide the repair process. Over a period of months a fibro-cartilaginous covering of the bone developed.

0077-8923/80/0353-0285 $01.75/0 © 1980, NYAS

This technically demanding procedure and long recovery period achieved good to excellent results in 65 to 80 percent of the patients.[2] The rate of deep wound infection was 1.2 percent but in only 28 percent did the metal mold need to be removed to control the problem.

Into this state of affairs came the new technique of total hip replacement, largely developed by Charnley, McKee-Farrar, and Ring in England. The method developed by Charnley has become the most widely accepted and requires replacement of the head and neck of the femur with a metallic prosthesis and insertion of a high density polyethylene liner into the acetabulum. Polymethylmethacrylate cement holds the two components in place. The joint is aneural; pain relief is prompt and almost uniformly complete. Restoration of function requires only the healing of the soft tissues and a modest rehabilitation program. Ninety-five percent of patients have complete or almost complete relief of pain and restoration of excellent function.

In England, during the period 1959 to 1961, 8.9 percent of patients undergoing Charnley total hip arthroplasty developed deep wound sepsis and although Charnley undertook a concerted and successful effort to reduce the rate of deep wound infection, the fact of success was not immediately apparent and needed to wait longitudinal follow up.[3] When his technique was first adopted in the United States, the rate of deep wound infection was higher.[4] For those patients developing infection, Charnley recommended removal of the total hip components and advised against any further attempt at reconstruction.

It can be well appreciated that orthopaedic surgeons faced a difficult choice between the two methods, when one was so dazzling in its rate of success, and the other, though less spectacular, so infrequently accompanied by the disaster of infection.

Charnley addressed the issue in numerous ways but believed the step most effective was the development of ultra-filtered, unidirectional air flow with multiple air changes per hour that essentially cleansed the environment over the operative site of particulate matter and the microorganisms clinging to it. As he reduced the number of viable colonies per hour recovered on his settle plates from 80 to 0, his rate of deep wound infection diminished from 8.9 to 1.3 percent.

The Peter Bent Brigham Hospital is old; it received its first patient in 1913. Its sister institution, the Robert Breck Brigham Hospital, is of the same vintage. The operating suites are antiquated; the ventilation system is not satisfactory and provides only 17 air changes per hour. If these institutions were to offer joint replacement surgery to their patient population in the 1970s, measures to reduce the threat of airborne contamination appeared essential. A new hospital complex to house the two institutions was already deep in the planning stages and the administration and trustees were not anxious to install expensive air-handling equipment requiring major modifications to operating facilities soon to be abandoned. Some approach other than the use of ultra-filtered air was required.

The published material from Duke University on the use by Hart and his coworkers of ultraviolet radiation to reduce the problem of surgical infections was available and reviewed. His employment of ultraviolet radiation well antedated the use of antibiotics to prevent and treat surgical wound infections. From 1930 to 1941, the combined rate of wound infection in clean operations performed in conventional operating rooms was 11.3 percent and 1.04 percent died of their infections. In 1936 he introduced ultraviolet radiation in some of the operating rooms and the combined infection rate in operations done in these dropped to 0.24 percent in clean cases and the death rate secondary to sepsis to 0 percent.[5]

His approach to the problem of preventing wound infection was not widely accepted and few favorable reports can be found in the medical literature. Overholt and Betz reduced the infection rate in thoracotomies from 13.8 percent to 2.7 percent; Penfield saw a reduction of infection in neurosurgical procedures in Montreal from 1.1 to 0.4 percent; and Wright and Burke reported a reduction in the infection rate of craniotomy and discectomy wounds at the Massachusetts General Hospital from 4.76 to .64 percent.[6-7] An adverse report was published in 1964, a prospective study combining the experience of five institutions by an Ad Hoc Committee, the Committee on Trauma, Division of Medical Sciences, National Academy of Sciences, National Research Council.[9] In the concluding paragraphs of this cooperative study, it was stated that the only surgical wound which seemed to benefit from the employment of ultraviolet radiation in the operating room was the refined clean wound and in these, the infection rate was reduced from 3.8 to 2.9 percent. The effect of this improvement appeared to be lost in the overall experience and concerned only 19 percent of all infections.

There were hazards to the use of ultraviolet radiation and these included the development of painful conjunctivitis in individuals whose eyes were not protected by some form of shielding and if exposure exceeded 2–3 minutes. Erythema of the skin followed exposure of more than 20–30 minutes.[10]

Hart published a rebuttal to this report, noting that the rate of improvement of infection in the participating institutions varied between 15 and 44 percent with those institutions having the highest rate of infection in rooms where radiation was not used, experiencing the greatest percent of improvement in the rooms where it was.[11] It was apparent that during the study the intensity of the radiation was less than the recommended optimum in 58 percent of the operating rooms and that it was less than recommended in the periphery of all of the operating rooms. It may have been 19 percent of the infections but it was 43 percent of the operations.

Our own review of this study suggests that the relationship between the humidity of the operating theatre and the effectiveness of ultraviolet radiation was not considered. This is an important factor, known and reported by Wells in 1940, and from data we obtained from the United States Weather Service could easily have entered into the results observed in the cooperative study in a negative fashion.[12]

Exogenous microbial contamination of surgical wounds is a recognized occurrence but few reports exist equating pathogens subsequently indicted as the cause of a post-operative infection as being within the environment at the time of surgery, on members of the operating team, or on the patient. Burke reported such a study in which 100 percent of 50 surgical wounds were found to contain organisms upon culture during the course of the operation.[13] Ninety-two percent of these wounds contained a coagulase-positive staphylococcus and the average number of strains of these staphylococci in each wound was 5.8. Two wound infections ensued. In one of these, the coagulase-positive staphylococcus responsible for the infection could, by phage typing, be identified as an organism present in the air in contact with the wound during the operation and in washings from the wound. Walter, Kundsin, Harding and Page have reported on the high incidence of *Staphylococcus aureus* carriers among operating room personnel and by phage typing identified four disseminating carriers as the source of 18 wound infections occurring at the Peter Bent Brigham Hospital.[14] By epidemiological evidence, they identified these four disseminating carriers as the source of 25 additional wound infections. Walter, Kundsin, and Brubaker in a separate study by phage typing identified again a known *Staphylococcus aureus* carrier as the source of two wound infections occurring in 169 clean operations, during which he was present in the room as a nonscrubbed member of the surgical team.[15] Walter and Kundsin have also identified by typing two anesthesiologists in different institutions as being the source of four post-operative *Staphylococcus aureus* infections occurring in 55 patients in one instance and the source of 13 beta hemolytic streptococcus Group A infections following 183 operations in the other. The infection rates in these three groups of patients are 1.2 percent, 7.3 percent and 7.1 percent respectively. A formula can be developed to show the probability of infection occurring in a patient operated upon in a hypothetical circumstance where these three individuals would participate. The probability is 14.4 percent. Such are the possibilities of exogenous contamination.

In 1973, ultraviolet lamps were installed in the two operatings of the Robert Breck Brigham Hospital and in four of the operating rooms of the Peter Bent Brigham Hospital. They are ceiling-mounted and located to produce an intensity of radiation at the level of the operating room table throughout the room in accordance with the criteria of Hart. This level of intensity is 25–30 microwatts per second per centimeter squared.[16] Soon after their installation, an experiment was carried out to assess their effectiveness.[17] Using an ultrasonic nebulizer, nonpathogenic *Escherichia coli* were nebulized into each of two operating rooms and a Well air centrifuge was used to determine the concentration of viable organisms. In the first room, 930 organisms per 5 cubic feet were recovered by the air centrifuge, but when the lamps were illuminated, even though the nebulizer was not turned off, no viable organisms could be recovered; in the second room, 310 viable organisms per 5 cubic feet could be recovered and when the same test of the lamps was used again, one viable organism per 5 cubic feet was recovered. In the first room, there was 100 percent removal; in the second, 99.7 percent removal of viable organisms.

Settle plates were then used to assess the number of viable particles landing on flat surfaces during the course of an actual procedure. Throughout the room with each minute of time, 4–8 viable particles could be recovered. The spectrum of organisms was varied including Bacillus species, *Staph epidermidis*, Micrococcus, diphtheroids, and Sarcina. When the lamps were illuminated during three unusual and difficult procedures lasting up to 5 hours, the number of viable particles recovered throughout the room dropped to 0.2 per square foot per minute. A culture of the face mask of one of the scrubbed members of the operating team which was made at the conclusion of the procedure by pressing it on a blood agar plate revealed innumerable *Staph epidermidis* and a few *Staph aureus* organisms. Volumetric air samples taken at multiple locations about the operating room including the region of the surgical wounds showed a drop in the number of viable particles from 7 per 5 cubic feet to an average of 1 with illumination of the lamps. *Staphylococcus aureus* was among the organisms recovered in this portion of the study.

Lastly Rodac agar contact plates were used to sample a large number of flat surfaces, both with and without the use of ultraviolet radiation. The findings from this method were quite interesting, particularly with reference to the overhead lights used to illuminate the operating field. Under the usual operating room circumstances, there was a gradual build-up of viable particles on the tops of these lamps from which they could easily be dislodged if the lamps were shifted to obtain better lighting of the operative field. With exposure to ultraviolet radiation, the top of these lights became bacteriologically sterile. The operating room floor of an unirradiated room had viable microorganisms too numerous to count, including pseudomonas but the floor of the irradiated room yielded no viable organisms. Rendered essentially free of viable organisms by ultraviolet radiation were the Mayo stand, open shelves, the top of the Bovie apparatus, the top of the anesthesia cart and exposed flat surfaces of basically any type. Organisms in profusion, however, could be recovered from the pedestral of an operating room lamp shielded from the radiation by the proximity of surgical drapes. Ultraviolet radiation then deals both with airborne organisms and those which have already settled on dry, flat surfaces.

Safe use of ultraviolet radiation has required the development of a protocol to protect the operating room personnel and patients from harmful side effects. The most unpleasant and disabling side effect is conjunctivitis which will occur after only 2–3 minutes of direct exposure but will also occur after indirect exposure over slightly longer periods. The eyes must be protected by shields of some sort. Ordinary eye glasses are impenetrable to 2537 A radiation, the electromagnetic frequency produced by the mercury vapor lamps. Reflected light, however, can reach the eyes at the sides. Industrial goggles or side shields are necessary in addition. Only specially formulated glass allows the passage of 2537A radiation so essentially any ordinary goggle of glass or plastic is protective. The skin should be protected from exposure of more than 15–20 minutes either by clothing or a sunscreen lotion containing benzophenone.

Cloth drapes, gowns, and hoods as well as disposable types are each protective against ultraviolet radiation. The patient's face can and should be protected by the drapes placed over the anesthesia screen. A disagreeable, superficial erythema with delayed scaling will result from over-exposure. 2537 A radiation is not a good tanning agent, as it does not penetrate deeply into the skin.

Because we have found the ultraviolet lamps so immediately effective in destroying airborne microorganisms, we have elected to turn the lamps on at the time of incision and off at the completion of wound closure. This makes the logistics of bringing the patient into the operating room, inducing anesthesia, prepping and draping much simpler than if the lamps were kept illuminated continuously.

Frequently the question has been raised by operating room personnel with respect to the possibility of skin malignancy being produced as a result of ultraviolet radiation exposure in the operating theatre. Although the Brigham experience comprises slightly less than 7 years of use, the experience at Duke University extends for a period greater than 30 years. They report no occasion of ultraviolet radiation induced malignancy in their personnel—physicians, patients or assistants—and experimentally it has not been possible to produce skin malignancy in mice with 2537 A radiation.[18]

The relative humidity is monitored in each operating room and should be kept below 60 percent. The effectiveness of the lamps drops off precipitously above this level, to become almost ineffectual at 80 or 90 percent. The intensity of the radiation is monitored during each operative procedure by the nursing service with a germicidal photometer which is portable, battery-operated, and easy to use. Based on the photometer reading, the power input to the lamps can be readily adjusted by a wall-mounted dimmer switch similar to that used for home lighting. Including the nursing service as part of the controlling team has made the monitoring process accurate, simple, easy, and frequent and the overall

TABLE 1

COMPARISON OF INFECTION RATES WITH AND WITHOUT ULTRAVIOLET RADIATION

Infections Hips		PBBH & RBBH		
Pre-UV Radiation				
Primary Ops	519	Infections	11 =	2.1%
Previous Ops	102	Infections	8 =	7.8%
	621		19	3.06%
With UV Radiation				
Primary Ops	1516	Infections	6 =	.4%
Previous Ops	196	Infections	3 =	1.5%
	1712		9	.53%

acceptance of the method much easier in an era when the very word "radiation" conjures up frightening visions.

Records have been kept of all patients undergoing total hip and knee arthroplasty at the two Brigham hospitals since June 1970 to the present and in assessing the patients with the problem of deep wound infection, none have been followed for shorter than a six-month period. The most recent follow-up study includes those patients operated upon through March, 1979. Records have also been kept on all those patients undergoing other types of total joint replacement as they were developed during this same period. Prior to the installation of the ultraviolet lamps in 1973, 621 patients had undergone total hip replacement and 19 deep wound infections followed; the infection rate was 3.06 percent (TABLE 1). Among this group of patients, 519 had primary surgery and 11 infections followed, a rate of 2.1 percent. One hundred two patients had had previous surgery on the same hip and 8 deep wound infections followed, a rate of 7.8 percent. Since the use of ultraviolet radiation, 1712 patients have undergone total hip replacement surgery and 9 infections followed, producing an inflection rate of 0.53 percent. Of these, 1516 were primary operations and followed by 6 infections, a rate of .4 percent. One hundred ninety-six patients had had previous surgery on the same hip and 3 infections followed, a rate of 1.5 percent. In our series, as well as in all other reported series, the rate of infection in hips previously operated has been 2–4 times as high as those without previous surgery, but where methods of air contamination control have been instituted, the deep wound infection rate in each category of patient has dropped.

The deep wound infection rate in total knee replacement surgery also improved during this same observation period (TABLE 2). Sixty-eight patients

TABLE 2

DEEP WOUND INFECTION RATE IN TOTAL KNEE REPLACEMENT SURGERY

Infections Knees		PBBH & RBBH		
Pre UV Radiation				
Primary Ops	63	Infections	6 =	9.52%
Previous Ops	5	Infections	1 =	20.0%
	68		7	10.3%
With UV Radiation				
Primary Ops	1424	Infections	4 =	.28%
Previous Ops	100	Infections	8 =	8.0%
	1524		12	.79%

TABLE 3

INFECTION RATE OF TOTAL ELBOW, SHOULDER AND ANKLE REPLACEMENT SURGERY
WITH ULTRAVIOLET RADIATION

Infections With UV Radiation	Elbow, Shoulder, Ankle		PBBH & RBBH	
Elbow	Primary Op	46	Infections	2 = 4.3%
	Previous Op	11	Infections	0 = 0
		57		2 3.5%
Shoulder	Primary Op	71	Infections	0 = 0
Ankle	Primary Op	58	Infections	0 = 0
		186		2 1.1%

underwent total knee replacement surgery without ultraviolet radiation in the operating room and 7 developed deep wound infection. Sixty-three had not had previous surgery on the same knee and 6 developed infection; 5 had had previous surgery and 1 developed infection. Since the use of ultraviolet radiation, 1524 patients have undergone knee replacement surgery; 12 have developed deep wound infection, a rate of .79 percent. Among the 1424 of these having primary surgery in the knee, 4 developed infection, a rate of .28 percent; of 100 having had previous knee surgery, 8 developed an infection, a rate of 8.0 percent.

The total elbow, shoulder, and ankle replacement surgery has come into being since the use of ultraviolet radiation was adopted at the Brighams and in 186 patients undergoing this type of surgery, deep wound infection occurred in 2, a rate of 1.1 percent (TABLE 3). Both of these infections occurred among 46 patients undergoing primary elbow arthroplasty. To date, none have occurred among the 11 patients undergoing elbow arthroplasty who had had previous surgery, or in 71 patients undergoing primary shoulder arthroplasty, or in 58 patients undergoing primary ankle arthroplasty.

J.P. Nelson reviewed much of the published literature on the problem of deep wound infection in patients undergoing total hip arthroplasty and by combining available data, found the problem to be as follows:[19]

If the patient had his hip replacement surgery in a conventional operating room and prophylactic antibiotics were not used, the infection rate was 5.8 percent (TABLE 4). If it was a regular operating room and antibiotics were used, the rate of 1.3 percent. If ultra-filtered air rapidly changed (a clean room) was employed but prophylactic antibiotics were not given, the rate was 0.7 percent. With a clean room and the use of prophylactic antibiotics, the rate was 0.6 percent. Our concurrently observed infection rate of 0.53 percent compares favorably.

TABLE 4

TOTAL HIP ARTHROPLASTY DEEP WOUND INFECTION RATES

		Total number of Patients	Infected Patients	
Regular or	No antibiotics	1880	109	5.8%
Regular or	Antibiotics	6791	90	1.3%
Clean room	No antibiotics	2730	18	0.7%
Clean room	Antibiotics	2754	17	0.6%
Ultraviolet	Antibiotics	1712	9	0.5%

The cost of equipping an operating room with ultraviolet radiation, at the time it was done at the two Brigham hospitals, was $1500 per room including the photometer. Assuming it to have doubled or tripled in cost in the interim, it still leaves the cost considerably below that for the installation of air-filtration techniques and the electrical consumption of the lamps is almost negligible. The lamps are completely out of the way of other equipment in the room and do not interfere with use of the room for cases other than joint replacement surgery. To date, our experience can be summarized by saying the equipment has been simple to install, easy to use, productive of minor inconvenience, effective, relatively inexpensive and with few complications.

REFERENCES

1. EFTEKHAR, N. S. 1978. Principles of Total Hip Arthroplasty. C.V. Mosby Co. St. Louis.
2. AUFRANC, O E. 1957. Constructive hip surgery with the vitallium mold: A report of 1000 cases of arthroplasty of the hip over a fifteen-year period. J. Bone Joint Surg. **39A:** 237–248.
3. CHARNLEY, J. & N. EFTEKHAR. 1969. Post operative infection in total hip prosthetic replacement arthroplasty of the hip joint with special reference to the bacterial content of the air of the operating room. Br. J. Surg. **56:** 641–649.
4. WILSON, P. D., Jr., H. C. AMSTUTZ, A. CZERNIECKI, E. A. SALVATI & D. G. MENDES. 1972. Total hip replacement with fixation by acrylic cement. J. Bone Joint Surg. **54A:** 207–236.
5. HART, D. 1960. Bactericidal ultraviolet radiation in the operating room. J. Am. Med. Assoc. **172:** 1019–1028.
6. OVERHOLT, R. H. & R. H. BETTS. 1940. A comparative report on infection of thoracoplasty wounds: Experience with ultraviolet irradiation of operating room air. J. Thorac. Surg. **9:** 520–529.
7. WOODHALL, B. R., et al. 1949. Ultraviolet radiation as an adjunct in the control of postoperative neurosurgical infection, II. Clinical experience 1938–1948. Ann. Surg. **129:** 820–825.
8. WRIGHT, R. L. & J. BURKE. 1969. Effect of ultraviolet radiation on postoperative neurosurgical sepsis. J. Neurosurg. **31:** 533–537.
9. AD HOC COMMITTEE OF THE COMMITTEE ON TRAUMA. 1964. Division of Medical Sciences. National Academy of Sciences-National Research Council. Postoperative wound infections: The influence of ultraviolet irradiation of the operating room and of various other factors. Ann. Surg. (Suppl) **160:** 1–192.
10. PARRISH, J. A., M. A. PATHAK & T. B. FITZPATRICK. 1972. Topical protection against germicidal radiation. Arch. Surg. **104:** 276.
11. HART, D., R. W. POSTLETHWAIT, I. W. BROWN, W. W. SMITH & P. A. JOHNSON. 1968. Post-operative wound infections: A further report on ultraviolet irradiation with comments on the recent (1964) National Research Council cooperative study report. Ann. Surg. **67:** 728.
12. WELLS, W. F. 1955. Airborne Contagion and Air Hygiene. Harvard University Press. Cambridge.
13. BURKE, J. F. 1963. Identification of the sources of staphylococci contaminating the surgical wound during operation. Ann. Surg. **158:** 898–904.
14. WALTER, C. W., R. B. KUNDSIN, A. L. HARDING & L. K. PAGE. 1967. The infector on the surgical team. Clin. Neurosurg. **14:** 361–379.
15. WALTER, C. W., R. B. KUNDSIN & M. N. BRUBAKER. 1963. The incidence of airborne wound infection during operation. J. Am. Med. Assoc. **186:** 903.
16. NAGY R. 1964. Application and measurement of ultraviolet radiation. Amer. Indust. Hygiene Assn. J. **25:** 274–281.
17. LOWELL, J. D. & R. B. KUNDSIN. 1977. Ultraviolet radiation: Its beneficial effect on the

operating room environment and the incidence of deep wound infection after total hip and total knee arthroplasty. **26:** 58–65. American Academy of Orthopaedic Surgeons Instructional Course Lectures. C.V. Mosby Co. St. Louis.

18. RUSCH H. P., B. E. KLINE & C. A. BAUMAN. 1941. Carcinogenesis by ultraviolet rays with reference to wave length and energy. Arch. Pathol. **31:** 135–146.

19. NELSON, J. P. 1977. The operating room environment and its influence on deep wound infection. The Hip Society. Proceedings of the Fifth Open Scientific Meeting of the Hip Society: 129–146. C.V. Mosby Co. St. Louis.

THE TREATMENT OF BURN PATIENTS IN A LAMINAR AIRFLOW ENVIRONMENT

Robert H. Demling

Department of Surgery
University of California, Davis
Sacramento, California 95817

Jeanne Maly

Burn Center of the University of Wisconsin
Madison, Wisconsin 53206

Infection is the major cause of death in the burn patient.[1] The burned skin is an ideal culture media for bacteria. This added to the severe immune depression seen after burn injury produces a patient very prone to infection.[2] Although endogenous bacteria readily colonize the wound, life threatening infections are frequently caused by exogenous hospital born organisms resistent to standard antibiotics.[3] These organisms are not only dangerous to the individual patient but can also infect other neighboring patients by cross-contamination. It is difficult to determine how significant infection by airborn transmission of these organisms, is as compared to contact spread by personnel. Laminar airflow techniques have been shown to significantly decrease infection rate in other infection prone patients which indicates airborn transmission to be an important source of infection.[4] As a result of a laminar airflow system, particles and bacteria in the air are rapidly removed producing a sterile air environment[5] (FIGURE 1).

The University of Wisconsin Burn Center constructed a four bed horizontal laminar airflow isolation unit in 1974 to be used exclusively for the care of the burn patients in order to decrease infection rate (FIGURES 2,3). Recently the burn center moved to a new university hospital where two isolation units with a total of seven beds, is being used. The rate of laminar air flow in the system can be adjusted between 60 and 90 feet per minute depending on activity. The air filters then remove 99.85 per cent of particles more than 0.3μ. The patient area in each unit measures 20×20 feet with no physical barrier between beds. This allows room for ambulation, therapy and burn care. The nurse's station, kitchen and storage are in an area outside of the laminar airflow system (LAF).

We reviewed our experience over a three year period (1975–1978) to determine the effectiveness of the system in decreasing infection and also to identifying any problems encountered with the system.[6]

METHODS

Burn patients with a high risk for infection were admitted to the LAF unit. These included patients with more than 15 percent body burn or with an inhalation injury irregardless of the size of the burn. Strict sterile techniques with the use of caps, masks, gowns, and gloves, were practiced at all times in the unit. No contact was made between patients, each having separate supplies, with personnel changing sterile clothing between patient treatments. All material, except food, entering the unit was sterilized or dipped in disinfectant. Food

0077-8923/80/0353-0294 $01.75/0 © 1980, NYAS

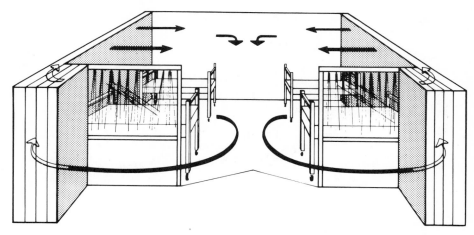

FIGURE 1. Design of 4-bed laminar airflow system is shown. Air is filtered in panels then recirculated in a horizontal nonturbulent manner at 60 to 90 feet per minute.

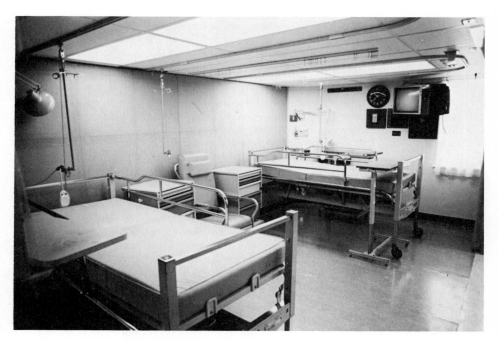

FIGURE 2. One-half of a 4-bed unit is shown. The laminar airflow panel is shown at the head of the beds. There is room for ambulation and patient activities within the unit.

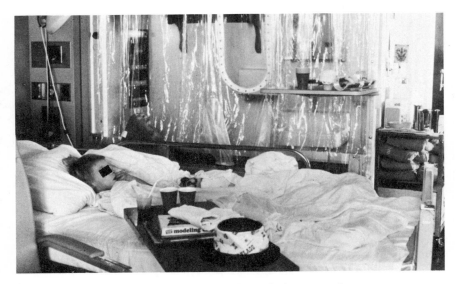

FIGURE 3. A burn patient is shown being cared for in the laminar airflow system.

underwent microwave treatment. Cultures, both surface and biopsy, from multiple sites were obtained on admission and twice weekly. Cultures were also obtained of air samples, surfaces, and the floor of the unit at least annually. Burn care consisted of daily debridements, with surface colonization controlled primarily with silver sulfadiazine (Silvidene) applications twice a day. No systemic antibiotics were used unless eschar biopsies had more than 10^5 organisms/gm or an infection was clearly determined by other culture data, namely sputum, blood, or urine. During the early part of our experience, patients were placed on a bowel sterilization routine using neomycin and erythromycin. This routine was discontinued in 1977. Burn care was initially performed in the patient's bed. This, however, proved to be unsatisfactory and in 1976 daily debridements in a portable hydrotherapy tank was instituted. Patients were removed from the unit only for major surgical procedures. Debridement of eschar was performed in the unit under Ketamine analgesia.[7]

We compared our experience with 135 patients treated in the LAF and 25 burn patients treated during the same time period in the medical-surgical intensive care unit. This occurred when the burn unit was filled or when staffing shortage necessitated the use of the intensive care unit. These patients were treated in isolation rooms with the same basic technic except without laminar airflow. The nursing staff were different between the two groups but the ICU nurses had spent training time in the burn unit.

RESULTS

The 135 patients studied in the LAF unit ranged in age between 10 months and 90 years. The ICU patients ranged between 17 and 85. Mortality rates were not compared statistically because of the small numbers of patients and the wide range of age and degree of burn. The severity of burn injury was comparable between patients in the burn unit and the ICU. Overall mortality rate for all patients was 16%.

Bacteriology

Air samples from the laminar airflow unit on all occasions were sterile. The ceiling and walls also showed no bacterial growth. Bed frames and patient cabinets on occasion showed scant growth of bacillus species, but no pathogens were isolated. This is in contradistinction to the medical-surgical intensive care unit where *Pseudomonas aeruginosa* was isolated from sinks and patient equipment on several occasions.

Patient data is summarized in the table. Sixty-five percent of the burn wound organisms isolated in the burn unit were gram positive whereas in the ICU, 70% were gram negative. Although *Staphylococcus aureus* was isolated from 60 percent of the patients, phage typing revealed these to be multiple types indicating that this was not a resident strain in the unit. All staphylococcus isolated were sensitive to methicillin. The gram negative organisms isolated in the LAF unit were all sensitive to standard antibiotics. Fifty percent of the pseudomonas isolated in the ICU were resistant to gentamycin. We were able to document only two cases of bacterial cross-contamination in the burn unit whereas 50% of the ICU burn patients developed infections with antibiotic resistant organisms found on other non-burn patients.

Patient Care

General patient management was accomplished equally well in both environments with ample room available for adequate physical and occupational therapy. Specific nursing functions were, however, more complicated in the LAF unit because of the need for the passage of supplies from the unsterile to the sterile environment. No supplies were stored in the sterile area because of space constraints. The need for nurses in both areas of the LAF unit also increased the nurse patient ratio to 1:1 during essentially all shifts. A 1:1 ratio was required in the ICU during the day shift but a 1:2 ratio was adequate during the other shifts. Patients in the LAF unit tended to remain in the unit for a longer period before transfer to the ward that did ICU patients who were moved to the general surgery floor when a bed was needed for a more critical patient. The average stay in the LAF unit was 30 days. The increased length of stay was based not only on the need for rapid turnover of beds in the ICU but as significant was the delayed separation of the burn eschar in the LAF unit due to less bacterial colonization of the wound. This prolonged isolation produced significant psychological problems for patients and not infrequently for nursing personnel. The efficiency of temporary nursing help, required because of increased census or sickness, was decreased in the LAF unit because of the longer time required for orientation to the more complex patient care environment. Precise time effort studies of nursing efficiency were, however, not performed.

TABLE 1

CULTURE DATA OF BURN WOUNDS TREATED IN THE LAF BURN UNIT AND THE ICU
(ISOLATION ROOMS)*

| | | Hospital Course | |
	Admission (n = 160)	LAF Unit (n = 135)	ICU (n = 25)
S aureus	15%	60%	40%
S epidermidis	20%	65%	30%
Str group A	4%	5%	4%
Enterococcus	10%	40%	30%
E coli	10%	30%	40%
Enterobacter	5%	15%	30%
P aeruginosa	8%	15%	80%
Klebsiella	0%	6%	60%
Proteus	0%	5%	60%
Serratia mar	0%	0%	15%

*Figures represent percentages of the patient population. LAF = laminar airflow; ICU = intensive care unit.

DISCUSSION

It is quite evident that the bacteriologic study was not well controlled because of the changes in the burn care protocol, during the course of the study, required to improve overall patient care. The bowel sterilization was discontinued when the side effects of diarrhea and abdominal cramps impaired nutritional support. Daily hydrotherapy was instituted to improve eschar removal. The low rate of cross-contamination and infection with resistant gram negative organisms did, however, demonstrate major benefit from the LAF system. We previously reported an extremely low rate of sepsis and sepsis related complications in the LAF unit.[6] Burke et al[3] using individual laminar airflow units also reported a significant decrease in infection rate after major burns. A major criticizm of the LAF system is that most infection in burn patients is felt to be from endogenous bacteria and laminar airflow only decreases airborn infection. Cross contamination is felt by many to be due to contact spread. Strict sterile technique preventing contact spread of bacteria is certainly extremely important. I am convinced that it is much easier to control the sterile technique of burn unit personnel in a laminar airflow unit where there are geographically well defined sterile and nonsterile areas than in an intensive care environment where less distinct separations are found. Our results, therefore, may be reflecting a more rigid sterile technique as much as the airflow system. A study controlling all aspects of burn care except for laminar airflow would, therefore, be very difficult.

An interesting comparison could be made between the open ward laminar airflow system versus the individual isolator used by Burke et al.[3] The open ward clearly provides more room for ambulation, physical therapy and contact with relatives, however, maintaining a warm temperature comfortable to the patient results in a very uncomfortable working environment for personnel wearing caps, masks, and gowns. The environment in the individual unit can be controlled to satisfy the patient without affecting the working environment of the personnel outside the isolator.

We did identify two problem areas with the LAF system which need to be evaluated further. First the nursing requirements appear to be increased due to the need for personnel both inside and outside the sterile air area to pass material back and forth so as to maintain the sterile environment. We required a nurse patient ratio of 1:1 exceeding the more standard ratios of 1:1.5 or 1:2 utilized in other units. This has not been sufficiently studied to determine the exact increase in personnel required. The second problem concerns the psychological disturbances produced in patients confined to a limited area for prolonged periods of time. A severe burn may be confined to the unit for several months except for grafting procedures when the patient is transported to the operating room. We attempted to solve this by earlier transfer out of the unit to the surgical floor and by increasing the variety of daily activities, however, this remains a significant problem which needs to be studied further.

With our four year experience we have, therefore, found the laminar airflow open ward system to be beneficial for controlling infection in burn patients due to a combination of strict sterile techniques and sterile airflow. We have not been able to determine the relative importance of these two factors. We have also identified several problems with the use of the system which needs further study.

REFERENCES

1.   ARTZ, C. P. 1978. Burns updated. J. Trauma **16:** 3.
2.   ALEXANDER, J. W., C. OGLE, J. D. STINNETT, & B. G. MACMILLAN. 1978. A sequential, prospective analysis of immunologic abnormalities and infection following severe thermal injury. Ann. Surg. **188:** 809.
3.   BURKE, J. F., W. C. QUINBY, C. C. BONDOI, et al. 1977. The contribution of a bacterially isolated environment in the prevention of infection in seriously burned patients. Ann. Surg. **186:** 377.
4.   LEVINE, S. A., S. E. SIEGEL, & A. D. SCHRUEBER. 1973. Protected environments and prophylactic antibiotics: A prospective controlled study of their utility in the therapy of acute leukemia. N. Eng. J. Med. **288:** 477.
5.   PEDERSON, P. D., W. Z. PENLAND, & K. A. UFFORD. 1974. Laminar flow patient isolation system in cancer treatment—current status. Proceed. Internat. Symp. Contamination Control. London.
6.   DEMLING, R. H., A. PEREA, & J. MALY. 1978. The use of a laminar airflow isolation system for the treatment of major burns. Am. J. Surg. **136:** 377.
7.   DEMLING, R. H., S. ELLERBE, & F. JARETT. 1978. Ketamine anesthesia for tangential excision of burn eschar: A burn unit procedure J. Trauma **18:** 269.

THE CONTRIBUTION OF A BACTERIALLY ISOLATED ENVIRONMENT TO THE PREVENTION OF INFECTIONS IN SERIOUSLY BURNED PATIENTS

Glenn E. Behringer

Massachusetts General Hospital
Boston, Massachusetts 02114

John F. Burke

Shriners Burns Institute
Boston, Massachusetts

The treatment of the severely burned patient by early excision of burned tissue and immediate wound closure with skin grafts has been shown to be effective in lowering mortality and morbidity.[1] This method of treatment in itself prevents the development of infection by promoting early wound healing. In massively burned patients, when multiple procedures are necessary before all burned areas are closed, special measures are required to prevent unexcised areas of necrotic tissue from becoming infected before excision and closure can be carried out. Topical agents of a bacteriostatic or bacteriocidal nature provide help in this regard but are not completely satisfactory, for their effectiveness is for a limited time only.

In an attempt to provide a better method of preventing sepsis in burn patients, a system of complete bacteriologic isolation was designed at the Massachusetts General Hospital, Boston, Mass. (MGH) and is currently in use at the Shriner's Burns Institute in Boston, (SBI).

This system is based on strict environmental control of a 6 × 10 foot area immediately surrounding the patient's bed. It affords the ability to deliver all medical care without entering the protected environment and maintain all monitoring, life support and I.V. equipment outside the controlled environment so that bacteria carried by the staff or equipment do not contaminate the patient, nor does the patient contaminate personnel or equipment. This patient protective area is called the Bacteria Controlled Nursing Unit (BCNU) and is an integral part of an overall plan for the surgical care of the seriously burned patient which involves prompt excision of the entire extent of the burn eschar and immediate wound closure, including immunosuppression and allograft closure of the most extensive injuries.

MATERIALS AND METHODS

The effectiveness of the BCNU in protecting patients from bacterial complication was investigated by recording the rate of bacterial contamination and its potential for invasive infection. These rates were then compared with rates of patient protection afforded by two other methods of isolation in common use: single room isolation on a strict isolation burn unit and isolation precautions on an open ward.

300

0077–8923/80/0353–0300 $01.75/0 © 1980, NYAS

Patient Groups Studied

Three groups of patients were studied, separated by the type of isolation procedure used.

Group 1. Patients who were admitted directly to the BCNU. Two hundred and sixty four patients were admitted to the Shriner's Burns Institute, Boston, with burns greater than 10 per cent of their body surface area (BSA), and who remained in the protected environment for more than one week. The average length of stay in the BCNU was 31 days. The ages of the patients ranged from 6 months to 16 years with an average age of 7 years. The average burn size was 42.6 per cent BSA.

Group 2. Two hundred and twenty two consecutive patients with burns greater than 10 per cent of body surface area were admitted directly to the open acute burn ward of the Shriner's Burns Institute, Boston, because the environmental control units were not available. The ages ranged from 2 months to 16 years with average burn size of 19.6 per cent BSA.

Groups 1 and 2 are made up of children of comparable age, but the burn size of those treated in the BCNU was considerably greater because the most severe injuries were placed in the controlled environment, if available, rather than the open ward.

Group 3. This group consists of 214 consecutive adult patients admitted to the burn service of the Massachusetts General Hospital, Boston, Mass., where the patients are cared for in single room isolation on a burn isolation floor. The ages ranged from 16 to 86 years and the average burn size was 39.2 per cent BSA.

Isolation Techniques and Facilities

The BCNU is a 6 × 10 foot area on an open ward separated from the ward by a clear plastic curtain wall. (Figures 1 and 2) The area within the curtain wall is continuously subject to a ceiling to floor flow of bacteria free air. The air temperature and humidity is controlled at about 31.5°C and 90 percent relative humidity. The side or access walls are constructed of two longitudinal overlapping sheets of plastic. The free edges of those panels overlap just above the level of the bed and are supported by an elastic cord. All medical and nursing care, monitoring and life support are carried out through this maze in the wall.

Four Bacteria Controlled Units are located a tone end of an open 12 bed, critical care ward, occupying no more space than four ordinary hospital beds. Staff and visitors are allowed on the floor without protective clothing. Medical and nursing care is administered to the patients by unit personnel, wearing protective aprons and shoulder length plastic gauntlets, through the overlapped access walls. The continuous flow of sterile air increases the effectiveness of the seal between the plastic panels by carrying any bacterial particle entering to the floor.

Wound dressings and all other medical care is delivered in the same way as would be done on an open ward except that it is carried out within the unit by personnel who are protected by plastic gauntlets. Inside the unit sterile packs are opened and sterile gloves put on before starting a procedure. Food and bed clothing are not sterilized. Wounds are protected by the use of sterile dressing techniques and topical $AgNO_3$.

All intravenous, monitoring and life support equipment remain outside the

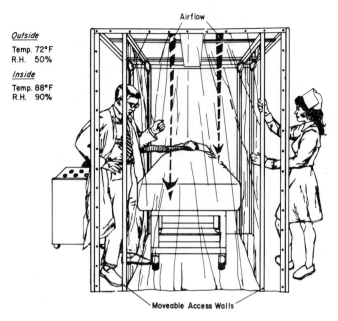

FIGURE 1. Drawing of the Bacteria Controlled Nursing Unit. Note the 6 × 10 foot area surrounding the bed which is enclosed by transparent curtain walls. The interior of the unit is continuously washed by a flow of bacteria free air. Temperature and humidity are controlled.

unit. Tubes, lines, EKG leads, etc. enter through a panel port at the head of the bed.

Group 2. Isolation facilities and techniques

These consist of the remaining eight beds on the 12-bed critical care ward at the Shriner's Burns Institute. Hand washing and toilet facilities are located between beds. Personnel and visitors wear caps and gowns or aprons in proximity to the patients. Sterile technique is used for all procedures.

Group 3. Isolation facilities and techniques

The adult burn ward is located on the top floor of the Massachusetts General Hospital. All patients are housed in single rooms, each with its own hand washing facility and toilet. Access is limited to staff and two patient visitors at a time.

All persons entering the ward don caps, masks and protective gowns or aprons. These are changed if personnel go from patient to patient. Dressings and procedures are carried out using sterile gloves and equipment. Patients with problems requiring intensive nursing care are nursed by a "special" nurse who remains in the room and has no contact with other patients.

Burn Treatment

All patients were treated by the same method and under the direction of the same medical staff.[2] One half percent silver nitrate solution was used as the topical agent to all body areas except the face and perineum which were treated with silver sulfadiazene. Surgical therapy consisted of prompt excision of burn eschar and immediate wound closure.[1] Most recipient sites were immediately closed with autografts. In patients who sustained burns in excess of 35 percent of BSA, initial wound closure was accomplished by a combination of skin autograft and allograft. The allografts were replaced by autografts 2 to 3 weeks later. Nineteen children who sustained burns of greater than 80 percent BSA and third degree component over 70 per cent BSA were treated by temporary skin transplantation and immunosuppression.[3,4] These patients were all nursed in the BCNU.

Antibiotic therapy of the acutely burned patient consisted of penicillin for the first three days following admission. No further antibiotics were given unless there was clinical evidence of bacterial invasion. Antibiotics were given in the

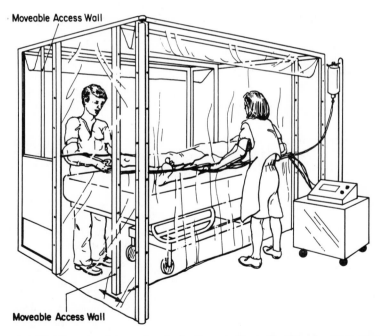

FIGURE 2. Nursing care of the patient in the Bacteria Controlled Nursing Unit. The nurse wears shoulder length plastic gauntlets and gains access to the patient through the overlap in the curtain wall. Intravenous and life support systems are located outside the unit.

perioperative period, (immediately pre-op and 24° post-op). The choice of agent was made on the basis of sensitivity studies of the wound flora.

Classification of Bacterial Contamination

Bacterial studies were carried out to determine the incidence of cross contamination and auto-contamination. Cross contamination is defined as bacterial contamination of the burn wound, respiratory or urinary tract with an organism different from those carried in any site by the patient on admission. Auto-infection is considered as the appearance in the same areas of a bacterial strain carried by the patient on admission. Bacterial contamination is defined as the isolation of bacteria from the burned area, respiratory or urinary tract and included those cases where there was evidence of bacterial invasion or inflam-

	Group 1 Bacteria Controlled Environment (BCNU–SBI)	Group 2 Open Ward (SBI)	Group 3 Single Room (MGH)
Total Patients	264	222	214
Age	6mos – 16yrs	2mos – 16yrs	16 – 86yrs
% BSA Burned	42.6	19.6	39.2
% 3° Component	26.7	6.8	26.0

FIGURE 3. Distribution of patients by type of isolation.

mation. Wound infection was said to be present when the patient demonstrated evidence of clinical deterioration, positive blood culture or evidence of bacterial invasion of viable layers of the wound.

RESULTS

The composition of the three study groups is outlined in FIGURE 3. There were 264 who remained for one week or more in the BCNU (Group 1). The length of stay was from seven to 86 days, the average being 31 days. The upper limit of the range for all three groups was considered to be the time when the burn wound was clinically beyond the risk of infection. Two hundred and twenty two patients were treated on the open burn ward of the S.B.I. (Group 2) from seven to 62 days, (average 22 days). Two hundred and fourteen patients were cared for in single room isolation (Group 3) for periods of seven to 112 days, (average 38 days). TABLE 1 shows that the age of the patients in Groups 1 and 2 are comparable but that the average burn size is double, (42.6% vs. 19.6%), and the third degree component is more than three times greater (26.7% vs. 6.8%) in Group 1

Group 1 Bacteria Controlled Environment (BCNU–SBI)		Group 2 Open Ward (SBI)		Group 3 Single Room (MGH)	
2 wks	4 wks	2 wks	4 wks	2 wks	4 wks
3.8*	8.0†	13.1*	22.7†	32.0	86.0

(row label: *% Cross Contamination*)

* ↔ * P<0.001
† ↔ † P<0.001

FIGURE 4. Rate of burn wound cross-contamination.

compared with Group 2. There is no significant difference between Group 1 and Group 3 patients with regard to burn size or 3° component.

FIGURE 4 demonstrates the rate of cross contamination for the first two weeks and the cumulative contamination over the first four weeks of hospitalization in each of the three groups of patients. In all groups contamination includes those wounds with a positive bacterial culture and those with bacterially infected wounds. Three and eight tenths percent of patients receiving treatment in the BCNU (Group 1) were cross contaminated during the first two weeks of hospitalization and 8 percent were cross contaminated at the end of four weeks. When these figures are compared with those of Groups 2 and 3, marked differences are seen. In comparing Groups 1 and 2, where the age of the patients is comparable, there is a significant increase in the rate seen in Group 2 (13.1% at two weeks and 22.7% at four weeks), over that seen in Group 1 (3.8% and 8%). Due to the differences in age of the populations in Groups 1 and 3, only broad conclusions can be drawn. However, the difference in the rate of cross contamination at two and four weeks between Group 1 (3.8% and 8.0%) and Group 2 (32% and 86%) is impressive.

The rate of burn wound auto-contamination is shown in FIGURE 5. It is apparent that auto-contamination did not follow the same pattern as cross contamination in that the marked reduction in cross contamination which was

Group 1 Bacteria Controlled Environment (BCNU)		Group 2 Open Ward (SBI)		Group 3 Single Room (MGH)	
2 wks	4 wks	2 wks	4 wks	2 wks	4 wks
14.1	75.8	15.8	67.0	18.0	88.0

(row label: *% Auto Contamination*)

FIGURE 5. Rate of burn wound auto-contamination.

observed in Group 1 was not present in the auto-contamination rate. Group 1 patients experience an auto-contamination rate of 14.1 percent in two weeks and 75.8 percent in four. In Group 2 patients, the rate was 15.8 percent in two weeks and 67.0 percent in four weeks. In Group 3, it was 18.0 percent and 88.0 percent respectively.

FIGURE 6 demonstrates the probability of developing an invasive wound infection following cross contamination as opposed to auto-contamination in patients treated in the BCNU. There was a significant increase in clinical wound infections following cross contamination (65%) over auto-contamination (39%) of the burn wound.

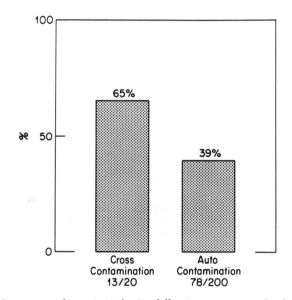

FIGURE 6. Percentage of invasive infection following cross contamination in B.C.N.U.

DISCUSSION

The problems of cross infections between hospitalized patients has long been recognized a serious threat to their care. No satisfactory solution to this problem has been developed. The "Isolation Procedures" to which each hospital adheres in an attempt to control this risk have been woefully lacking in their ability to protect the small group of patients at risk of acquiring bacterial disease during their hospital stay. Severely burned patients are numbered among this group.

The work reported is an assessment of the value of a system designed to protect highly susceptible patients from cross infection. This system incorporates a highly effective environmental control of the areas surrounding the patient's bed with the ability to deliver all medical care and to maintain all monitoring and life support systems outside the controlled environment.

The use of topical antibacterial therapy has improved the rate of burn wound sepsis and mortality for the moderate sized burn injury,[5,6] but in the massively burned patient it has not solved the problem of inevitable cross contamination of the burn wound,[7,8] nor has it made burn care more effective as judged by the length of hospital stay.

The closed system of environmental control has been shown to reduce greatly the rate of cross contamination (Group 1) as compared with patients on an open ward (Group 2) or in single rooms on an isolated burn unit (Group 3). The decrease in cross contamination between Groups 1 and 2 is even more impressive when it is emphasized that patients in Group 1 (BCNU) have much more extensive burn injuries than those in Group 2. Although Groups 1 and 3 are not comparable because of differences in age, it does not appear that the rate of bacterial cross infection differs greatly between adults and children when treated in a similar manner.

TABLE 4 indicates that a burn wound is almost twice as likely to become clinically infected if the source of the organism was from cross contamination rather than auto-contamination. The exact reason for this is unknown but presumably host resistance is more effective against the patient's native flora than to contaminating strains which his immunologic system does not recognize.

All of the patients studied were treated by primary excision of burn eschar and immediate wound closure. Multiple procedures were required in large injuries. It is not possible to determine what portion of cross contamination occurred when the patients were moved from the BCNU to the operating room and back again, and this may be significant. However, all cross contamination was considered to have occurred within the unit.

The data concerning the effectiveness of the BCNU and the clinical experience gained through its use indicate that it is of extreme importance in the care of the severely burned patient. It has allowed the safe application of prompt excision of burned tissue and immediate wound closure which has been shown to reduce the length of hospital stay and the mortality of the injury.[6] It has also allowed lthe expansion of these techniques to massively burned patients using temporary allograft transplantation and immunosuppression which can be employed without the threat of bacterial infection in the immunologically suppressed patient.

BIBLIOGRAPHY

1. BURKE, J. F., C. C. BONDOC & W. C. QUINBY. 1974. Primary burn excision and prompt grafting as routine therapy. J. Trauma **14 (5)**: 389–394.
2. BURKE, J. F., W. C. QUINBY, JR. & C. C. BONDOC. 1976. Primary excision and prompt grafting as routine therapy for the treatment of thermal burns in children. Surg. Clin. North Amer. **56 (2)**: 477.
3. BURKE, J. F., J. W. MAY, JR. & N. ALBRIGHT. 1974. Temporary skin transplantation and immunosuppression for extensive burns. N. Engl. J. Med. **56 (5)**: 269.
4. BURKE, J. F., W. C. QUINBY, & C. C. BONDOC. 1975. Immunosuppression and temporary skin transplantation in the treatment of massive third degree burns. Ann. Surg., **182 (3)**: 183.
5. MONCREIF, J. A. 1968. The status of topical antibacterial therapy in the treatment of burns. Surgery **63**: 862.
6. MOYER, C. A., L. BRENTANO, & D. L. GRAVENS. 1965. Treatment of large human burns with 0.5% silver nitrate solution. Arch. Surg. **90**: 812.
7. MONCREIF, JR., J. A., R. B. LINDBERG, W. E. SWITZER & B. A. PRUITT, JR. 1966. Use of topical antibacterial therapy in the treatment of the burn wound. Arch. Surg. **92**: 558.
8. POLK, M. C., JR., W. W. MONAFO, JR. & C. A. MOYER. 1969. Human burn survival. Arch. Surg., **98**: 262.

SPECULATIONS ON THE POSSIBLE EFFECTS OF THE INDOOR AIR ON AIRBORNE CONTAGION

Donald F. Proctor

Department of Environmental Health Sciences
Johns Hopkins School of Hygiene and Public Health
Baltimore, Maryland 21205

Since 1937, some 42 years ago, I have been involved in the clinical practice of otolaryngology. During those years one development after another was believed to herald an era when airborne infections would cease to be a major public health problem. As far as I can see that era never arrived. From the perspective of those years I believe that our best chance of bringing this ubiquitous threat to human health, airborne disease, under control may lie in an improved understanding of our own natural defenses.

Since 1970 I have worked with Dr. Ib Andersen and his colleagues in Aarhus, Denmark in a series of investigations of the effects of the indoor air on human health. Although our major interests were directed at the effects upon upper airway physiology in healthy young adults, we could not help but speculate on how these influences might affect the incidence of airborne infection. Most of us most of the time are indoors and most airborne infections are probably contracted indoors. It seems justifiable to suggest that, if respiratory defense mechanisms may be impaired by certain ambient air conditions, that impairment might in turn affect airborne infection susceptibility.

A number of animal experiments, and epidemiological studies in man, have indicated that air pollution exposure can alter the susceptibility to and the severity of respiratory infections.[1,2] As one example, a 1966 report from England[3] pointed out, in comparing children living in relatively polluted and nonpolluted regions, that while there was no difference in the incidence of upper respiratory infections, lower respiratory complications were more prevalent in the polluted area. Such studies fail to clearly identify the responsible pollutants or to cast light on the pathogenetic mechanisms involved. It has been our objective to study the specific effects of various characteristics of ambient air on upper airway defenses in carefully controlled conditions in an environmental chamber.

The nasal airways are the site of a number of physiological defense mechanisms.[4] During nasal passage the temperature and water vapor content of inspired air are adjusted and a large portion of pollutant gases and dusts are removed. In addition the fluid covering of the epithelium serves as a barrier separating deposited noxious materials from underlying cells. Although a number of facets of nasal physiology are involved in these processes, the *sine qua non* for their maintenance is the mucociliary system which provides a continually refreshed layer of airway secretions as well as continual clearance of their contaminated surfaces. With that in mind, our chief efforts have been directed at accurately measuring nasal mucociliary clearance (as one index of the efficacy of nasal defenses) and investigating the effect of ambient air on this system.

Our studies have been carried out in the environmental chambers of the Institute of Hygiene at the University of Aarhus, Denmark. Our method for measuring nasal mucociliary clearance involves the external detection of the motion of a small particle tagged with $3\mu c$ technetium.

0077-8923/80/0353-0308 $01.75/0 © 1980, NYAS

After determination of the range of such clearance in clean air at 23° C and 70 % R.H. in healthy subjects we next studied the effect of dry air. There was no detrimental effect of exposure to air at 23° C and 9 % R.H. for 78 hours.[5] From this we conclude that attempts to artificially moisten indoor air have no justification from the standpoint of nasal health. This conclusion is substantiated by a number of studies comparing the health of office workers and schoolchildren in humidified vs nonhumidified rooms. For instance, Sataloff and Menduke[6] showed this in schoolchildren in 1963.

Our next study investigated the effects of ambient temperatures between 7 and 39° C.[7] Although nasal clearance was reduced in going either up or down from 23° C, the change was of little physiological significance. Numerous studies (such as that of Douglas et al[8] in 1968) have shown that exposure to cold has no effect upon the susceptibility to the common cold.[9] But, I should point out a factor which has been neglected in this connection. Many experimental studies of the transmissibility of respiratory viral infections involve the instillation of a solution containing virus into the upper portion of the nasal cavity. Fair tests of environmental conditions on viral infection susceptibility should involve the inhalation of virus as an aerosol, thus simulating natural conditions and delivering the virus to the same region of the nose as that which is exposed to the possible adverse effects of inspired ambient air.

We then turned to the effects of SO_2 in otherwise clean air and found a very significant deterioration in clearance at 5 ppm.[10] Following that investigation we measured the effects of an inert dust.[11] Even at a level of 25 mg/m^3 no unfavorable effect could be detected. On exposing subjects to SO_2 in a dusty atmosphere we found the reduction in mucociliary clearance to be similar to that with SO_2 alone (unpublished data).

From these studies we conclude that neither dry air, nor air within the temperature range of 7 to 39° C, nor dusty air (at least with an inert dust) significantly impair nasal defenses in healthy subjects; but that SO_2 has a definitely harmful effect. Thus the expenditure of energy and money on artificial air humidification in homes and offices seems unjustifiable.

In each of our studies we have also measured nasal airflow resistance. Obviously, as far as the lungs are concerned, nasal defense mechanisms have no effect on air inspired through the mouth. Especially in certain occupational situations, where heavy work is involved, the ability to maintain nasal breathing is a function of the resistance to airflow at relatively high ventilation rates. Fortunately during exercise in most individuals there is a nasal vasoconstriction resulting in a fall in nasal airflow resistance and a rise in the capacity to continue nasal breathing in the face of high ventilatory demand. Unfortunately we do not know how varying degrees of nasal mucosal shrinkage may affect the efficacy of nasal defenses. Also, to my knowledge, no attempts have been made to evaluate nasal airflow resistance and its response to exercise in workers exposed to hazardous ambient air conditions.

We do know that exposure to cold air or to SO_2 (at a level of 5 ppm) will cause an increase in nasal airflow resistance and therefore a relative inability to continue nasal breathing. How many other factors in the indoor air of our homes or work places may have a similar effect we do not know. But we are all familiar with the sense of nasal stuffiness we note in some unpleasant indoor air conditions. This question of the influences which alter our nasal airflow capacity is a badly neglected area in need of further research. It is of special importance in connection with certain occupationally related hazardous atmospheres; but it could also play a part in the transmissibility of airborne contagion in our homes, schools, and offices.

Another factor involved in these considerations has attracted Dr. Andersen's attention. With Dr. Lars Mølhave he has been studying both the effect of building materials on indoor ventilation and the capacity of building materials to gas-off pollutants into the atmosphere. While the studies just described were progressing they began a systematic survey of the chemicals to be found in the indoor air. Indoor air of course includes that in our work places (offices and industry), in meeting places, schools, and our homes. We spend a great deal of money controlling the physical conditions of the indoor air. Today, in addition to the cost in money of this endeavor, we must add the very significant cost in energy. It is important to identify to what degree these costs are related to protection of human health in contradistinction to providing human comfort.

To conserve energy and cost there is an all out effort to make our buildings as nearly as possible airtight, that is to reduce exchange between indoor and outdoor air to a minimum. In some respects this is good since these efforts can reduce the contamination of indoor air with pollutants from the outdoors. But two other considerations are important. First, many air pollutants have their origin indoors and their concentration is increased when exchange with outdoor air is reduced. Among these pollutants must be included droplet nuclei carrying infectious microorganisms. Second, building materials themselves can both reduce some indoor air pollution by absorption into surfaces, and conversely, many building materials will gas-off pollutants into the indoor air.[12]

The group in Aarhus have compared the air of new unoccupied flats (usually constructed with concrete walls) with that of older flats (frequently with brick walls). The ventilation rate thorugh the latter (brick) has been found to be 50 times higher than through the former (concrete). The concentration of organic gases and vapors was on the average 1.3 mg/m^3; but in the new flats it averaged 6.2 mg/m^3 compared to 0.4 mg/m^3 in the older flats, a fifteen fold difference. The minimum concentration in the new flats was 0.5 mg/m^3, about four times the U. S. standard for hydrocarbons in outdoor air. They found ventilation rates of only 0.3 changes per hour in the new flats compared with 1.3 per hour in the older flats, a four fold difference. They conclude that the difference in concentration of organic gases was caused equally by differences in ventilation rates and in the sources of gases and vapors.[13]

Their study of building materials as such sources has resulted in the identification of some 48 different chemical compounds in their gas-off. One of their earlier studies revealed high levels of formaldehyde in homes with pressed wood walls. Consequent alterations in the nature of that material have already reduced that hazard in Danish homes.[14,15]

Using similar methods they have also begun analysis of air in work places. In the printing industry, for instance, they have thus far identified 32 airborne chemicals. Of course there are many other sources of indoor air pollution including cooking, heating, smoking, cleaning materials, etc. One report has shown that levels of 500 to 3000 micrograms of NO_2/m^3 can arise from cooking with gas.

An immense amount of work remains to be done. At the moment there is little but suggestive evidence pointing toward a possible relationship between indoor air problems and respiratory infections. Comparing families in the older (well ventilated and less polluted) homes with those living in the newer (less ventilated and more polluted) homes, the total morbidity of the youngest child and the mother was significantly higher in the newer homes.

As mentioned earlier, building materials not only influence indoor air ventilation rate and may gas-off pollutants into rooms, but they may also serve a useful purpose in absorbing air pollutants. Some of the materials used for indoor walls (such as cinder block) are very efficient absorbers for SO_2.

Obviously speculations are about all I have offered on these important questions. But, in conclusion let me reemphasize certain points:

1. In our anxiety to conserve energy today let us not overlook the importance of the public health.

2. We can save energy by increasing insulation but such action should be accompanied by identification of those pollutants of indoor origin which may be harmful to our health and make every effort to control them.

3. To arrive at appropriate conclusions and decide on necessary actions epidemiological studies, further measurements of the pollutants in our indoor air, and, when indicated, human volunteer investigations are necessary.

Although the case for indoor air being a factor in airborne contagion is as yet a weak one I, for one, do not believe we can afford to overlook the possibility.

REFERENCES

1. EHRLICH, R. 1963. Effect of air pollutants on respiratory infection. Arch. Environ. Health **6:** 638–642.
2. LAVE, L. B. & E. P. SEESKIN. 1972. Air pollution, climate, and home heating: their effects on U.S. mortality rates. Am. J. Public Health **62:** 909–916.
3. DOUGLAS, J. W. & R. E. WALLER. 1966. Air pollution and respiratory infection in children. Br. J. Prevent. Soc. Med. **20:** 1–8.
4. PROCTOR, D. F. 1977. The upper airways I. Am. Rev. Respir. Dis. **115:** 97–130.
5. ANDERSEN, I., G. LUNDQVIST, P. L. JENSEN, & D. F. PROCTOR. 1974. Human response to 78 hours exposure to dry air. Arch Environ. Health **19:** 319–324.
6. SATALOFF, J. & H. MENDUKE. 1963. Humidity studies and respiratory infections in a public school. Clin. Pediatrics **2:** 119–121.
7. POCTOR, D. F., I. ANDERSEN & G. LUNDQVIST. 1977. Human nasal mucosal function at controlled temperatures. Respir Physiol **30:** 109–124.
8 DOUGLAS, R. G., K. M. LINDGREN & R. B. COUCH. Exposure to cold environment and rhinovirus common cold. N. Engl. J. Med. **279:** 742–747.
9. DOWLING, H. F., G. G. JACKSON & G. INOUYE. 1958. Transmission of the experimental common cold to volunteers under controlled conditions. III. The effect of chilling the subjects upon susceptibility. Am. J. Hyg. **68:** 59–65.
10. ANDERSEN, I., G. LUNDQVIST, P. L. JENSEN & D. F. PROCTOR. 1974. Human response to controlled levels of sulfur dioxide. Arch. Environ. Health **28:** 31–39.
11. ANDERSEN, I., G. LUNDQVIST, D. F. PROCTOR & D. L. SWIFT. 1979. Human response to controlled levels of inert dust. Am. Rev. Respir. Dis. **119:** 619–628.
12. KIRSCH, H. 1978. Comparison of SO_2 concentration inside and outside of buildings. Z. Ges. Hyg. **24:** 910–912.
13. MØLHAVE, L., J. MOLLER & I. ANDERSEN. 1979. Luftens indhold af gasarter, dampe og stov in nyere boliger. Ugeskr f Laeger **141:** 956–961.
14. ANDERSEN, I., G. LUNDQVIST & L. MØLHAVE. 1975. Indoor air pollution due to chipboard used as a construction material. Atmos. environ. **9:** 1121–1127.
15. ANDERSEN, I., G. LUNDQVIST & L. MØLHAVE. 1979. Formaldehyd i boligluft. Ugeskr f Laeger **141:** 966–971.

PREVENTION AND CONTROL OF AIRBORNE
INFECTION IN HOSPITALS

Carl W. Walter*

*25 Shattuck Street
Boston, Massachusetts 02115*

The preceding papers in this annual are superb presentations of the complex mix of problems that must be solved to prevent postoperative wound infection in clean cases. The results express success in terms of morbidity and mortality of patients exposed to the severe stress of prosthetic hip surgery or massive burns. The authors illustrate the extraordinary resources of intellect and conviction available to a hospital administration that is determined to make hospitals safe for patient care whatever the cause of their hospitalization. The best standards of care should apply to all patients. Indeed, neglect in any facet of patient care becomes the nidus whence infection eventually spreads throughout a hospital. There must be an end to rationalization, compromise and debate that ignores the fact that some hospitals—or rather parts of some hospitals—practice and describe superb performance while others wallow in professional discord, administrative ambiguity, and patient sepsis.

Hence, I have chosen five areas of major importance to outline some illustrative and challenging problems. These concern: 1) ventilation, 2) detection and control of carriers, 3) effective isolation technic, 4) the need for good hospital practices in the institutional care of patients, and 5) administrative responsibility for control of nosocomial and postoperative wound infection.

Ventilation

Air conditioning is the modern misnomer for ventilation, a more important function that controls pollution, odors, fumes, microbes and smoke. Moving air, whether by natural convection or forced, is used additionally for heating, cooling and humidity control. System designs have evolved to encompass climatic, cultural and medical concepts.

The energy crisis and public apprehension over Legionnaire's Disease prompt a critical review of the design of air conditioning. Mr. Mallison described the microbial contamination of air sucked into ventilating systems as an important factor in the dissemination of *Legionella pneumophila*.[1] He illustrated a common fault in the design of ventilating systems—improper location of the air intake. Too often it is located at ground level, under eaves or on the roof where exhaust ducts, sanitary systems, or evaporative coolers are vented.

The air intake must be vertical to avoid lee eddies that trap airborne particulates, and located out of the strike path of plumes of exhaust or vent air. The intake plenum must be protected from vines, birds, and chimney smoke.

Because ventilating systems have the potential of spreading microbes as described by Drs. Edward Riley and Gundermann, careful maintenance is

---

*Clinical Professor of Surgery, Emeritus, Harvard Medical School; and Surgeon, Emeritus, Peter Bent Brigham Hospital, Boston.

0077–8923/80/0353–0312 $01.75/0 © 1980, NYAS

essential.[2,3] Yet, neglect best characterizes the maintenance of many hospital systems I have inspected over the years. Several illustrations of faulty design and neglect suffice to make my point.

The first example is a new state university hospital of 310 beds. The design provided for heating, cooling and humidity control. In aseptic areas and nurseries, 100 percent primary air, cleaned by coarse filters and electrostatic precipitators, was used. Clinics and patient areas received 5 to 15 percent primary air, which was filtered through metal mesh filters and distributed to induction type air conditioners located above the hung ceiling in each room. Exhaust air was removed through toilets and corridors. The kitchen was supplied with 100 percent primary air filtered through mesh filters. A separate high rate exhaust system maintained negative pressure in the cooking areas.

The air intake was through an underground plenum in an area-way with the intake extending 8 feet above ground. A common intake plenum was used for primary air for the entire hospital including the kitchen and vents from the hospital were through cupolas on the roof ten stories above ground.

Cross infection handicapped operation of the facility almost from the first day. There were several extensive outbreaks of gram negative postoperative wound infection. Clostridial umphalitis occurred. Clostridia were demonstrable in aseptic areas; pseudomonas in clinical areas. The air conditioning louvers in the nursing units became slimy and green. Kitchen and incinerator odors permeated the hospital at night. A severe epidemic of hepatitis occurred.

Inspection of the ventilating system revealed that the screen behind the ground level intake louvers was choked with trash, leaves and wood chips from manure that had been spread over the unplanted courtyard. Fragments of similar debris had accumulated on the floor of the intake plenum. There was a high negative pressure in the plenum, enough to cause violent turbulence in the dozen or more blowers that fed from it. The water in the recirculating spray scrubber system was murky, and the refrigerating coils were slimy.

The kitchen opened on a service corridor terminating at one end at the receiving platform, at the other at the incinerator and trash collection rooms (FIGURE 1).[4] The soiled linen room adjoined that for trash collection. The latter were located beneath laundry and trash chutes respectively. A sorting room, contiguous with the linen room, was ventilated by a small exhaust fan mounted in a window opening on an areaway. The door between these rooms had been removed; the door from the sorting room to the corridor was wired open to improve working conditions. An open belt conveyor had been installed in the corridor between the trash room and the incinerator so that the trash could be scavenged.

Performance of the air conditioning and ventilating systems was satisfactory when the hospital first opened. However, ventilation gradually became ineffective and odor control became difficult. Conditions were much worse at night.

Aside from the faulty maintenance of the intake louvers, plenum and scrubber that resulted in marginal air flow, no other defects were noted until late in the evening. Then quite suddenly ventilation throughout the hospital improved and concomitantly kitchen odors became offensive. Inspection revealed that the kitchen ventilators had been shut down. The high negative pressure in the common intake plenum caused reverse flow through the kitchen air ducts. The double acting doors between the service corridor and the kitchen opened under the pressure gradient to suck in air from the corridor. This air was drawn from the soiled laundry, trash and incinerator areas.

Several defects in ventilation of epidemiologic significance were demon-

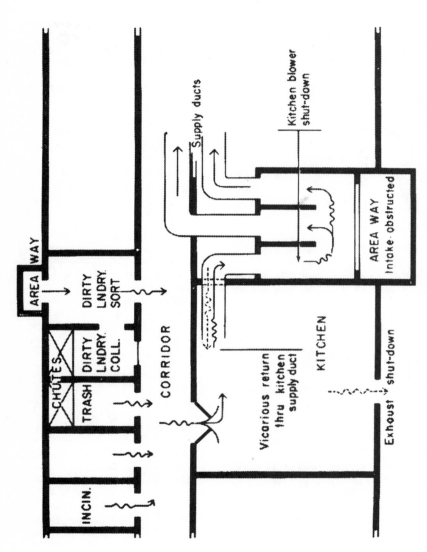

FIGURE 1. Condition at shut-down of kitchen ventilation. (From Walter.[4] By permission of ASHRAE Journal.)

strated:

1. Reverse flow through the kitchen air conditioning ducts sucked odors from the kitchen when that system was shut down. Even the high rate kitchen exhaust system became an air supply duct.
2. Contamination from soiled linen and trash was sucked into the kitchen from the sorting and scavenging operations to contaminate food.
3. Smoke and odor from the incinerator were drawn from the service corridor through the kitchen air conditioning duct and distributed throughout the hospital.
4. *Pseudomonas* from soiled linen and trash were carried by the primary air to contaminate the induction type air conditioners in each hospital room.

The system was corrected by compartmentizing the intake plenum to isolate the air supply of each blower. The intake louver was elevated 10 feet off the ground and its capacity quadrupled. A corrosion-inhibiting germicide dispenser was installed in the recirculating water system for the scrubbers.

The *clostridia* that pervaded the hospital were not eliminated until birds, predominantly pigeons, were prevented from nesting in the exposed trusses supporting the roof of the sunbelt style open-sided laundry located several blocks away. Dust, emanating from bird droppings, contaminated the clean linens to a hazardous degree.

The second example is a Veterans Administration Hospital that historically experienced mixed clostridial and gram negative wound infections. These were believed to characterize the essentially rural patient population. The causative organisms, plus fungi, were found in environmental cultures, on settle plates, and dust taken from diffusors. Inspection revealed pigeons roosting in the intake plenum of the air conditioning system. Eight inches of guano and the decomposed carcasses of a half dozen birds littered the floor. The filters, laden with molding dust, had dropped out of their frames and the refrigerating coils were a confluent mass of slime and mold.

The third example is a university hospital where miliary abscesses of the lung and fungemia were noted 16 to 18 weeks following placement of prosthetic aortic valves. Some patients had noted painful chronic infections in the nail beds. There had been several instances of panophthamitis due to fungi. Extensive investigation of the operating room and its personnel showed no source for the fungus or the *Staphylococcus epidermidis* that were found in blood cultures. Volume air samples from the cardiac catheterization laboratory showed heavy contamination with *aspergillis* and *S. epidermidis* (FIGURE 2).[5] The laboratory had been built in the basement as an afterthought in a relatively new hospital. It was air-conditioned by a domestic type window unit that projected over a trash compactor. Its filter was moldy. Its refrigeration coils and fan were slimy. Personnel in the laboratory reported little illness—perhaps because they wore masks as part of an elaborate program of asepsis. Fungi were cultured on settle plates exposed on aseptic fields and from angiographic catheters taken from the instrument table after removal from patients.

These examples emphasize the need for a critical review of the design of ventilating systems in hospitals and the need for an active weekly program of preventive maintenance.

Ulrich[6] has shown the bacteriologic effectiveness and efficiency of recirculation of air at 29 air changes per hour. Filters are available that make recirculation safe. The dust-free air can be sterilized by a bank of ultraviolet lamps in the

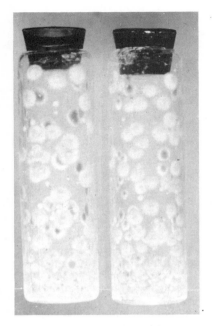 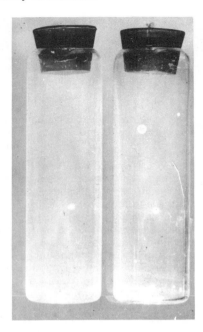

FIGURE 2. Airborne bacteria in volume air samples taken in cardiac catheterization laboratory (left), and operating room (right) show marked contrast in hygiene. Chronic postoperative *Candida* and *S. epidermidis* infection reflect endogenous infections brought to operating room by patient. (From Walter.[5] By permission of *Clinical Neurosurgery*.)

ducts. Sanitary threshold ventilation is economically and technically feasible with recirculation of 85 percent of the air.

Carriers

Recognition of the infected patient and the carrier as the in-house source of the microbes that cause postoperative wound infection is of paramount importance in the control of cross infections. Dr. Kundsin described the role of the carrier in disseminating pathogens.[7] Consider the infected patient as the fundamental source.[8]

The following observations on the shedding of staphylococci by a healthy appearing patient with three small carbuncles provide background for an understanding of the dynamics of hospital cross infection. Although the study was published 20 years ago, its import for control of cross infection is still ignored.

An overtly healthy 58-year old widowed telegrapher and grandmother presented herself for treatment of three small carbuncles. These had formed successively at intervals of two to three weeks in the skin over the angle of the right scapula, behind the left elbow, and below the areola of the right breast. The initial carbuncle on the back was a shallow granulating crater; the center of the lesion at the left elbow was necrotic with minimal induration and swelling; the most recently developed carbuncle on the breast had the typical appearance with draining central sinuses, peripheral pustules, and a red, swollen, indurated margin.

A history of a decade of recurrent attacks of skin infection was elicited. These were described as "crops of boils" in the armpits or groins, pimples around the belt line and beneath pendulous breasts, pussy dermatitis and single boils in various areas of the body. Studies had been done that eliminated diabetes, "bad blood," and abscessed teeth as possible causes for the recurrent infections. Antibiotics had been used to treat the earlier infections, but the occurrence of diffuse dermatitis ascribed to penicillin discouraged further antibiotic therapy.

Family history revealed that the patient had cared for her husband during the terminal phase of multiple myeloma. He had developed a boil on his ankle, the infection had spread, and he died of septicemia after several months' hospitalization.

Prior to admission, the patient's single hospital room was disinfected. The walls were sprayed with a germicidal detergent and squeegeed dry. The furniture was washed with germicide. The floor was flooded with a detergent germicide and the residual was picked up by a wet vacuum cleaner. The upholstered furniture and bedding were sterilized by ethylene oxide. At the end of the process, the floor, bedding, and air were cultured to determine the bacteriology of the environment. Periodically during her hospital stay the bedding, floor, air and room dust were cultured.

Cultures were also made of the patient's nasopharynx, skin of the hands and feet, anus, gastric juice, urine and each of the carbuncles. The organism recovered from all sources except the gastric juice, which was sterile, was of epidemiologic interest because it was atypical and alien to the hospital. Cultural characteristics were distinctive, colonies were minute, pigmentation occurred late, mannitol did not ferment, plasma coagulated. The staphylococci were phage type Group I, type 79, and were susceptible to all antibiotics.

The bacteriologic studies illustrate two important concepts too little appreciated by physicians: (1) The patient's carbuncles were local manifestations of systemic staphylococcal disease. (2) Despite "adequate" dry sterile dressings, staphylococci were shed to her environment.

Because the staphylococci were atypical of those in the hospital, they could be traced as they were shed. Cultures obtained from the sheet and pillow cases when the bed was clean and after it had been used for fourteen hours are shown

TABLE 1

CLEAN AND USED BEDDING—BACTERIA PER SQUARE FOOT*

	Clean Linen	Linen Used 20 Hours
Bottom sheet	340 (0 Staph.)	24,000 (18,000 Staph. 79)
Top sheet	20 (0 Staph.)	16,000 (12,000 Staph. 79)
Pillowcase	140 (0 Staph.)	16,000 (14,000 Staph. 79)
Bedspread	0 (0 Staph.)	360 (280 Staph. 79)

*(From Walter.[9])

in TABLE 1.[9] Colony-producing particles in volume air samples from air in the unoccupied room are shown on the right in FIGURE 3;[8] on the left from the air after the patient occupied the room overnight.

Cultures made from dust on the windowsill in this patient's room are shown in FIGURE 4.[8] Note the colonies of staphylococci scattered throughout. The source of these organisms proved to be the patient.

FIGURE 5[9] illustrates the shedding of bacteria to the room. Bacteria are whisked into the air in sufficient numbers by activity such as bedmaking to inoculate the nasopharynx of anyone entering the area. The accumulation of

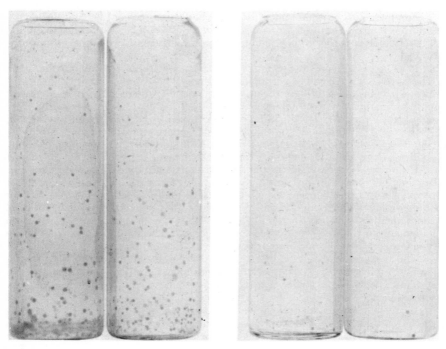

FIGURE 3. Well's air centrifuge tubes exposed to five cubic feet of air prior to admission (right) and during bedmaking on the morning following admission (left). (From Walter et al.[8] By permission of Medical Encyclopedia.)

bacteria on successive days makes the environment increasingly hazardous (TABLE 2).[9]

The patient was only inconvenienced by her infection. She appeared healthy and if left to her own devices, would have joined in ward activities. Such patients often assist with tray service, distribute mail, or help with other small chores. TABLE 3[9] shows the bacteriology of the patient's hands. Obviously everything she touched became contaminated.

The outer layers of dry dressings are customarily thought to be sterile. This is not so. Bacteria can be picked up by pressing a blood agar plate against the outer

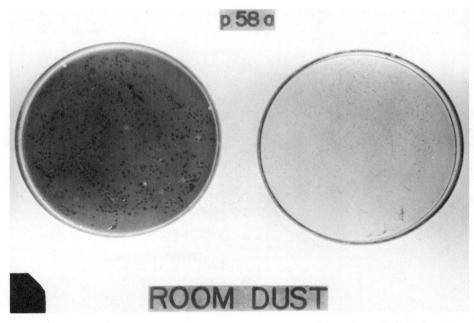

FIGURE 4. Cultures made by swabbing a demarked area of the window sill: (left) after 14 hours' occupancy; (right) before occupancy. (From Walter et al.[8] By permission of Medical Encyclopedia.)

layer of a dry dressing. Wound discharges carried into the dressing material by capillarity dry and deposit bacteria in the outer layer of the dressing. Patients often contaminate their fingers on the dressings, or, what is more probable, wound bacteria establish themselves on the skin. It is obvious that personnel readily contaminate themselves while caring for the patient (FIGURE 6).[10]

Sincere efforts at control of cross infections require that patients with

TABLE 2
FLOOR CULTURES—ORGANISMS/CM.^{2}*

Date	Right Side of Bed	Left Side of Bed	Foot of Bed	Center of Room	Average
1958					
Jan. 2†	2	2	6	14	6
Jan. 3	17	69	92	50	57
Jan. 6	69	18	19	12	30
Jan. 8	100	84	68	73	81
Jan. 9	22	65	96	26	52
		Floor Cleaned			
Jan. 9	6	7	46	3	16

*(From Walter.[9])
†Patient admitted

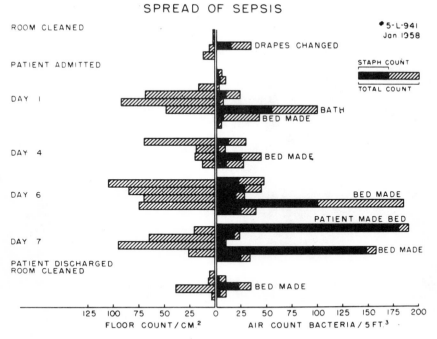

FIGURE 5. Bacterial counts of floor and room air while patient was being cared for under isolation technique. Staphylococci recovered from air after drapes were changed were untypeable; the remainder were type 79. This type persisted in the room following routine cleaning on discharge. (From Walter.[9])

infection be isolated by physical bounds rather than by "dry sterile dressings" and subjective definitions.

The septic patient then is the source of the bacteria. He must be effectively isolated. This is difficult to achieve in routine hospital practice. The ambulatory convalescent patient is an extreme hazard unless he is bacteriologically safe.

Similar studies on patients with infection due to traceable bacteria support construction of the schematic presented in FIGURE 7.[11] It presents the dynamics of

TABLE 3

GLOVE JUICE COUNTS—TOTAL NUMBER OF BACTERIA RECOVERED PER HAND*

Date	Right Hand	Left Hand	Average
1958			
Jan. 6	5,600	19,000	12,000
Feb. 28	2,900	5,400	4,200
April 7	1,300	800	1,100†

*(From Walter.[9]) Rubber gloves are worn for two hours. The interiors are rinsed with 100 ml. of sterile water, of which 1 ml. is plated out in duplicate.

†Patient on chloramphenicol.

airborne contagion, a neglected consideration in discussions of cross infection that emphasize traditional concepts of contact infection. The ventilation vortex swirls about everyone and is patterned by ventilation practices in each room and building. Only still air in an uninhabited closed space is free from dust and bacteria.[12] Any motion sets up air currents that sweep up settled dust. Imperceptible currents of sterile air raise dust. Human activity scuffs dust from the floor and dislodges it from skin, hair and clothing. Airborne bacteria and dust particles are inhaled with the 0.3 cubic foot of air inspired per minute. Most of these particles are trapped in the nasal passages; the smaller penetrate the bronchial tree to the alveoli.[13]

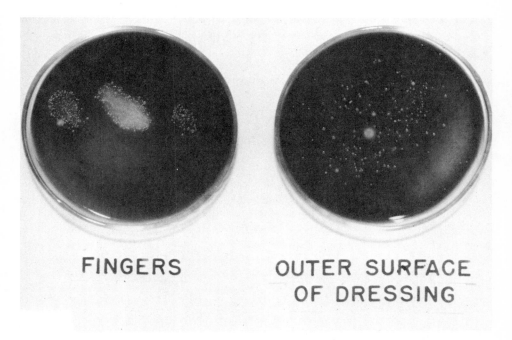

FINGERS OUTER SURFACE OF DRESSING

FIGURE 6. (left) bacteria imprinted on blood agar by tips of fingers that had removed a gauze dressing over the granulating crater of carbuncle; (right) impression plate made on outer layer of dressing to illustrate bacteria left on surface by evaporation of wound secretion. (From Walter.[10] By permission of the *Rhode Island Medical Journal*.)

Colonization of the nasopharynx may occur either by inhalation or by finger contact. In work areas where aseptic technic demands disinfection of the hands and masking, colonization rates are low. Sixty-seven weeks of exposure are required to establish the carrier state in the average worker in these areas in contrast to twenty-two weeks' of exposure on surgical wards.[14] The latter figure approximates the twenty weeks' exposure demonstrated to be necessary to convert 63 percent of the student nurses caring for tuberculous patients eight hours a day to positive tuberculin reactors. Guinea pigs developed a single tubercle by breathing approximately the same volume of air exhausted from the tuberculosis ward that was inhaled by the nurses.[15]

Patients occupying a ward continuously receive at least six times the exposure to ward air as do personnel. The importance of the nasopharynx as a portal of entry has been demonstrated. In this study, an unmasked attendant making the bed inhaled at least two hundred particles laden with staphylococci.[16] Because she worked in the trajectory of the bacteria being whisked into the air, many times this number of staphylococci reached her nostrils. Implantation of airborne tracer staphylococci can be demonstrated by occluding one nostril during bedmaking. Cultures show environmental bacteria in the patent nostril in contrast to the occluded control.

Longitudinal study of the carrier state in hospital personnel and bacteriologic

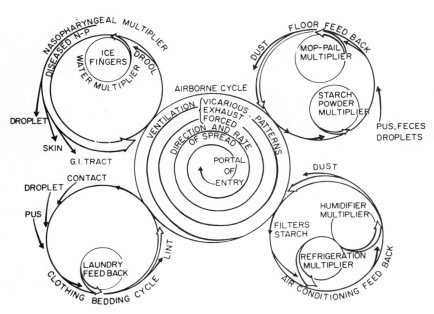

FIGURE 7. Vortex of environmental sepsis.

surveillance of wound infection over five years provided data that identified a startling epidemiologic pattern.

Several carriers, a resident, an anesthetist, and a nurse, were studied prospectively to discover their impact on patients. Eighteen infections resulted from the participation of four disseminating carriers on the surgical team (TABLE 4).[5] Complete data were not obtainable on the intern and nurse; detailed information was obtained on the anesthetist and resident. Twenty-five additional neurosurgical infections were epidemiologically associated with the same carriers, but the bacteriologic evidence was inconclusive because the data were not completely distinctive (FIGURE 8).[5]

An anesthetist was epidemiologically associated with 13 infections. This

CHRONOLOGIC LISTING OF S. AUREUS INFECTIONS BACTERIOLOGICALLY
LINKED TO FOUR DISSEMINATING CARRIERS*

Date		Operation	Infector	Phage†
1963	February	Craniotomy	Resident	U
		Craniotomy		U
		Hypophysectomy		U
	May	Craniotomy	Nurse	Y
	June	Laminectomy	Intern	Z
	July	Cranioplasty	Anesthetist	T
1964	June	Open reduction shoulder	Anesthetist	T
1965	March	Thoracotomy	Anesthetist	T
	June	Hiatus herniorrhaphy		T
	July	Hip nailing		T
		Mammary artery implant		T
		Pyelolithotomy		T
	August	Craniotomy	Resident	V
	November	Laminectomy		V
		Craniotomy		V
	December	Laminectomy	Anesthetist	T
1966	July	Carotid endarterectomy	Anesthetist	T
		Hip nailing		T

*(From Walter et al.[5] By permission of Clinical Neurosurgery.)
†Phage designation: U, 52/52A/79/7/73/75/80/82; Y, 52A/79; Z, 53/77; T, 83A/6/7/42E/47/54/73/75/42B/83B/UC-18/81/82; V, 52/52A/80/81.

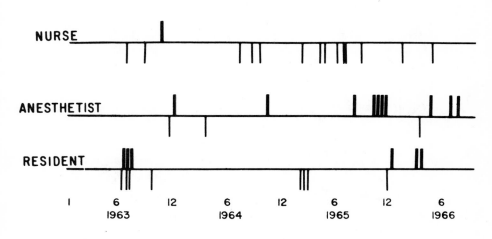

FIGURE 8. Epidemiological association of postoperative sepsis with disseminating carrier on team. Standing bold bars indicate bacteriologic incrimination; dangling light bars indicate epidemiologic association. During 1964 and the last six months of 1965, the resident worked elsewhere. (From Walter et al.[5] By permission of Clinical Neurosurgery.)

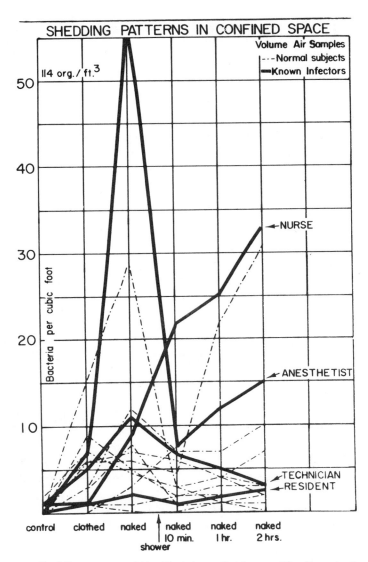

FIGURE 9. Shedding patterns of 14 subjects in confined space. The disseminating carriers have been accentuated. Note that two, the anesthetist and nurse, are predominantly skin shedders; the resident and technician disseminate from the throat. (From Walter et al.[5] By permission of Clinical Neurosurgery.)

TABLE 5

COLONIZATION BY THE SURGICAL TEAM—*S. AUREUS* IN 73 HIGH SCHOOL STUDENTS*

Time	Bacteria Present
Before 4 hr. in surgical ward	49
After 4 hr. in surgical ward	58

*Seventy-three high school girls with no recent contact with the hospital environment sat around a table in the center of a square 16-bed open ward for 4 hours during the period when beds were being made. S. aureus of the phage patterns prevalent in the environment and wounds of 2 patients with septic hips isolated by barrier nursing, were cultured from the nasopharynx of seven. Carriage of S. aureus increased 12 per cent. The high rate of carriage is typical of the teenage population. (From Walter et al.[5] By permission of *Clinical Neurosurgery*.).

woman was an overtly healthy, fastidious individual. She had psoriasis of the scalp with several blotches on extensor surfaces of the extremities. Onychomycosis involved the majority of the nails of both hands and feet. The skin of the hands was inflammed, rough, and scaly. *Staphylococcus epidermidis* was cultured from the psoriatic areas. *Klebsiella pneumonia* (Type 21) was recovered from the subungual spaces of the fingers. *Staphylococcus aureus* (83A/6/7/42E/47/54/73/75/42B/83B/UC-18/81/82) was recovered repeatedly from her nostrils, throat, hands and perineum.

A neurosurgical resident was epidemiologically associated with 14 infections. This man carried three different types of S. aureus in sequence, two of them were recovered from infections. The initial series of three infections in 1963 was due to S. aureus (52/52A/79/7/73/75/80/82) recovered from his nostrils. In 1965 three infections were due to a different type (52/52A/80/81) that was isolated from his throat.

The disseminating characteristics of the four carriers incriminated in postoperative sepsis were studied by determining the bacterial contamination of a confined volume of air during a standard exercise program. Ten overtly healthy hospital employees were also studied. All 14 subjects were daily bathers and had grossly clean skin. Volume air samples (FIGURE 9)[5] and settling plates demonstrated the number and size of the bacteria-laden particles shed.

The data show that two (the resident and technician) of the carriers implicated in wound infections were predominantly throat disseminators; the other two (the anesthetist and the nurse) were both throat and skin dispersers. Shedding by the anesthetist was controlled by showering, whereas dispersal by the nurse was enhanced by showering.

The import of shedding by the anesthetist was revealed by a review of 2,000 consecutive patients she had attended. Two hundred fifty-six postoperative infections were associated with her presence.

Dust particles may settle onto burns, open wounds, or other susceptible tissue such as that of a tracheostomy or unhealed umbilicus. Of greater epidemiological import is the fact that they are inhaled and inoculate the mucous membranes of the upper respiratory tract. Colonization results and the subsequent attenuated infection is known as the carrier state (TABLE 5).[5]

Disseminating carriers lend ubiquity and continuity to the spread of bacteria by expelling, wherever they go, droplets and droplet nuclei which may be sprayed directly into wounds or be inhaled by others. Droplets settle on skin, clothing, and other surfaces, eventually giving rise to bacteria-laden lint and dust.

TABLE 6

CLINICAL NEUROSURGERY—*STAPHYLOCOCCUS AUREUS* CARRIERS AMONG
OPERATING ROOM PERSONNEL*

Carriers	Staphylococcus Aureus
OR Nurses	21%
Surgeons	33%
Anesthetists	57%
Orderlies	71%

*The carrier rate is low among the nurses who are protected by masking while working in a hygienic environment. The higher rate among surgeons reflects the hazard of entering the general hospital environment. The occupational hazard of intimate contact with patients and bedding is illustrated by the higher rate among anesthesiologists and orderlies. Faulty aseptic technique and lack of training intensify the hazard. (From Walter et al.[5] By permission of *Clinical Neurosurgery*.)

Members of the surgical team are the couriers in the transmission of hospital-based infection to the aseptic field, for they, too, share the occupational hazard of the hospital environment (Table 6).[5] Personnel remain the chief source of exogenous bacteria in the properly managed operating room.

A study of patients, personnel, and environment of 250 operations described the bacterial exposure of the patient during surgery. The postoperative wound infection rate was 8.4 percent. Four-fifths resulted from endogenous seeding; one-fifth was due to exogenous bacteria (Table 7).[10] The sources of these bacteria were several staphylococcus carriers.

ISOLATION

Despite the evidence that the patient with infection is the source of bacteria that establish the carrier state, it is difficult to achieve effective isolation in routine hospital practice. Isolation of patients with infection becomes a contro-

TABLE 7

BACTERIA IN 21 POSTOPERATIVE WOUND INFECTIONS FOLLOWING 250 OPERATIONS*

	Staphylococcus Aureus	Streptococcus Pyogenes	Gram-Negative	Mixed
Exogenous				
Personnel Carrier	4			
Endogenous				
Patient Nasopharangeal Carrier	3			
Surgical Specimen	1	1	2	
Urine	1		3	
Previous Wound	1		3	1
Surgical Error			1	

*The bacterial exposure of 250 individual patients scheduled randomly for surgery at 9:00 a.m. on Tuesdays and Thursdays over 20 months. Twenty-one postoperative infections were discovered; a rate of 8.4 per cent. The source and kind of bacteria are tabulated. (From Walter.[10] By permission of the *Rhode Island Medical Journal*.)

versial subject. The one extreme is conventional isolation by nursing technique, isolation by definition rather than by physical barriers. The opposite extreme is the Federal requirement of air control in hospital isolation areas.[17] A basic obstacle is the physician's denial that his patient with overt infection is a hazard.

I wish to present a system used in the intensive care unit at the Peter Bent Brigham Hospital. It evolved after many years of failure to contain sepsis by

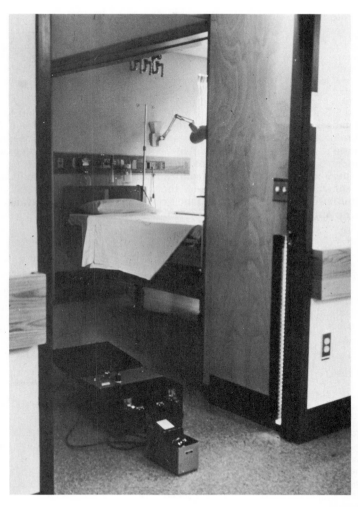

FIGURE 10. A barrier of ultraviolet radiation (254nm) from lamps at the top and side of the doorway stops spread of microbes. The temperature gradient between the room and corridor causes convection amounting to 10 air changes per hour in the room. Die-away studies of an aerosol of E. coli demonstrated threshold sanitary ventilation. The ultraviolet meter on the floor emphasizes the need to maintain the energy level at $25\mu W/cm^2$. (From Walter.[20] By permission of Medical Instrumentation.)

TABLE 8

RESULTS OF ULTRAVIOLET BARRIER INSTALLATION

Prior to May 1966	After May 1966
Crowding—Four Bed Room	Single Room
Recirculating Air Conditioner	Threshold Sanitary Ventilation
	Ultraviolet Barriers
	Alcohol Hand Wash
42 Patients—25 Deaths = 60%	194 Patients—58 Deaths = 30%
70% Deaths Due to Sepsis	7% Deaths Due to Sepsis
R.N. Carriage of S. Aureus = 60%	R.N. Carriage of S. Aureus = 15%

conventional technic. It gained acceptance because crowding causes unacceptable levels of cross infection. Each patient has a single room equipped with a germicide dispenser* for disinfection of the hands.[18] Each room is ventilated with 17 air changes, with the return air drifting through the open door to be exhausted from the corridor near the nurses' station. Eighty-five percent of the air is recirculated; humidity is controlled at 50 percent. An ultraviolet barrier as demonstrated by Robertson[19] at each door accomplishes two objectives (FIGURE 10).[10] It sterilizes the convection currents through the doorway—equivalent to 10 changes of air per room per hour due to the temperature differential between the room and the corridor, and sterilizes the net volume of ventilating air leaving the room. The results are illustrated in TABLE 8.[21,22]

Good Hospital Practice

Dr. Alexander Langmuir emphasized the importance of dust suppression in the control of airborne contagion.[23] Dr. Lloyd Herman demonstrated the accumulation of fungi as the cause of asthma and infection.[24]

There is little difference in expense between slipshod housekeeping and that required to suppress microbe-laden dust other than when and how it is done.[25] Dust is either redistributed or removed and the surfaces disinfected. Well organized negligence, as with the maintenance of air conditioners, is indefensible even when justified by the popularly held conviction that airborne contagion does not occur.

It becomes obvious that the bioburden in hospitals must be considered in any program of infection control. Environmental monitoring and suppression of bioburden would seem to be as an essential quality control measure in hospitals as it has become in industries that produce sterile products under the FDA's Good Manufacturing Practices.

TABLE 9[25] lists the bacteriologic critiera (bioburden) that should be enforced in hospital practice.

*Zephiran 12.8 percent	10 cc.
Cetyl Alcohol	5.0 gm.
Isopropyl Alcohol	500 cc.
Water q.s. to	1000 cc.

TABLE 9

SUMMARY TO TOTAL COUNTS OF BACTERIA CULTURED FROM THE
ENVIRONMENT IN 169 OPERATIONS*

Type of Culture	Mean
Settling Plates	
on Aseptic Field	3.3 (± 1.9) organisms/ft.^{2}/min.
Settling Plates on Floor	4.3 (± 1.9) organisms/ft.^{2}/min.
Volume Air Samples	3.7 (± 2.7) organisms/ft.^{3}
Floor Cultures	2.6 (± 2.6)† organisms/cm.^{2}

*(From Walter et al.[26] By permission of American Medical Association Journal.)
†Geometric mean.

Administrative Responsibilities

The complexities of monitoring a successful program for the control of nosocomial and postoperative wound infections demands administrative attention. Indeed only comprehensive responsibility can coordinate the many facets of infection control. The medical staff must be involved in promulgation of policy. The clinicians chosen must have the driving interest of this morning's speakers. Each infection control program must fit the individual hospital, its structure, its staff, its patient load, its practices. The larger and more complex the hospital the greater the need for a definitive program.

The services of an epidemiologist are essential to interpret the surveillance data to identify outbreaks and disclose carriers. Epidemiologic implication is a valuable tool. A microbiologist must be depended upon to accumulate data that permits bacteriologic incrimination.

All this expensive, time-consuming activity is unrewarding unless action results. Files of data on infected patients and lists of carriers are of no avail unless something is done to define problems and achieve their resolution. That is an administrative responsibility unique to each hospital and can no longer be evaded.

REFERENCES

1. MALLISON, G. F. 1980. Legionellosis: Evidence of airborne transmission. This annal.
2. RILEY, E. C. 1980. The role of ventilation in the spread of measles in an elementary school. This annal.
3. GUNDERMANN, K-O. 1980. Spread of microorganisms by air conditioning systems especially in hospitals. This annal.
4. WALTER, C. W. 1966. Cross-infection in hospitals. ASHRAE J.: 41–45. October.
5. WALTER, C. W., R. B. KUNDSIN, L. PAGE & A. L. HARDING. 1967. The Infector on the Surgical Team. Clin. Neurosurg. 14: 361–379. Williams and Wilkins. Baltimore.
6. ULRICH, J. A., B. E. CRIBBS & B. E. MICHAELSEN. 1976. Recirculation of air in operating rooms. Med. Instrum. 10: 282–286.
7. KUNDSIN, R. B. 1980. Documentation of airborne infection during surgery. This annal.
8. WALTER, C. W., R. B. KUNDSIN, M. A. SHILKRET & M. M. DAY. 1958–1959. The spread of staphylococci to the environment. Antibiot. Annu.: 952–957. Medical Encyclopedia. New York, N. Y.
9. WALTER, C. W. 1958. Cross Infection in Hospitals. Becton, Dickson Lectures on Sterilization. Seton Hall College of Medicine: 65–77. October.

10. WALTER, C. W. 1977. 36th Annual Charles V. Chapin Oration: The Physician's Role in Cross Infection. R. I. Med. J. **60:** (11) 534–548. November.
11. WALTER, C. W. 1958. Environmental sepsis. Mod. Hosp. **91**(6): 69–78. December.
12. FLUGGE, C. 1897. Uber luftinfection. Zeitschrift fur Hygiene und Infektionskrankheiten. **25:** 179.
13. WELLS, W. F. 1955. Airborne Contagion and Air Hygiene. Harvard University Press. Cambridge.
14. DUNCAN, I. B., A. M. COLLINS, E. M. NEELIN & T. E. ROY. 1957. Nasal carriage of staphylococcus pyogenes by student nurses. Can. Med. Assoc. J. **11:** 1001.
15. RILEY, R. L. 1957. Aerial dissemination of pulmonary tuberculosis. The American Review of Tuberculosis and Pulmonary Diseases. **76:** 931. December.
16. WILLIAMS, R. E. O. 1956. The progress of ideas on hospital infection. Bull. Hyg. **31:** 965. October.
17. COMMENTARY. 1979. Inappropriate federal requirements for air control in hospital isolation rooms. J. Am. Med. Assoc. **242:** 1971–1972.
18. WALTER, C. W. 1960. The problem of recurrent staphylococcal infections in our modern hospitals. Anesth. Analg. **39:** 81.
19. ROBERTSON, E. C., E. C. DOYLE & F. F. TISDALL. 1943. Use of ultraviolet radiation in reduction of respiratory cross infections. J. Am. Med. Assoc. 908–914.
20. WALTER, C. W. 1978. The surgeon's responsibility for asepsis. Med. Instrum. 12: 149–157.
21. LITTON, A., C. W. WALTER & R. B. KUNDSIN. 1965. Septic Shock and Terminal Sepsis in Critically Ill Surgical Patients. In Proceedings of Workshop. Committee on Shock of the National Academy of Science-National Research Council. September 1964. National Academy of Science-National Research Council. Washington.
22. MOORE, F. D. et al. 1969. Post-traumatic Pulmonary Insufficiency: 3. Saunders. Philadelphia.
23. LANGMUIR, A. D. 1980. Changing concepts of airborne infection of acute contagious disease: A reconsideration of classic epidemiologic theory. This annal.
24. HERMAN, L. G. 1980. Aspergillus in patient care areas. This annal.
25. WALTER, C. W. & R. B. KUNDSIN. 1960. The floor as a reservoir of hospital infections. Surg. Gynecol. Obstet. **111:** 412.
26. WALTER, C. W., R. B. KUNDSIN & M. M. BRUBAKER. 1963. Incidence of airborne wound infection during operation. J. Am. Med. Assoc. **186:** 908.

PREVENTION AND CONTROL OF AIRBORNE INFECTION IN THE COMMUNITY

Richard L. Riley

Petersham, Massachusetts 01366

In presenting the historical background of airborne contagion earlier, I mentioned several attempts at control in the community by air disinfection and pointed out that all except one were failures. I should like now to analyze these studies in more detail and to attempt a more general consideration of the requirements for community-wide control. Finally, I shall suggest practical steps which can be taken in moving toward control of airborne contagion in the community.

Definition of "Community"

For purposes of this discussion I will use the term "community" to refer to people who are free to move about and take part in all their normal activities. This excludes hospital patients and military personnel, but includes school children.

Historically, efforts to control airborne contagion by air disinfection have focused on schools because, in small communities, they provide a common indoor environment in which the youthful segment of the community congregates. Furthermore, many childhood contagions, measles in particular, are both airborne and productive of lasting immunity. Schools thus provide the simplest and most promising point of attack on the immensely complicated problem of airborne contagion in the community.

Past Attempts at Control in the Community: Germantown Friends School and Swarthmore Public Schools

The control of measles by Wells, Wells, and Wilder (1942)[1] was both the first and the most successful example of control by disinfection of the air. The degree of success can be visualized in the following two slides showing, for measles, weekly attack rates among susceptibles in UV irradiated and unirradiated classrooms, first for Germantown Friends School and then for Swarthmore Public Schools, during the epidemic of 1941–42. There were more susceptible children in the primary grades so that, without UV irradiation, the attack rates would be expected to be higher in the primary grades and not lower, as observed. Though not as dramatic, the study also showed a reduction in mumps and chickenpox in the children attending the UV irradiated classrooms, indicating that much of the spread of these diseases was airborne and occurred in school. The prevention of airborne infection among intermittent aggregations necessitates both an effective means of air disinfection and the employment of that means within the particular atmosphere in which the infections actually were transferred. Wells knew that the UV lights were effective in disinfecting the air because he tested them *in situ* against airborne test organisms. The schools were

0077–8923/80/0353–0331 $01.75/0 © 1980, NYAS

the particular atmospheres in which infections were transferred because, in Germantown and Swarthmore in the early forties, there were relatively few opportunities for transfer of infection among children outside of school.

During the five years following the epidemic of 1941–42 the percentage of children who were susceptible to measles was continuously higher in the UV irradiated classes than in the nonirradiated classes (Figures 1 and 2). This indicates that fewer children caught measles in the irradiated classes. The density of susceptibles varied from year to year, depending on the balance between the number of endemic cases and the number of susceptibles entering the school population. The horizontal lines, drawn through the average percentage of susceptibles in the irradiated and nonirradiated groups, represent the threshold density of susceptibles for each group. Epidemics occur when the density of susceptibles exceeds the threshold, and the severity of the epidemic depends on the amount by which the actual density of susceptibles exceeds the threshold. The UV lights increased the number of susceptibles that could occupy the irradiated classrooms without causing an outbreak of measles, hence, they raised the epidemic threshold. UV lights, which raise the threshold density, and vaccination, which lowers the actual density, both serve to reduce the probability that the actual density of susceptibles will exceed the epidemic threshold.

Mexico and Cato-Meridian Schools

Perkins, Bahlke and Silverman (1947)[2] were aware of the technical and epidemiological requirements of a good study and attempted to satisfy them by UV irradiating the centralized Cato-Meridian School, located on the boundary between these two rural communities in upstate New York. All might have been well but for the fact that 97 percent of the children reached school by bus. The endemic pattern of measles in UV irradiated Cato-Meridian School contrasted with the peaked epidemic pattern in the nonirradiated Mexico School, as shown in slide 3, but the total attack rate of measles was not reduced by UV irradiation. All signs indicate that measles was propagated in the school buses at a slow rate, accounting for the large number of cases even though exposure to measles was probably controlled by UV in the classrooms. This is the public health version of the surgeon's claim that the operation was a success even though the patient died. In Wells' language: "Effective sanitary ventilation in the school does not guarantee adequate air hygiene among school children exposed outside of school."

Southall, England

The major English study of childhood contagion, carried out under the auspices of the Medical Research Council (1954)[3] failed to satisfy either of Wells' requirements. Adequate air disinfection was not demonstrated in the school that was chosen, and, being located in the Southall district of London, there were many opportunities for exposures outside of school. The British failed to heed their own R. M. F. Picken, who, in the Proceedings of the Royal Society of Medicine had said: "Clearly it would be difficult to control an epidemic of the latter (urban) type by efforts directed at the school. Random infection (outside of school) plays too large a part. On the other hand, the epidemic traced in Chart I (a rural epidemic) indicates that control through schools may be possible." This extraordinary insight was dated 1921.[4]

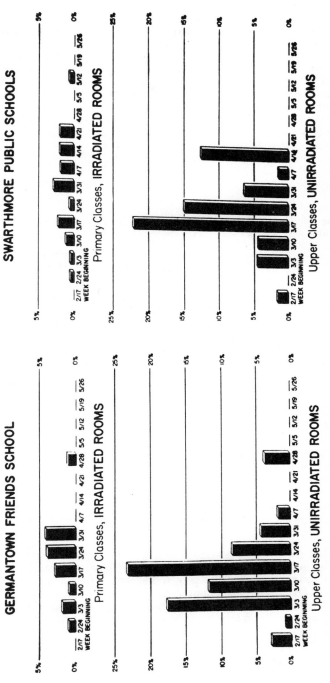

FIGURE 1. Measles epidemic in Philadelphia, 1941. Weekly attack rate among susceptibles (home secondaries excluded).

Pleasantville and Mt. Kisco

Wells, from whom I lifted the quote by Picken, was well aware of the difficulties of environmental control of contagion in urban, and even suburban, communities. Nevertheless, Mildred W. Wells, William F. Wells' epidemiologist wife, undertook, with W. A. Holla, to irradiate with UV many of the indoor atmospheres in which contagion spread throughout the town of Pleasantville.[13] This study bears so directly on the subject of this presentation that I will quote two entire paragraphs in which William F. Wells (1955) discusses the work.[4]

"The primary purpose of the study was to demonstrate the feasibility of

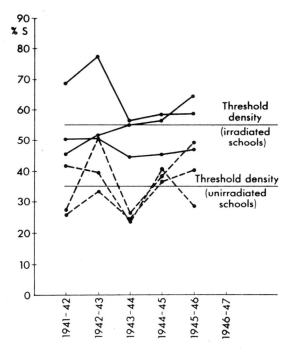

FIGURE 2. Percentages of children susceptible to measles in three irradiated and three unirradiated schools in suburban Philadelphia during the five-year period following the epidemic of 1941.

environmental control of epidemic childhood contagion in a suburban community—to determine how extensive need be the radiant disinfection of atmospheres breathed by children of a community to control contagious disease. Since, however, the relative importance of atmospheres breathed outside the school must be surveyed, the study becomes a survey of the channels of commerce in contagion, using radiant disinfection of air as a tool of ecological analysis.

"When these channels of infection have been traced, and the vital foci of propagation of contagious diseases of childhood have been located, then—and not until then—will it be feasible to consider the study of prevention of the spread of colds and influenza in which adults as well as children contribute to the vast reservoir of contagion. Control of all airborne contagion is theoretically possible, but the practicability of such measures must be proven before a general art of air hygiene can be established."

In the Pleasantville study, air disinfection shifted the channels of infection but, as in the Perkins (1947)[2] study, the total number of cases was not reduced. Wells concluded: "The true significance of these studies lies rather in recognizing that analysis of the sources of infection is a necessary preliminary to effective environmental control."[4]

Lessons from Past Studies

We are not likely to get a clearer statement of the problem. However, with increased urbanization, tracing channels of airborne infection, using air disinfection as a tool, has become almost impossible due to the mobility of the population. For practical reasons we must forego this "necessary preliminary." Furthermore, we cannot expect environment control alone to be adequate using existing techniques of air disinfection.

The Nature of the Solution

Godfrey, in 1932, made the way out of this dilemma sound easy: "The absence of airborne epidemics among ecological populations is merely a matter of raising threshold density by sanitary ventilation or air disinfection, or of lowering susceptible density by immunization."[4] Translated, this means that you can reduce the likelihood of infectious exposure of susceptibles either by air disinfection or by immunization. As a guide for action, I would change only one word. We must employ both air disinfection and immunization. These two approaches are not in competition; they are synergistic. They supplement each other in approaching the common objective of reducing the likelihood of exposure of susceptibles, and thus controlling epidemic respiratory contagion by keeping below the threshold density of susceptibles. In the simplest terms, this means reducing the likelihood of infectious exposures of susceptibles to the point where, on the average, each case begets less than one new case.

The Immunological Approach

The two parts of Godfrey's proposal are environmental and immunological. Immunization has been the traditional approach to the prevention of many airborne diseases. It has been widely applied in connection with measles, mumps, smallpox, tuberculosis and other respiratory tract infections. Immunization is of proven value, particularly in childhood, but its effectiveness in preventing some of the common airborne infections, such as colds and influenza, is limited. Even in the case of measles, it should be recalled that the explosive outbreak, reported by Dr. Edward Riley on the first day of this conference, occurred in a school where 97 percent of the children had been vaccinated.[5] Measles immunization has since been improved and progress is being made with other vaccines, but fundamental difficulties with mass immunization remain, as shown at the time of the threatened epidemic of "swine flu."

The unprecedented elimination of smallpox from the face of the earth is the ultimate in control of airborne contagion in the community.[14] This was accomplished by intense world-wide surveillance and containment of foci of infection by isolation of each case and vaccination of potential contacts within a given radius of the case. The success of this approach in controlling smallpox suggests its application to other forms of airborne contagion for which an effective vaccine is available. Isolation of the infectious case removes airborne organisms from the air breathed by others and is thus a form of environmental control. Viewed in this light, the eradication of smallpox was accomplished by a combination of immunological and environmental measures, with immunological measures dominant.

The Environmental Approach

Isolation of the patient as a means of improving the environment for others should be encouraged in relation to all forms of contagion. However, for this occasion I shall consider the possibility of disinfecting air that the patient has already infected. In the measles outbreak reported by my brother, disinfection of air recirculated throughout the school would have prevented, by calculation, 26 of the 28 second generation cases.[6] Immunization without air disinfection permitted the density of susceptibles to exceed the epidemic threshold. With air disinfection these same susceptibles would have been well below the raised threshold density, and epidemic spread would not have occurred. This result is hypothetical, but it exemplifies what Godfrey meant by raising the threshold density of susceptibles by air disinfection.

Techniques of Air Disinfection

If raising sanitary ventilation or air disinfection is a desirable thing to do, what are some of the ways of doing it? Conceptually the simplest way is to increase ventilation, the mass movement of air, to the point where infectious droplet nuclei are diluted so much that on the average each case begets less than one new case. This is the air hygienist's application of the old axiom: the solution to pollution is dilution. Ventilation of such an amount is too expensive to apply in buildings that have to be heated or cooled. It may be supplied by nature when windows are opened in the summer months, increasing ventilation enough to account for the reduced amount of respiratory contagion in the summer.[7] A second way to rid air of infection is to filter out the infectious particles. This is possible, but since the droplet nuclei transmitting infection are in the one to three micrometer size range, a good filter is required and much energy must be expended in moving the air through the filter. Standard filters used in ventilating systems take out less than 30 percent of the small respirable particles.[5] A third possibility is electrostatic precipitation of airborne particles. This is expensive and requires considerable maintenance. A fourth possibility is the use of glycol vapors. These were tried in the 1940s and found to be difficult to manage because they required exact control of humidity.[4] A fifth possibility is ultraviolet radiation. With all its difficulties, it is more effective and economically feasible than any of the other approaches.[4]

Method of Applying UV

Although UV barriers of various sorts have been used in special situations, there are two principal ways of applying UV: upper air irradiation and duct irradiation. Upper air irradiation is provided by either wall fixtures or fixtures suspended from the ceiling at about the seven foot level. Baffles prevent downward radiation and thus protect occupants of the room from direct exposure to UV. The air in the lower part of the room is purified by mixing with the disinfected air in the upper part of the room. The efficiency of the system depends upon the speed of mixing as well as the completeness of disinfection of the upper air. A good installation reduces the concentration of airborne organisms in the breathing zone to between a tenth and a fifth of the concentration that would exist in the absence of UV.[8] Upper air irradiation is well suited to fairly large rooms with high ceilings, such as classrooms, and Wells' success in blocking the spread of measles indicates that inactivation of measles virus with UV is possible. Improved UV fixtures are currently under development, but the modern trend toward low ceilings seriously limits the applicability of upper air irradiation.

UV irradiation of air in ventilating ducts is technically easy because intense radiation can be used without hazard to people. The amount of radiation required depends on the size of the ducts and the volume flow of air.[9,10] Duct irradiation assumes importance when forced air ventilation with recirculation of air is used for heating or air conditioning. Recirculated air is distributed to all parts of the building supplied by the forced air system, and infectious droplet nuclei are carried by this air. The measles epidemic described by my brother was propagated primarily by recirculated air which carried infectious droplet nuclei throughout the distribution of the forced air heating system. Many new buildings, from homes to hotels, office buildings, and hospitals, use forced air systems with recirculation. Disinfection of air in central distributing ducts would prevent distribution of airborne organisms throughout the areas supplied by the system. Duct irradiation would not stop the spread of infection in individual rooms occupied by infectious cases. In these rooms the concentration of infectious droplet nuclei is relatively high and dilution by ventilation of, say, five air changes an hour is insufficient to interrupt transmission, no matter how pure the incoming air. It is difficult to estimate the health benefits of duct irradiation in recirculation systems because it ranges from very effective with a single index case to very ineffective in an established community-wide epidemic.[6] Much would depend on how many buildings used duct irradiation. The installation of UV lights in ducts is a simple and inexpensive procedure, so that a building code requiring its use is not out of the question.

Magnitude of the Problem

In a 9½ year study of 85 families in Cleveland, Ohio, Dingle[11] found that 63 percent of all illnesses were respiratory, and the National Health Survey finds that more than half of all acute conditions are respiratory.[12] There can be little doubt that most acute respiratory conditions are infectious, and in my opinion most of them are caused by airborne viruses. If airborne contagion is the greatest cause of loss of time from work and from school, it ranks among the most important public health problems. To reduce the economic loss alone, a significant effort to improve on the present situation is justified.

Specific Suggestions

Believing that immunological and environmental approaches must go hand in hand, I recommend supplementing present immunological efforts with wide application of the most cost effective environmental efforts. At the moment, this might well be duct irradiation in all large buildings with forced air ventilation. Such installations could be introduced into existing systems without major expense and could be required in new buildings. Individual room installations should be recommended in special situations such as hospitals, where many patients have suppressed immunological responses, and in schools. In spite of past failures, there can be no doubt that schools are among the principal places of association for children, and, in any attempt at community-wide control, schools must be given special attention. Buses, trains and airplanes, which are often crowded, should be protected, probably by high ventilation rates with air that is disinfected in ducts. Although beyond the scope of this meeting, it should be added that better housing to reduce crowding in slum areas also reduces the density of susceptibles and hence the likelihood of epidemic respiratory contagion.

CONCLUSIONS

Three new considerations add urgency to a renewed effort to control airborne contagion. The first of these is the vast increase in the use of forced air systems for heating and air conditioning. The second is the urgent need for energy conservation by making tighter buildings. Inescapably this will mean less dilution of airborne organisms and other indoor pollutants, as discussed by Dr. Proctor. The third is the inordinate cost, in terms of both medical care and reduced productivity, for the victims of airborne contagion.

We know that to prevent epidemic spread we need only keep below the threshold density of susceptibles; it is not necessary to eliminate all airborne contagion. We know that air disinfection will rechannel infection to unprotected atmospheres, producing a more endemic pattern of infection but not necessarily reducing the number of cases. We also know that air disinfection will serve in this way to identify places that remain to be controlled and thus, with perseverance, lead on to success. In short, we know we can control airborne epidemics by raising the threshold density of susceptibles by air disinfection and lowering the actual density of susceptibles by immunization. All that remains is to do it.

REFERENCES

1. WELLS, W. F., M. W. WELLS & T. S. WILDER. 1942. The environmental control of epidemic contagion. I. An epidemiologic study of radiant disinfection of air in day schools. Am. J. Hygiene **35**(1): 97–121.
2. PERKINS, J. E., A. M. BAHLKE & H. F. SILVERMAN. 1947. Effect of ultraviolet irradiation of classrooms on the spread of measles in large rural central schools. Am. J. Public Health **37**: 529–537.

3. MEDICAL RESEARCH COUNCIL. 1954. Air disinfection with ultraviolet irradiation; its effect on illness among school children. Special Report Series No. 283. London, England.

4. WELLS, W. F. 1955. Airborne Contagion and Air Hygiene. Harvard University Press, Cambridge, Mass.

5. RILEY, E. C., G. MURPHY & R. L. RILEY. 1978. Airborne spread of measles in a suburban elementary school. Am. J. Epidem. **107:** 421–432.

6. RILEY, R. L. 1979. Indoor spread of respiratory infection by recirculation of air. Bull. Européen de Physiopathol. Resp. **15:** 699–705.

7. WELLS, M. W. 1944. The seasonal patterns of measles and chickenpox. Am. J. Hygiene **40:** 279–317.

8. RILEY, R. L. 1974. Airborne infection. Am. J. Med. **57:** 466–475.

9. WESTINGHOUSE LAMP DIVISION. Two new dimensions in forced air heating and air conditioning. ASC-170 Rev., Westinghouse Electric Corp., Bloomfield, N.J.

10. BUTTOLPH, L. J. & H. HAYNES. 1950. Ultraviolet air sanitation. LD-11, General Electric Engineering Division, Lamp Department. Cleveland, Ohio.

11. DINGLE, J. H. 1959. An epidemiological study of illness in families. Harvey Lectures **53:** 1–24.

12. NATIONAL HEALTH SURVEY. 1975. Acute conditions: incidence and associated disability, United States, July 1973–June 1974. Series 10, Number 102. USDHEW/PHS, National Center for Health Statistics. Rockville, Maryland.

13. WELLS, M. W. & W. A. HOLLA. 1950. Ventilation in flow of measles and chickenpox through community: Progress report, Jan. 1, 1946 to June 15, 1949, airborne infection study, Westchester County Department of Health. J. Am. Med. Assoc. **142:** 1337–1344.

14. HENDERSON, D. A. 1976. The eradication of smallpox. Sci. Am. **235:** 25–33.

Index of Contributors